This book is due for return not later than the
last date stamped below, unless recalled sooner.

THE COMPARATIVE PSYCHOLOGY
PSYCHOLOGY
OF AUDITION:
Perceiving Complex Sounds

THE COMPARATIVE PSYCHOLOGY OF AUDITION:
Perceiving Complex Sounds

Edited by

ROBERT J. DOOLING
The University of Maryland

STEWART H. HULSE
Johns Hopkins University

LEA LAWRENCE ERLBAUM ASSOCIATES, PUBLISHERS
1989   Hillsdale, New Jersey   Hove and London

Lawrence Erlbaum Associates, Inc., Publishers
365 Broadway
Hillsdale, New Jersey 07642

Library of Congress Cataloging-in-Publication Data

The comparative psychology of audition.

Bibliography: p.
Includes index.
1. Auditory perception. 2. Psychology, Comparative.
I. Dooling, Robert J. II. Hulse, Stewart H.
BF251.C66   1989   156'.215   88-33576
ISBN 0-8058-0020-4
ISBN 0-8058-0384-X (pbk.)

Printed in the United States of America
10 9 8 7 6 5 4 3 2 1

Contents

8.   Species Differences in Auditory Responsiveness in Early Vocal Learning   243

Peter Marler and Susan Peters

9.   Individual Recognition by Voice in Swallows: Signal or Perceptual Adaptation?   277

Michael D. Beecher, Patricia Loesche, Philip K. Stoddard, and Mandy B. Medvin

Preface

We have organized this book around several interleaved themes with a heavy emphasis on the "comparative" and the "complex" in auditory perception. The first theme is, roughly speaking, that of "bottom-up" versus "top-down" processing. From the bottom-up perspective there are chapters by Ehret (Chapter 1) and Saunders and Henry (Chapter 2) relating psychoacoustic data to peripheral mechanisms in mammalian and avian auditory systems. From the top-down perspective there are chapters by Espinoza-Varas and Watson (Chapter 3), Mullennix and Pisoni (Chapter 4), and Carterette and Kendall (Chapter 5), all of which review compelling evidence for the operation of central, cognitive, and integrative mechanisms in the perception of complex tonal patterns, speech, and music.

The second theme, in many ways the most central, is that of species comparisons involving species-specific vocal signals. Here ecological considerations are prominent and these chapters involve a creative blend of field and laboratory methodologies. The comparative approach to complex stimulus perception is viewed in the light of larger issues of learning, development, communication, and adaptation in chapters by Gerhardt (Chapter 6), Brown (Chapter 7), Marler and Peters (Chapter 8), Beecher, Loesche, Stoddard, and Medvin (Chapter 9), and Ralston and Herman (Chapter 10).

The third theme also focuses on a variety of species comparisons but now draws distinctions and parallels either explicitly or implicitly between animals and humans tested in the laboratory on the perception of complex acoustic signals. Comparisons are made between animals and humans on the perception of such complex acoustic signals as tone patterns, speech sounds, and bird calls in the chapters by Hulse (Chapter 11), Moody and Stebbins (Chapter 12), Kuhl (Chapter 13), Dooling (Chapter 14), and Sinnott (Chapter 15).

Our intention was to bring together people from different disciplines and perspectives who are studying the perception of complex sounds. They are psychologists, psychophysicists, speech scientists, biologists, and ethologists. What emerges from these pages is a set of common subthemes and crosscurrents. Each chapter, for instance, has touched on issues related to the use of natural versus synthetic acoustic stimuli, data obtained under natural environments (ecologically valid) versus controlled, artificial testing environments (the laboratory), whether an organism is using "special" versus "general" processing mechanisms in perceiving complex sounds, and, directly or indirectly, the necessity of a comparative approach for a full understanding of the perception of complex sounds by humans.

Finally, the diversity of contributions in this volume reflect the richness of modern day comparative psychology. No longer a discipline preoccupied with the laboratory rat, modern comparative psychology increasingly concerns itself with learning, development, and perception in the context of innate predispositions, ecological variables and the natural history of behavior. Only against this backdrop will we reach a full understanding of behavior including the perception of complex acoustic stimuli.

Robert J. Dooling
Stewart H. Hulse

Editor's Comments on Ehret

The processing of complex sounds begins at the auditory periphery. No matter what central nervous system processes contribute to our final perception of complex sounds, the auditory periphery delivers the raw encoded information upon which these processes must act. It is the mammalian auditory system with which many of the chapters in this volume are concerned and for this reason a discussion of the levels of processing in a mammalian auditory system is needed. Along with humans, there are several other mammals which have become favorite subjects for modern auditory research.

In this chapter, Ehret describes what is known about hearing in the house mouse with special emphasis on the stages of peripheral processing. From simple audibility constraints to temporal and spectral filtering mechanisms, the early stages of auditory processing exert a profound influence on what features of a complex acoustic stimulus are encoded by the auditory system and available for higher order processing. Ehret does a superb job of relating data from mouse from work with simple sounds describing basic processing capabilities to data on the processing of complex, biologically relevant acoustic stimuli.

1 Hearing in the Mouse

Günter Ehret*
Universitat Konstanz, Federal Republic of Germany

INTRODUCTION

Over the last 15 years, knowledge on hearing in the mouse has grown extensively, now including not only aspects of what and how the mouse can hear (see e.g., Willott, 1983) but also strategies to perceive communication sounds and cognitive processes to evaluate their meaning. In this review, I concentrate on relationships between hearing abilities and their physiological bases and will relate to other subjects and points where comparisons become useful and stimulating.

The substrates of complex acoustic perception are complex sounds. Starting with a continuous pure tone, the most simple sound, one can increase complexity in three dimensions (spatial aspects are not considered here):

a. in the spectral domain by adding other tones higher or lower in frequency and same or different in intensity with the result of a harmonic or nonharmonic or noisy spectrum,

b. in the temporal domain by making the tone discontinuous and thus generating a temporal pattern or rhythm,

c. in the spectro-temporal domain by introducing modulations of frequency and/or intensity with the result of a time-dependent frequency spectrum and time-varying intensity distribution across the frequency components.

*Present address: Abteilung Vergleichende Neurobiologie, Universität Ulm, M25/5, Postfach 4066, D-7900 Ulm, F.R.G.

Natural sounds such as many animal calls and songs and speech are complex with regard to all three dimensions. And, most important, relevant information about a sender is often encoded by spectral, temporal, and spectro-temporal aspects of the sound, so that the auditory system of the receiver, primarily a conspecific individual, must be designed to analyze in all three dimensions in order to make the information available. Because an appropriate analysis is the prerequisite for sound recognition, i.e., the release of an adequate response in the receiver—the goal of all communication loops—we can expect mechanisms of complex sound perception matching with the sounds to be analyzed in all vocal animals.

In the following, hearing in the mouse is discussed with regard to analysis in all three sound dimensions. Data are used for pointing out general factors of analysis, perception and recognition of animal calls.

I.   ANALYSIS IN THE SPECTRAL DOMAIN

Peripheral Filtering

The result of the most peripheral sound analysis in the auditory system is the absolute auditory threshold curve (Ehret, 1977). The shape of the threshold curves of the mouse shown in Fig. 1.1 (Ehret, 1974, 1976a; Heffner & Masterton, 1980; Schleidt & Kickert-Magg, 1979) is typical for mammals and birds (see also Saunders & Henry, this volume). They show a bandpass characteristic and thus define the frequency range of hearing. This bandpass is established by properties of the outer, middle, and inner ear.

The sensitivity optimum in the range of 15–20 kHz is the result of resonances of the ear canal which increase the sound pressure level within this frequency

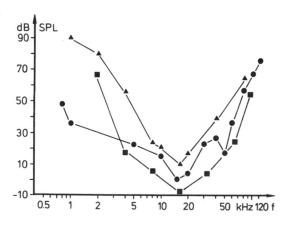

FIG. 1.1. Three absolute auditory threshold curves of house mice measured by different conditioning techniques. All show a sensitivity optimum between 15 and 20 kHz and good hearing in the ultrasonic range. Squares: feral mice, conditioned suppression (Heffner & Masterton, 1980); circles: albino laboratory mice NMRI outbred strain, operant reward and eyeblink response (Ehret, 1974, 1976a); triangles: albino laboratory mice, shock avoidance (Schleidt & Kickert-Magg, 1979).

range at the tympanum by about 16 dB (Saunders & Garfinkle, 1983). Resonance frequencies of the ear canal and sensitivity optima of hearing coincide in many mammals (Shaw, 1974).

The low-frequency slope of the threshold curve is determined mainly by the size and mechanical properties of the tympanum and the oval window through which sound waves enter the cochlea (e.g., Dallos, 1973; Saunders & Garfinkle, 1983) and by the size of the helicotrema at the apex of the cochlea (Dallos, 1970). The bigger the area of the eardrum and the smaller the helicotrema are, the better is the low-frequency sensitivity and the lower is the cutoff frequency of the bandpass at the low side. Because the tympanum and the helicotrema are not specialized in the mouse (Ehret, 1977; Saunders & Garfinkle, 1983) auditory sensitivity decreases (thresholds increase) rapidly with decreasing frequency below the sensitivity optimum. The low-frequency limit of hearing may not be far below 500 Hz.

The high-frequency sensitivity and the upper frequency limit of hearing are determined by the moment of inertia and frictional losses of the osseous chain of the middle ear (Dallos, 1973; Henson, 1974) and by the construction of the cochlea at its base (near the stapes) (e.g., Bruns, 1976a; Eldredge, 1974). The mouse has a "microtype" middle ear (Fleischer, 1978; Saunders & Garfinkle, 1983) with good transmission of sound energy in the high-frequency range and a rather thick and narrow basilar membrane within the cochlea (Ehret & Frankenreiter, 1977), which is optimally suited to vibrate at high frequencies. Thus, the upper frequency limit of hearing in the mouse is beyond 100 kHz.

The absolute sensitivity level shown by the threshold curve is influenced by animal-inherent factors (anatomy and physiology of the ear) and, of course, by psychoacoustical methods of measurement. The efficiency of sound transfer through the middle ear is one major determinant. Pressure amplification by the middle ear necessary for overcoming the high input impedance of the fluid-filled cochlea is about 1:22 in man, 1:86 in the cat (Khanna & Tonndorf, 1972) and 1:30 in the mouse (Saunders & Garfinkle, 1983). This corresponds well with the differences in behavioral absolute sensitivity among these three species measured at the sensitivity optimum. With −18 dB absolute threshold level, the cat is by far the most sensitive mammal (Miller, Watson, & Covell, 1963). The threshold of the feral mouse is 10 dB higher (−8 dB; Heffner & Masterton, 1980). Because cat and mouse differ in middle ear amplification by a factor of 2.9, the mouse should be 20 log 2.9 = 9,2 dB less sensitive than the cat and this is almost exactly the case. Similarly, the −4 dB absolute threshold of man (ISO-Rec., 1961) can be calculated from the difference of middle ear amplification compared with mouse and cat.

This close agreement between relative sensitivity measurements based solely on physical properties of the outer and middle ear and relative behavioral sensitivities measured at the output of the whole auditory and motor systems of mouse, cat, and man raises an important point. The psychophysical threshold determinations obviously did justice to their name, namely, they measured the absolute *sensory* thresholds that directly depend on the physical properties of the systems and were not dominated by some behavioral *response* threshold governed by the methods of measurement (including motivational, attentional, and paradigm-dependent factors in addition to sensory ones). Every method of psychophysical threshold determination leads, under otherwise identical conditions, to its own threshold values which ideally are identical to those of the sensory system but often reflect thresholds of valuation of sensory input in the central nervous system or thresholds of the motor response. Thus, it is not surprising that seven different methods of estimation of absolute auditory threshold in the mouse produced seven basically different threshold curves (Ehret, 1983a). It follows that those measurements leading to the lowest thresholds (highest sensitivities) can be regarded as the closest approximations to the true sensory thresholds. Measurements leading to higher than absolute-threshold values are not useless because they may throw light on processes that value the contribution of sound for the release of behavior in different behavioral settings. Method-dependent threshold values are not restricted to absolute sensitivity but can be found in measurements of all sorts of auditory capabilities including difference limens, frequency and temporal resolution, and pattern recognition. We look at these perceptual abilities later.

Cochlear Filtering and the Origin of Frequency Resolution

Sound entering the cochlea via stapes motion forms traveling waves running along the fluid spaces towards the apex of the cochlea (e.g., v.Békésy, 1960). By the traveling-wave displacement of the basilar membrane, sound frequency is transformed into cochlear place. That is, sensory hair cells sitting in the organ of Corti on the basilar membrane at a certain distance from the base of the cochlea are stimulated best by sound frequencies corresponding to that place. In mammals like the mouse without prominent anatomical specialization in the cochlea, the frequency-place-transformation is proportional to a regular stiffness change of the basilar membrane from stiff (thick and narrow) at the base to elastic (thin and wide) at the apex (Ehret, 1978, 1983b; Ehret & Frankenreiter, 1977).

The frequency-place-transformation in the cochlea is the starting point for the frequency selectivity (within the hearing range) of the whole auditory system. It has been shown for the cat that the tuning of the basilar membrane displacement is as sharp as the tuning measured by tuning curves of single fibers of the auditory nerve (Khanna & Leonard, 1982, 1986). There are two populations of sensory cells in mammals, the inner hair cells (one row) and the outer hair cells (three rows) by which the tuning of the basilar membrane is transformed into response sensitivity and tuning of the auditory nerve fibers. The two hair cell populations contribute differently to information coding in the auditory nerve:

Hearing is established by the function of inner hair cells (Deol & Gluecksohn-Waelsch, 1979). Also, tuning and frequency selectivity of the auditory nerve fibers are mediated by the inner hair cells (Dallos & Harris, 1978; Russel & Sellick, 1978) from which, by divergent innervation, more than 90% of the afferents in the auditory nerve originate in the mouse (Ehret, 1979a) and in other mammals (e.g., Bohne, Kenworthy, & Carr, 1982; Spoendlin, 1972). Psychophysically determined frequency selectivity deteriorates if inner hair cells are damaged but is completely normal if the outer hair cells are absent (Nienhuys & Clark, 1979; Ryan, Dallos, & McGee, 1979). Outer hair cells contribute significantly (about 30–60 dB) to the absolute sensitivity of hearing (e.g., Ehret, 1979b; Liberman, 1984; Liberman & Beil, 1979; Ryan & Dallos, 1975) and to the shape of the tuning curves of auditory nerve fibers (Dallos & Harris, 1978; Liberman & Dodds, 1984).

Thus it appears that the inner hair cells act as the elements where cochlear filtering is transformed into neural filtering making available the frequency selectivity of the cochlear place code to the central nervous system. The outer hair cells seem not to assess the bandwidths of the filters. However, they do contribute to filter shapes and control the amount of energy passed through and integrated by them (Ehret, 1979b). The result of cochlear filtering is an array of nerve fibers leaving the cochlea as filters tuned to frequencies corresponding to their place of innervation in the cochlea. Thus frequency selectivity gets a *spatial* dimension which is important to recognize when we consider frequency resolution of complex sound signals as the result of frequency selectivity of the cochlea.

Frequency Resolution and the Critical Band Concept of Spectral Analysis

In 1940, Fletcher conducted psychoacoustical experiments on the perception of tones in noise. He found that noise energy within certain bandwidths around the test tone contributed to masking the detection of the tone while energy outside the bandwidths did not influence tone perception. Fletcher assumed that these "critical bandwidths" of masking reflect the acuity of frequency resolution in the auditory system which is accomplished by a bank of bandpass filters with continuously variable center frequencies. Obviously, the bandwidths of the proposed filters are the critical quantities that determine the frequency resolving power of the whole system. Hence, these internal filters of the auditory system are called "critical bands" or "critical bandwidths" if they are measured with procedures in which frequency is a variable as shown in Fig. 1.2, or "critical ratios" (CR-bands) if they are determined indirectly by comparison of signal intensity (I_{tone}) and spectral intensity of the noise ($I_{noise/Hz}$) at the masked threshold of a tone in broadband white noise as demonstrated in Fig. 1.3:

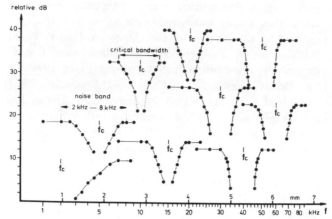

FIG. 1.2. Psychophysical measurement of frequency resolution (critical band estimation, see text) in the mouse. Tone bursts at the center frequency (f_c) of a band of white noise are masked by that noise of constant spectral intensity and masked tonal thresholds (ordinate: arbitrary dB) are determined as a function of the noise bandwidth. The results are filter curves (measured at various f_c) that demonstrate the frequency bandwidths (critical bandwidths) within which sound energy is integrated to mask the tone at f_c. The abscissa gives two scales: the length of the basilar membrane and the frequency representation on it. Modified from Ehret (1976b).

FIG. 1.3. Masked tonal thresholds (ordinate) for the mouse (closed circles). Masker is a broadband white noise at the 4 different spectrum levels shown. Critical ratio bandwidths (CR-bands) can be calculated from tone and noise levels at the masked thresholds (Eq. 2). Open squares show the absolute thresholds for comparison. Modified from Ehret (1975a).

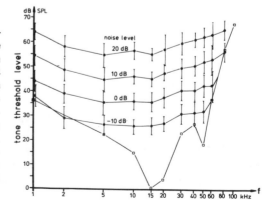

8

$$\text{CR-band (Hz)} = I_{\text{tone}}/I_{\text{noise}/\text{Hz}} \tag{1}$$

A transformation of the intensity ratio into a difference of sound pressure levels (L_{tone}, l_{noise} = spectrum level of noise) leads to the CR-band expressed in dB:

$$\text{CR-band (dB)} = L_{\text{tone}} - l_{\text{noise}} \tag{2}$$

Since Fletcher's (1940) classical study, numerous psychophysical investigations have confirmed the foundations of the critical band concept and expanded it to *the* filter theory of the auditory system (summaries in Scharf, 1970; Zwicker & Feldtkeller, 1967). Critical bandwidths have been defined in various sound detection tasks as filters that divide a complex sound into units of perception. In Fig. 1.2, an experiment of bandwidth measurement is shown for the mouse (Ehret, 1976b). Relative tone levels from masked tonal thresholds are plotted as a function of the bandlimits of a masking noise of constant spectrum level. Masked tonal thresholds increase with increasing noise bandwidth up to a certain break point at which a further bandwidth increase has no further effect on the masked threshold. The bandwidth at the breakpoint defines the critical bandwidth of a filter within which noise energy contributes to tone-masking and outside of which noise energy does not influence tone perception. Thus, Fig. 1.2 demonstrates filter bandwidths and filter shapes at various center frequencies. In general, the perceived sound quality determined by the output of a certain critical band filter changes whenever the sound energy passing the filter is changed but remains constant when sound components outside the filter bandwidth are altered. In the foreward to Scharf's (1970) chapter on Critical Bands, the general significance of the critical band concept is clearly expressed:

> Nowhere in auditory theory or in acoustic psychophysiological practice is there anything more ubiquitous than the critical band. It turns up in the measurement of pitch, in the study of loudness, in the examination of acoustic annoyance, in the investigation of the intelligibility of speech, in the analysis of masking and fatiguing signals, in the perception of phase, and even in the determination of the pleasantness of music. And likely, in one way or the other, it will be part of our final understanding of how and why we perceive anything that reaches our ears. (p. 157)

In a pioneering study, Greenwood (1961) demonstrated that the cochlear frequency map and the critical bandwidths of frequency resolution are closely related to each other in various mammals and in man. Spatial frequency representation in the cochlea is such that critical bandwidths cover about equal distances on the basilar membrane. Later, direct physiological measurements of the frequency map in the cochlea of the cat (Liberman, 1982), together with data on bandwidths of CR-bands and critical bands of the cat (Costalupes, 1983; Nienhuys & Clark, 1979; Pickles, 1975; Watson, 1963), supported the remarkable notion that filter bandwidths of complex sound perception are related to equal distances on the peripheral sensory epithelium.

FIG. 1.4. The dashed line with squares shows the relationship between cochlear place (in mm from the apex, left ordinate) and representation of frequency (abscissa). The other two curves indicate the critical bandwidths (circles) and the CR-bandwidths (triangles) at various center frequencies (abscissa). The similar and nearly parallel course of the curves suggests that critical bands and CR-bands cover constant distances on the basilar membrane. Data from Ehret (1975a, 1976b).

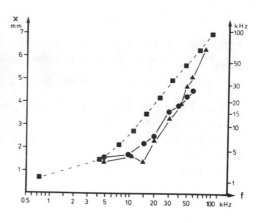

Figures 1.2 and 1.4 show the relationship between cochlear length, frequency representation, and critical bandwidths and CR-bandwidths for the mouse (Ehret, 1975a, 1976b, 1977; Ehret & Frankenreiter, 1977). In Fig. 1.5 the maximum number of CR-bands and critical bands which can be positioned on the basilar membrane without overlap are indicated. A maximum of 10 CR-bands each about 0,7 mm wide fit to the 6.8 mm length of the basilar membrane. This means that the mouse can resolve and process separately a maximum of 10 and a minimum of 7 pure tones with CR-band wide spacings, which *simultaneously* are transduced into the cochlea as a complex sound. In view of the rather broad frequency range of hearing of the mouse, which covers about eight octaves between 0,5 and 120 kHz (Fig. 1.1), this seems to be a poor resolution. In fact, it is the poorest frequency resolution found in all mammals for which appropriate data are available (Ehret, 1983a). If we use the frequency resolution index (Rf = the maximum number of CR-bands that can be formed simultaneously without overlap divided by the audible range in octaves; Ehret, 1983a) as a comparative measure of frequency resolution, Rf in the mouse is 2.5, 4.5 and 5.3 times smaller (the frequency resolution is worse) compared with cat, man and dolphin

FIG. 1.5. Scales of frequency representation, CR-bands and critical bands on the basilar membrane of the mouse. CR-bands and critical bands are arranged in a way that a maximum number of non-overlapping bandwidths could simultaneously be placed on the basilar membrane. Data from Ehret (1975a, 1976b).

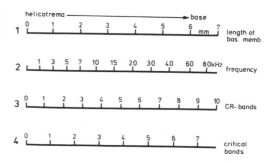

(*Tursiops truncatus*) respectively. A comparably short basilar membrane in combination with a considerable frequency range of hearing (Fig. 1.5) prevents the cochlear frequency analyzer from yielding a high resolution, because the sharpness of frequency selectivity of the basilar membrane plus hair cells is normally restricted to a filter bandwidth of about 0.7 mm. Improvement of frequency resolution can be achieved by the extension of the basilar membrane (e.g., dolphin: 39 mm; man: 32 mm) and by reduction of the frequency range of hearing (e.g., horseshoe bat: 4.5 octaves) (compare Ehret, 1977).

The close relationship between length of the basilar membrane, frequency representation, and frequency resolution, which become evident in the parallel functions shown in Fig. 1.4, apply only to cochleae following Greenwood's (1961) equation of frequency-place transformation:

$$f = A (10^{ax} - 1) \qquad (3)$$

f = frequency; x = distance on the basilar membrane in mm from the helicotrema (apex); A,a are species-specific constants. In mammals like horseshoe bats with discontinuities of basilar membrane stiffness and other specialization of the cochlea (Bruns, 1976a, 1976b; Vater & Duifhuis, 1986), frequency resolution deviates considerably from the function shown in Fig. 1.4 (Long, 1977) and is much improved at the reference frequency of the bats echolocating system. Deviations from the relationship between frequency and frequency resolution (Fig. 1.4) are also found in the parakeet (Dooling, 1980), which has a surprisingly good frequency resolution in the frequency range of best hearing. Whether mammals differ from birds in systematic ways what peripheral frequency resolution is concerned needs further investigation (see Saunders & Henry, this volume).

Neural Coding in the Spectral Domain

We have seen that critical bands are the central mechanism of spectral analysis in the auditory system. They operate whenever a complex frequency spectrum is perceived. Hence, neuronal coding in the spectral domain means searching for neural correlates of critical band (CR-band) processing. What features of critical bands (CR-bands), do we have to look for?

1. The species-specific frequency dependence of critical bandwidths (CR-bandwidths) (compare Figs. 1.4, 1.5).

2. Intensity independence of critical bandwidths (CR-bandwidths). Measurements of CR-bands and various determination of critical bands show that the filter bandwidths performing the spectral analysis are constant over a broad intensitiy range, often up to 70–80 dB above the detection threshold of sound (e.g., Ehret, 1975a; Hawkins & Stevens, 1950; Scharf, 1970; Scharf & Meiselman, 1977; Zwicker & Feldkeller, 1967). In Fig. 1.3, masked thresholds of tone

perception of the mouse (Ehret, 1975a) are shown at four spectrum levels of broadband white noise. Obviously, a 10 dB increase of the noise level leads to a 10 dB increase of the masked threshold. This mean that, according to Eq. 2, CR-bands remain constant while sound intensity is changed. Such an independence of spectral analysis of sound intensity is essential for the generation of perceptual constancy in the frequency domain which guarantees that animals and man can recognize the *meaning* of a sound independent of its loudness.

3. Spectral integration, independent of the kind of sound passing the critical band filters. Besides filtering in the frequency domain (Fig. 1.2), sound energy is integrated within the filter bandpass to form the unit of perception.

Tests of neural CR-bands and critical bands have to be designed that replicate psychophysical measurements on the neuronal level and reveal bandwidths, spectral integration, and intensity characteristics. In view of the close relationships between length of the basilar membrane, frequency representation and width of CR-bands and critical bands (Figs. 1.4, 1.5), we can predict that at least the frequency dependence of these filters as evaluated in psychophysical tests is present already in the auditory nerve.

Ehret and Moffat (1984) performed CR-band measurements in auditory nerve fibers and single neurons of the cochlear nucleus of the mouse in the same way as done behaviorally (Ehret, 1975a). The response of single units to tone bursts in broadband white noise was recorded. At a given tone level, the spectrum level of the noise was varied until the tone response, defined by a discharge-rate criterion, was just masked and the neuron responded only to the noise. Once the masked threshold of auditory nerve fibers or cochlear nucleus neurons was determined, the difference of tone level and spectrum level of the noise could be used to define the CR-bandwidths according to Eq. 2.

Average neural (cochlear nerve and ventral cochlear nucleus) and behavioral CR-bandwidths are shown in Fig. 1.6 as a function of frequency. Neural values were obtained at a tone level 20 dB above the units' tone response thresholds. Three aspects are important. First, the frequency dependence of neural and behavioral means is roughly similar which is in agreement with the hypothesis of the cochlear origin of the filters. Second, filter bandwidths derived from cochlear nucleus units are, on the average, considerably smaller than those of auditory nerve fibers measured at the same sound intensities. This means that spectral filtering and frequency resolution of complex sound is improved in the cochlear nucleus compared to the auditory nerve. Third, the bandwidths of the neuronal filters increase with increasing sound intensity. A variation of filter size over a tone intensity of 40 dB above threshold is indicated by vertical bars with arrow heads pointing to an expected further extension at even higher tone intensities. Because CR-bandwidths determined psychophysically in the same type of experiment are constant over a broad range of sound intensity (Fig. 1.3), we recognize an important difference between spectral analysis in the auditory nerve

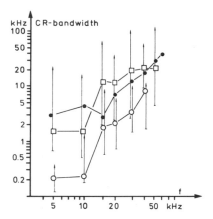

FIG. 1.6. A comparison of average CR-bandwidths (ordinate) at various center frequencies (abscissa) from neurons in the auditory nerve (open squares) and ventral cochlear nucleus (open circles) of the mouse (data from Ehret & Moffat, 1984) with average behavioral CR-bands (closed circles; Ehret 1975a). Neural data were obtained 20 dB above tone response thresholds of the neurons. The horizontal bars with arrowheads show the bandwidth variation of neural values for a tone level variation of 40 dB. Behavioral CR-bands are independent of sound intensity.

and ventral cochlear nucleus and frequency resolution in the perception test. We have to conclude that a major characteristic of sound analysis in the spectral domain, the intensity independence, is not yet realized at the level of the auditory nerve and ventral cochlear nucleus and thus must arise from further processing in higher auditory centers.

The neural data presented in Fig. 1.6 suggest a widening of filter bandwidths with increasing intensity. This, however, must not be the case because cutoff frequencies of the filters were estimated by an indirect method (intensity comparison at the masked threshold, Eqs. 1, 2). A different interpretation considers a possible deviation of linear filtering with increasing sound intensity. Linear filtering means that all sound energy passing a filter is treated equally and gives rise to the same kind of response, i.e., is reflected in the same way in the rate profile of a neuron's response (response rate was used to define masked neuronal thresholds; Ehret & Moffat, 1984). Hence, a decreasing effectiveness in masking tone responses of neurons by noise with increasing tone level (Ehret & Moffat, 1984) could mean an intensity dependent nonlinear integration of spectral energy in the CR-band filters instead of a widening of the bandwidths. On the basis of the present physiological data, which support both a deterioration of tuning in the presence of broadband sound at moderate and higher intensities (Evans, 1977; Møller, 1981; Pickles, 1982) and a nonlinearity of discharge rate to tones and noise (e.g., Costalupes, Young, & Gibson, 1984; Gibson, Young, & Costalupes, 1985; Palmer & Evans, 1980; Sachs & Abbas, 1974) in auditory nerve fibers, we cannot decide whether spectral analysis in the auditory nerve suffers from intensity dependent filter bandwidths or nonlinear integration of sound energy in the filters or both.

Direct measurements of filter bandwidth (e.g., critical band determinations by narrow band noise with variable bandwidths) at various sound intensities have to be carried out in order to clarify the issue at the level of the auditory nerve. A study on critical bandwidth coding in the inferior colliculus of the auditory midbrain of the cat has shown (Ehret & Merzenich, 1985, 1988) that all features of psychophysical frequency resolution as measured in critical band tests (appropriate, intensity-independent bandwidths of the filter, linear spectral integration) can be found in the discharges of the majority of neurons of the central nucleus. Sound analysis in the spectral domain, therefore, is realized in a behaviorally and perceptually relevant way in single neurons of the auditory midbrain.

II. ANALYSIS IN THE TEMPORAL DOMAIN

Temporal analysis has often been related to pitch coding and perception (e.g., de Boer, 1976; Langner, 1983; Nordmark, 1970). There are no data available for the mouse on this topic and I shall refer to Hulse (this volume) for a further discussion with regard to other animals. Here, we direct our attention to time constants of temporal summation and to the discrimination of sound duration. The detection of temporal variations of frequency and intensity is discussed in the next section.

Temporal summation for tones and white noise was determined in behavioral tests at the absolute auditory threshold of the mouse (Ehret, 1976a). This threshold was measured at signal durations between 1 and 3000 ms. Figure 1.7 shows that for sound durations shorter than a certain critical duration t_c threshold levels increase with decreasing length of sound bursts. This relationship can be expressed by the function (for $t \leq t_c$):

$$L = L_{tc} + |a| \log_{10} (t_c/t) \tag{4}$$

L = threshold level at the signal duration t, L_{tc} is the absolute threshold for long durations ($t \geq t_c$), and $|a|$ is the slope of the regression line. If expressed in sound intensity, Eq.4 leads to (Ehret, 1976a)

$$I \cdot t^b = \text{constant} \tag{5}$$

This means that for signal durations shorter than t_c, sound intensity is proportional to a power of signal duration. The exponent b is equal to $|a|/10$ so that a slope of 10 of the regression lines in Fig. 1.7 would lead to b = 1 and thus to an equivalence of the influence of duration and intensity on the detection threshold. Because measured slope values are always smaller than 10 (4.6 < $|a|$ < 8.6;

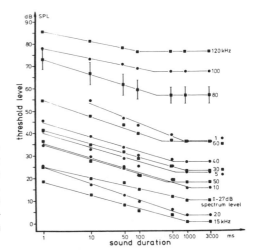

FIG. 1.7. Relation between absolute auditory thresholds for tones (kHz) and white noise (WN) and the signal duration. The break points of the broken lines define the critical durations (tc) (Eq. 4). Modified from Ehret (1976a).

Ehret, 1976a), we can suggest that the auditory system is not able to integrate sound energy over the whole signal duration or make use of all sound energy of a short tone that is, the integration process operates at a loss at short signal durations.

Figure 1.7 shows that the critical durations t_c depend on the frequency of the tone bursts. This can be described for frequencies between 10 and 100 kHz by

$$t_c = 2140 \, / \, f^{0.78} \tag{6}$$

This means that the higher the frequencies are, the shorter are the time constants of temporal summation.

Temporal summation as described by Eqs. 4, 5 and 6 is a general feature of the auditory systems of man (e.g., Feldtkeller & Oetinger, 1956; Plomp & Bouman, 1959; Zwislocki, 1960) and mammals (Clack, 1966; Costalupes, 1983; Henderson, 1969; Johnson, 1968a) and birds (Dooling, 1980). Implications for sound perception are obvious since rather short sounds require higher sound pressure levels to be detected and resolved, especially at low frequencies.

Discrimination of sound duration was tested in mice in the course of a study on acoustic features of ultrasounds of mouse pups necessary for the release of maternal behavior in their mothers (Ehret & Haack, 1982). Synthetic ultrasounds, i.e., tone bursts of 60 kHz frequency and 100 ms (including 10 ms rise and fall times) duration had to be discriminated in a nonconditioned seminatural situation from tone bursts of the same frequency but different duration. Figure 1.8 shows how the ratio of the responses to the standard versus the test stimulus depends on the duration of the test stimulus (20–40 ms stimuli had 5 ms rise and fall times). The data indicate that the duration continuum of the test tones can be divided into two classes of stimuli: those with durations between 30 and 270 ms

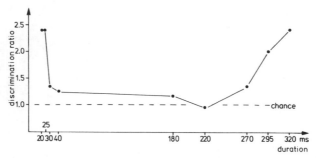

FIG. 1.8. Results of an experiment on unconditioned discrimination of tone burst durations in mice (Ehret & Haack, 1982). 60 kHz tone bursts of 80 ms duration had to be discriminated from 60 kHz bursts of the durations indicated on the abscissa. No discrimination (chance level) is seen at a discrimination ratio close to 1.0 (ordinate), significant discrimination is reached by a discrimination ratio larger than 2.0. A sharp border from discrimination to non-discrimination is evident between 25 and 30 ms. Modified from Ehret (1987a).

that are not discriminated from the standard 100 ms tone, and others shorter than 30 ms and longer than 270 ms which are well discriminated. The sharp transition from discrimination to nondiscrimination when the sound duration is increased from 25 to 30 ms or from 270 to 320 ms may indicate that the mouse is able to discriminate these similar sound durations although a direct discrimination test has not been performed. A 5 ms and 50 ms duration discrimination limen at 25 and 270 ms respectively can be expressed as a Weber fraction $\Delta d/d$. The similarity of the resulting $\Delta d/d$ values (0.2 and 0.19) suggest that relative temporal resolution is constant over a broad range of sound duration.

The $\Delta d/d$ values of the mouse are in good agreement with those of man and parakeet (Dooling & Haskell, 1978), which are between 0.1 and 0.2 for tone durations in the range of 25 to 300 ms. This similarity of relative resolution may be taken to indicate that the mouse reached the absolute limits of temporal resolution in an unconditioned situation in which communication relevant key-stimuli had to be discriminated from other sounds.

III.   ANALYSIS IN THE SPECTRO-TEMPORAL DOMAIN

Simultaneous variations in the spectral and temporal domain can be introduced to a continuous sound by frequency and/or intensity modulations or by making the sound discontinuous, and attributing different frequencies and/or intensities to the sound bursts. Intensity modulation and sound bursts in a series with a certain repetition rate produce side bands to the frequency components in a modulated or bursted sound. The side band components are equal to the carrier frequency ±

the modulation frequency (repetition rate). Thus rapid intensity variations in a sound create correlates in the spectral domain.

The detection of modulations in a continuous sound and of frequency and intensity differences in a series of sound bursts are different tasks with probably different mechanisms of analysis involved (e.g., Moore & Glasberg, 1986). For difference detection in a series of sound bursts memory of the features or some lasting influence of one burst when the next is evaluated has to be assumed. Thus, the just noticeable difference between two sound sensations is measured. In the case of modulation detection the listener has to notice a just audible amount of change in *one* sound sensation. Frequency and intensity discrimination of tones were tested in the mouse with the burst-series method of tone presentation (Ehret, 1975b).

Frequency Discrimination

Just noticeable frequency differences (Δf) between tone bursts of a repetition rate of 4,5 Hz were obtained with an operant-reward conditioning procedure in laboratory mice (strain NMRI; Ehret, 1975b). A few data are available from feral mice (Heffner, Heffner, & Masterton, cited in Heffner et al., 1971) which will, however, not be considered here because information about procedures and acoustic conditions are not given. Figure 1.9 shows how Δf depends on the

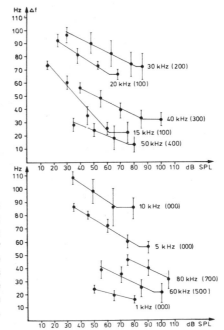

FIG. 1.9. The just noticeable frequency difference (Δf) as a function of the sound pressure level of the test tones with their frequencies as parameters. The Δf value at a given frequency is equal to the sum of the ordinate value and the number in brackets behind the frequency. Modified from Ehret (1975b).

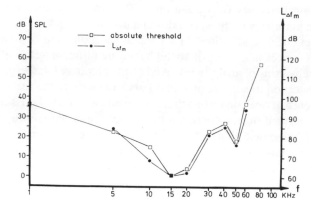

FIG. 1.10. A comparison of the absolute threshold levels (left ordinate) with the tone levels at which the minimum noticeable frequency
differences ($L_{\Delta fm}$, right ordinate) are reached at given frequencies (abscissa). Both levels differ by about 60 dB irrespective of frequency.
Modified from Ehret (1975b).

sound pressure level of the tones with frequency as parameter. A clear dependence of Δf on SPL and frequency is evident. Data points at each frequency
(except 1 and 80 kHz) can be approximated by two lines, one following the
decrease of Δf with increasing SPL and the other indicating the constant minimum Δf at highest SPLs tested. When we plot the SPLs at the intersections of the
two lines as a function of frequency and compare the curve with the auditory
threshold curve of the mouse (Fig. 1.10), a surprising similarity in shape is seen.
In fact, both curves become almost identical if one shifts the ordinate scale of the
SPL at minimum Δf ($L_{\Delta fm}$) for 60 dB so that 0 dB SPL equals 60 dB $L_{\Delta fm}$ (Fig.
1.10). This means that the just noticeable frequency difference becomes smallest
at 60 dB suprathreshold level independent of the test frequency. Thus we find
that equal amounts of excitation in the auditory system are necessary for smallest
difference thresholds to be reached over the major frequency range of hearing.
Similar findings are available from measurements in humans (Shower & Biddulph, 1931; Wier, Jesteadt, & Green, 1977) where at 60–80 dB above threshold
level (sensation level) the minimum Δf is approached.

The slopes of the regression lines in Fig. 1.9 depend on the frequency at
which the discrimination test is performed. Figure 1.11 shows that the steepest
slopes occur at 15 kHz and decrease for both higher and lower frequencies. In the
same figure, the numbers of nerve fibers leaving the cochlea over its length are
also plotted. The functional implications of nerve fiber density on frequency
discrimination are evaluated below in a model of frequency and intensity
discrimination.

Figure 1.9 demonstrates that Δf changes with frequency. This relationship,

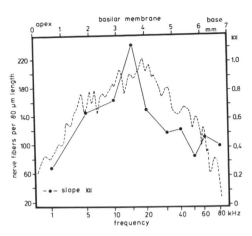

FIG. 1.11. Numerical values of the slopes /a/ of the regression lines in Fig. 9 (right ordinate) plotted against frequency (lower abscissa). Also, the density of nerve fibers (left ordinate) leaving the cochlea at various places corresponding to a certain position on the basilar membrane (upper abscissa) is shown. Modified from Ehret (1983b).

which is a general one and found in all mammals tested so far, is shown in Fig. 1.12. Except for very low frequencies in the species' hearing ranges where Δf is rather constant, Δf increases with increasing frequency which means that Δf/f is constant. Above about 10 kHz the just noticeable frequency difference in the mouse is nearly 0.85% of a given frequency. Humans are much more sensitive to frequency changes and reach a Δf/f value of about 0,23% (Shower & Biddulph, 1931), dolphin of about 0.5% (Jacobs, 1972), cats however, of only 1% (Elliott, Stein, & Harrison, 1960). Birds like parakeet (Dooling & Saunders, 1975a),

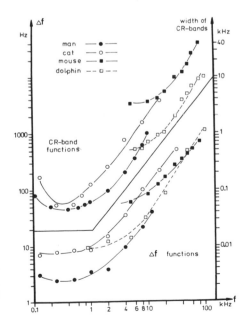

FIG. 1.12. Frequency dependence of the CR-bandwidths (right ordinate) and of the just noticeable frequency differences for man (Hawkins & Stevens, 1950; Shower & Biddulph, 1931), cat (Watson, 1963; Elliott et al., 1960), mouse (Ehret, 1975a, 1975b), and dolphin (Johnson, 1968b; Jacobs, 1972). Modified from Ehret (1977).

cowbird, and red-winged blackbird (Sinnott, Sachs, & Hienz, 1980) reach values close to 1% with curve shapes similar (except at very low frequencies) to those shown in Fig. 1.12 .

An interesting correspondence is evident in Fig. 1.12 between the frequency dependencies of the ability to resolve frequency components of a complex spectrum (CR-bandwidths) and to discriminate between frequencies that sequentially reach the ear Δf-values . The two sets of curves run parallel (except at the low-frequency end) for all species shown. A consequence is that the just noticeable frequency difference is a constant fraction of the frequency resolution power of the auditory system expressed by the CR-bandwidths (or critical bandwidths). The ratio between the CR-bands in Herz and the widths of the minimum Δf is 38 in house mice, 17 in cats, and 24 in humans. The ratio indicates that the analytical capacity of the ear of the mouse is 38 times better for the discrimination of the tone frequency in a sequence of bursts than for the resolution of a complex sound. In general, much smaller frequency differences in sequential acoustic events can be detected by mammals compared with frequency distances of simultaneously present components in a complex sound. This is true also for birds (Dooling, 1980).

Intensity Discrimination

With the same method described for frequency discrimination tests, data on just noticeable intensity differences were obtained in the mouse (Ehret, 1975b). Figure 1.13 shows a plot of difference thresholds (ΔL) versus supra-threshold

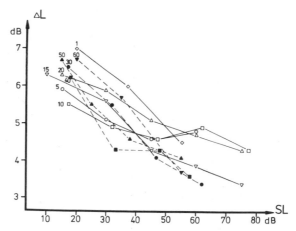

FIG. 1.13.   Just noticeable differences of sound pressure level (ΔL) as a function of the supra-threshold tone level (SL = sensation level) with frequency as parameter. Modified from Ehret (1975b).

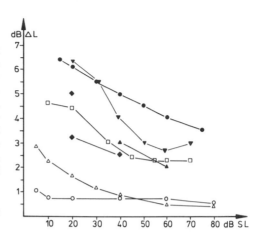

FIG. 1.14. A comparison of just noticeable intensity differences (averaged across frequencies) for various species. Man (open symbols): squares (Dimmick & Olson, 1941), circles (experiment I), triangles (experiment III, Harris, 1963); cat: triangles (Raab & Ades, 1946; Elliott & McGee, 1965); rat: diamond (Henry, 1938; Hack, 1971); mouse: circles (Ehret, 1975b); parakeet: inversed triangles (Dooling & Saunders, 1975b).

tone level (sensation level, SL) with frequency as parameter. At all tone frequencies, ΔL decreases rather steadily with increasing tone level. By taking the average of all curves shown in Fig. 1.13, the decrease can be expressed as:

$$\Delta L = -0.05 \text{ SL} + 7 \qquad (7)$$

or in terms of sound intensity as

$$\Delta I = 4 \cdot I^{0.95} \qquad (8)$$

The exponent of 0.95 in Eq. 8 indicates a "near miss" of Weber's law ($\Delta I/I =$ constant), which is a common characteristic found in several studies on humans. Exponents in human tests range between 0.875 and 0.965 with an average of 0.918 calculated from Table IV in Jesteadt, Wier, & Green, (1977) and from data of McGill and Goldberg (1968a, 1968b). Because the average exponent for humans is smaller than that for the mouse, intensitiy discrimination in the mouse is closer to Weber's law than in man.

A comparison of just noticeable intensity differences in Fig. 1.14 demonstrates that the difference thresholds of the mouse are the highest of the few mammalian species tested and are similar only to those obtained in the parakeet (Dooling & Saunders, 1975b). Procedures of testing as well as species-specific factors influencing intensity discrimination may be the reason for the discrepancies of difference thresholds among species (Fig. 1.14). Some possible factors are discussed below in a descriptive model of frequency and intensity discrimination.

Modeling Frequency and Intensity Discrimination

The cochlear frequency-place-transformation implies that a frequency shift or a variation of tone intensity in successive tone bursts will lead to a corresponding

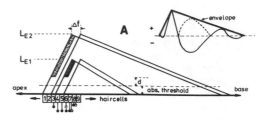

FIG. 1.15. A model of frequency (A) and intensity (B) discrimination based on the displacement of the basilar membrane
and the resulting excitation patterns of the cochlear hair cells
(compare text). From Ehret
(1977, 1983a).

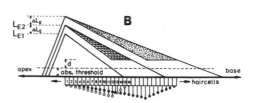

shift of the exitation maximum or to a variation of the spread of extation respectively along the basilar membrane. Based on this, Maiwald (1967) developed a
model in which frequency and intensity discrimination are related to shifts of
excitation along the basilar membrane. Figure 1.15 shows a modified and extended version of this model taken from Ehret (1977, 1983a) in order to make
clear how psychophysically determined difference thresholds may directly depend on features of sound processing within the cochlea. Thus, the model summarizes various peripheral factors that may contribute differently in different
species to the determination of frequency and intensity difference limens.

Traveling waves in the cochlea in response to a single tone have a triangular
envelope (see inset to Fig. 1.15A) which constitutes the half-way-rectified
amount of excitation that stimulates hair cell receptors at different places along
the basilar membrane. If the excitation level (L_E) is above a certain absolute
threshold, hair cells will respond to the sound. Likewise, a change of excitation
will be detected and will become apparent in a change of discharge rates of
auditory nerve fibers associated with the hair cells when a certain relative threshold of response change (d) is reached. The amount of response change of hair
cells and afferent fibers is indicated by the lengths of the bars with open (low
excitation level L_{E1}) or closed (higher excitation level L_{E2}) circles on top at the
hair cells. Thus changes of detectable excitation (dotted and cross-hatched areas)
due to a frequency shift Δf (A) or to an intensity increase ΔL_E (B) lead to
corresponding changes in the responses of only a few hair cells at a low excitation level L_{E1} and of considerably more hair cells at a higher level L_{E2}.

If we assume that the central nervous system uses a criterion for the detection
of a frequency shift or an intensity variation based on a *constant* amount of
change of hair cell responses in the cochlea independent of sound intensity, then
this criterion may be reached by the output of hair cells 6, 7 and 8 to a shift of Δf

at L_{E1} (Fig. 1.15A). At the higher excitation level (L_{E2}) the same Δf produces a response change in more hair cells which means that for the central nervous system to detect this change with a constant criterion, Δf can be smaller at L_{E2} compared to L_{E1}. Thus, the model (Fig. 1.15A) predicts a decrease of the just detectable frequency difference with increasing sound intensity. This decrease can continue until Δf corresponds to d. The experimental data shown in Figs. 1.9, 1.10 and the results from human studies (e.g., Shower & Biddulph, 1931; Wier et al., 1977) are in perfect agreement with these predictions. The just detectable frequency difference decreases with increasing SPL (Fig. 1.9) and reaches a minimum detectable difference at a constant 60dB supra-threshold level, independent of frequency (Fig. 1.10).

The model also predicts that the decrease of Δf with increasing sound intensity will be most pronounced (largest numerical slope) in the cochlear range of the highest hair cell and afferent innervation density. This is because we assumed a constant amount of response change necessary for reaching a central detection criterion. Hence, the more hair cells and afferent fibers are present at a certain cochlear place and are able to respond to a frequency shift the more rapid will be the decrease of the just noticeable Δf with increasing L_E. The data on the density of afferent fiber innervation in the cochlea of the mouse (Ehret, 1979a) and on the slopes of the Δf decreases (Ehret, 1975b) shown in Fig. 1.11 demonstrate by the close correspondence between the two curves that they follow the predictions of the model (Fig. 1.15). In addition, hair cell densities have a maximum right in the middle of the cochlea (Ehret & Frankenreiter, 1977) so that, in fact, the largest improvement of frequency discrimination with increasing sound intensity is found where hair cell and innervation densities in the cochlea are highest. The minimum Δf that can be reached equals an average shift of 18 μm along the basilar membrane (Ehret, 1975b, 1983), which is the distance covered by about two hair cells (Ehret, 1977). Thus, under the assumptions made, a remarkably small shift of excitation along the basilar membrane, that involves detectable response changes of only about two hair cells, produces the minimum detectable Δf.

Figure 1.15 shows a nonlinearity of the basilar membrane displacement which is an overproportional extension of the excitation toward the base with increasing sound intensity (e.g., v. Békésy, 1960; Zwicker & Feldtkeller, 1967). This nonlinearity is responsible for an extension of the range of hair cells together with the afferent nerve fibers that change their responses when the sound intensity is increased by a certain ΔL_E (Fig. 1.15B). When we again assume a constant, intensity independent amount of response change necessary for reaching a central detection criterion for ΔL_E, then the just noticeable intensity difference should be lowest in species with the most pronounced nonlinearity. This prediction is substantiated by the intensity discrimination data of man and mouse. Man has much smaller just noticeable intensity differences (Fig. 1.14) and a considerably smaller exponent in Eq. 8 indicating a greater nonlinearity compared with the mouse.

In summary, Fig. 1.15 can explain how just noticeable frequency and intensity differences depend on properties of the cochlea and are encoded by a small group of hair cells with their afferent nerve supply. Research on human intensity discrimination at high frequencies (Viemeister, 1983) indicates that difference thresholds can, in fact, be encoded by the response changes of only a few auditory nerve fibers. Then, difference thresholds among species could vary on the basis of a different hair cell and nerve fiber density in the cochlea, of different shapes and slopes of the travelling wave displacement patterns, a different amount of intensity dependent nonlinear extension of excitation toward the base of the cochlea, and different thresholds for the detection of excitation and of excitation change (d).

IV. HEARING ABILITIES AND COMPLEX SOUND PERCEPTION

The importance of sound analysis in the auditory system and of discrimination ability becomes immediately evident, for example, when sound communication is established as an important factor of intraspecies social behavior. Anurans, birds, and mammals communicate with a variety of calls and sounds so that mechanisms must have evolved to distinguish the auditory patterns of different sounds of relevance in order to produce an adaptive response behavior. Among these mechanisms are

1. those peripheral ones mentioned in the previous section that provide the audible frequency range and absolute sensitivity and the cochlear steps for frequency resolution and frequency and intensity discrimination;

2. more central auditory mechanisms being involved, for example, in critical band processing (Ehret & Merzenich, 1985, 1988), categorical perception (e.g., Ehret, 1987a; Macmillan, Kaplan, & Creelman, 1977) and auditory Gestalt perception (see Carterette, Watson, Pisoni, & Mullennix, this volume);

3. discriminations on the basis of learned acoustic information (e.g., Miyawaki et al., 1975; Spiegel & Watson, 1981; see also Marler, this volume);

4. interactive processes in higher brain centers between presentation of auditory information and attentive and motivational states (e.g., Beecher et al., 1979; Ehret, 1987b; Ehret et al., 1987; Glass & Wollberg, 1979);

5. nonoverlap in several acoustic parameters among calls of a species so that distinct qualities can be easily perceived.

In the following, the mouse is used as an example to show that mechanisms mentioned under points 1, 2, 4, and 5 contribute significantly to hearing and discrimination of species-specific calls.

FIG. 1.16. The frequency range of hearing of the mouse as illustrated by the extension of the absolute auditory threshold curve (Ehret, 1974) and the frequency ranges of the major spectral components of the calls of young (lower part) and adult (upper part) house mice. The calls shown are all used in intraspecies communication (Haack et al., 1983; Whitney & Nyby, 1983; Ehret & Bernecker, 1986.)

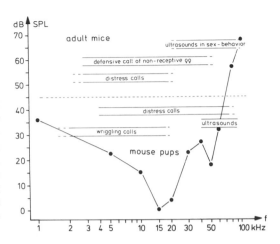

Figure 1.16 demonstrates that the frequency ranges of all mouse calls with significance in communication (Ehret, 1975; Ehret & Bernecker, 1986; Haack, Markl & Ehret, 1983; Whitney & Nyby, 1983) fall into the hearing range of the adult mouse. This and the occurrence of a relative sensitivity maximum of hearing near 50 kHz ensures that all call spectra are sufficiently audible. It is also obvious that the calls divide into three groups according to their frequency ranges: low-frequency calls (wriggling calls of pups and distress calls of adults), high-frequency calls (ultrasounds of young and adults), and broadband calls covering the entire midfrequency, high-sensitivity range (distress calls of young and defensive calls of nonreceptive females). Each of these groups contains one call type of pups and one of adults. This separation of calls by the frequency ranges of the spectra and by communicators offers a very simple mechanism for call discrimination and recognition. Calls will primarily be perceived as belonging to one of the three groups by their frequency ranges. At the same time, the motivational state of the receiver will be the deciding factor for the release of an appropriate behavioral response (recognition of the call) inasmuch as motivation will determine whether a perceived call is interpreted as coming from a young or an adult mouse. In a state of parental motivation (while caring for pups), sounds are related to pups and will elicit appropriate caretaking behavior; in a state of agonistic or sexual motivation with other adult mice close to the receiver of the calls, the calls will elicit an appropriate behavior that is directed towards adult mice. This hypothesis about the control of sound communication among house mice involves sound perception and analysis in the frequency domain and behavioral context perception (motivational adjustment) and a coincidence of both for the generation of adaptive response behavior. With regard to intraspecific communication, sound analysis in the frequency domain would be the main task of the auditory system.

FIG. 1.17. Analysis and perception of ultrasonic calls and wriggling calls of mouse pups by the critical band mechanism of the ear as shown by Ehret and Haack (1982) and Ehret and Riecke (to be published). The critical bandwidths are indicated by dotted lines running parallel to the call elements and harmonics (compare text). Abscissa: call duration, ordinate: frequency.

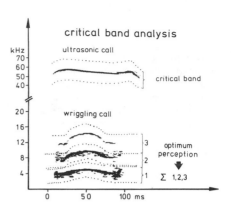

Measurements on the perception, identification and discrimination of two calls of the mouse repertoire, the ultrasounds and wriggling calls of pups (Fig. 1.17) strengthen the significance of spectral cues and their evaluation by the critical band mechanism and demonstrate the relative unimportance of temporal and spectro-temporal analysis in this case (Ehret & Haack, 1982; Ehret & Riecke, unpublished data). Figure 1.8 shows that a very wide window of call durations is accepted in ultrasound perception. The window in the frequency domain is just one critical bandwidth wide (Fig. 1.17) that is, for example, 23 kHz bandwidth at a center frequency of 50 kHz (compare Figs. 1.2, 1.4), with the further requirement that spectral components just outside the decisive critical band must be at least 20 dB down compared with those inside. Frequency modulations, which always occur in the ultrasounds (Fig. 1.17) and intensity changes both well above perception thresholds (Figs. 1.12, 1.13) are unimportant for call recognition. Interestingly, the windows in the spectral and temporal domain cover all the natural variability occurring in pup ultrasounds so that the close matching of perceptual strategies with the substrate of analysis becomes evident. It is important to notice that the perceptual strategy is to disregard information about the variability of individual calls, which the auditory system automatically supplies by its analysis, and to rely only on features common to all natural calls.

The strategy for wriggling call perception is tuned to the basically harmonic structure of this low-frequency call (Fig. 1.17). Most often it consists of 2–4 frequency modulated harmonics with various degress of intensity modulation visible in the sonagrams as side bands to the harmonics or as noisy components. Call recognition tests with synthetized calls under natural communicative conditions show that an optimum response release is achieved with a nonfrequency, nonintensity modulated three-component call in which the harmonics fall into three separate critical band widths (Fig. 1.17). The attractiveness of the call can be increased stepwise by starting with one harmonic and adding a second and third one, whereby the first harmonic near 4 kHz contributes most. Besides the number of harmonics, their spacing is most important. The presentation of a three-component call in which two or all three components fall within one critical bandwidth of frequency resolution (Figs. 1.2, 1.4) reduces the occurrence of response behavior significantly. This shows that in the perception of wriggling calls the frequency resolution power of the auditory system is fully exploited while spectro-temporal analysis seems to play no role at all. Again, information about variabilities of individual calls, mostly expressed in the kind of frequency and intensity modulation, is disregarded and recognition is based on more general call features which are available from analysis in the spectral domain.

These two examples of call perception and recognition (ultrasounds and wriggling calls of mouse pups) demonstrate clearly the discrepancy between what the auditory system is able to detect, analyze, resolve, and discriminate and what finally becomes significant as acoustic key-features controlling the response behavior to a given sound. Thus, the study of mechanisms of complex sound analysis in the auditory system and of the psychophysics of perceptual abilities is essential but not sufficient for the understanding of the perceptual strategies that govern auditory response behavior in animals. Only the releasing capabilities of natural calls and of various synthetized models thereof can indicate the significance of certain sound parameters in the perception of a given call. By its analytical capacity the auditory system offers possibilities, but the animal has to choose.

REFERENCES

Beecher, M. D., Petersen, M. R., Zoloth, S. R., Moody, D. B., & Stebbins, W. C. (1979). Perception of conspecific vocalizations by Japanese macaques. Evidence for selective attention and neural lateralization. *Brain Behavior & Evolution, 16*, 443–460.

Békésy, G. v. (1960). *Experiments in hearing.* New York: McGraw-Hill.

Bohne, B. A., Kenworthy, A., & Carr, C. D. (1982). Density of myelinated nerve fibers in the chinchilla cochlea. *Journal of the Acoustical Society of America, 72*, 102–107.

Bruns, V. (1976a). Peripheral auditory tuning for fine frequency analysis by the Cf-FM bat, *Rhinolophus ferrumequinum.* I. Mechanical specializations of the cochlea. *Journal of Comparative Physiology, 106*, 77–86.

Bruns, V. (1976b). Peripheral auditory tuning for fine frequency analysis by the Cf-FM bat, *Rhinolophus ferrumequinum.* II. Frequency mapping in the cochlea. *Journal of Comparative Physiology, 106*, 87–97.

Clack, T. D. (1966). Effect of signal duration on the auditory sensitivity of humans and monkeys (*Macaca mulatta*). *Journal of the Acoustical Society of America, 40*, 1140–1146.

Costalupes, J. A. (1983). Temporal integration of pure tones in the cat. *Hearing Research, 9*, 43–54.

Costalupes, J. A., Young, E. D., & Gibson, D. J. (1984). Effects of continuous noise backgrounds on rate response of auditory nerve fibers in cat. *Journal of Neurophysiology, 51*, 1326–1344.

Dallos, P. (1970). Low-frequency auditory characteristics: Species dependence. *Journal of the Acoustical Society of America, 48*, 489–499.

Dallos, P. (1973). *The auditory periphery.* New York: Academic Press.

Dallos, P., & Harris, D. (1978). Properties of auditory nerve responses in the absence of outer hair cells. *Journal of Neurophysiology, 41*, 365–383.

de Boer, E. (1976). On the "residue" and auditory pitch perception. In W. D. Keidel & W. D. Neff (Eds.), *Handbook of sensory physiology, Vol. V/3, Auditory system, clinical and special topics* (pp. 479–583). Berlin: Springer-Verlag.

Deol, M. S., & Gluecksohn-Waelsch, S. (1979). The role of inner hair cells in hearing. *Nature, 278,* 250–252.

Dimmick, F. L., & Olson, R. M. (1941). The intensive difference limen in audition. *Journal of Acoustical Society of America, 12,* 517–525.

Dooling, R. J. (1980). Behavior and psychophysics of hearing in birds. In A. N. Popper & R. R. Fay (Eds.), *Comparative studies of hearing in vertebrates* (pp. 261–288). New York: Springer-Verlag.

Dooling, R. J., & Haskell, R. J. (1978). Auditory duration discrimination in the parakeet (*Melopsittacus undulatus*). *Journal of the Acoustical Society of America, 63,* 1640–1642.

Dooling, R. J., & Saunders, J. C. (1975a). Hearing in the parakeet (*Melopsittacus undulatus*): Absolute thresholds, critical ratios, frequency difference limens, and vocalizations. *Journal of Comparative and Physiological Psychology, 88,* 1–20.

Dooling, R. J., & Saunders, J. C. (1975b). Auditory intensity discrimination in the parakeet (*Melopsittacus undulatus*). *Journal of the Acoustical Society of America, 58,* 1308–1310.

Ehret, G. (1974). Age-dependent hearing loss in normal hearing mice. *Naturwissenschaften, 61,* 506.

Ehret, G. (1975a). Masked auditory thresholds, critical ratios, and scales of the basilar membrane of the house mouse (*Mus musculus*). *Journal of Comparative Physiology, 103,* 329–341.

Ehret, G. (1975b). Frequency and intensity difference limens and nonlinearities in the ear of the house mouse (*Mus musculus*). *Journal of Comparative Physiology, 102,* 321–336.

Ehret, G. (1976a). Temporal auditory summation for pure tones and white noise in the house mouse (*Mus musculus*). *Journal of the Acoustical Society of America, 59,* 1421–1427.

Ehret, G. (1976b). Critical bands and filter characteristics in the ear of the house mouse. *Biological Cybernetics, 24,* 35–42.

Ehret, G. (1977). Comparative psychoacoustics: Perspectives of peripheral sound analysis in mammals. *Naturwissenschaften, 64,* 461–470.

Ehret, G. (1978). Stiffness gradient along the basilar membrane as a basis for spatial frequency analysis within the cochlea. *Journal of the Acoustical Society of America, 64,* 1723–1726.

Ehret, G. (1979a). Quantitative analysis of nerve fiber densities in the cochlea of the house mouse (*Mus musculus*). *Journal of Comparative Neurology, 183,* 73–88.

Ehret, G. (1979b). Correlations between cochlear hair cell loss and shifts of masked and absolute behavioral auditory thresholds in the house mouse. *Acta Otolaryngology, 87,* 28–38.

Ehret, G. (1983a). Psychoacoustics. In J. F. Willott (Ed.), *The auditory psychobiology of the mouse* (pp. 13–56). Springfield, IL: Charles C. Thomas.

Ehret, G. (1983b). Peripheral anatomy and physiology II. In J. F. Willott (Ed.), *The auditory psychobiology of the mouse* (pp. 169–200). Springfield, IL: Charles C. Thomas.

Ehret, G. (1987a). Categorical perception of sound signals: Facts and hypotheses from animal studies. In S. Harnad (Ed.), *Categorial perception* (pp. 301–331). Cambridge, England: Cambridge University Press.

Ehret, G. (1987b). Left hemisphere advantage in the mouse brain for recognizing ultrasonic communication calls. *Nature, 325,* 249–251.

Ehret, G., & Bernecker, C. (1986). Low-frequency sound communication by mouse pups (*Mus musculus*): Wriggling calls release maternal behaviour. *Animal Behaviour, 34,* 821–830.

Ehret, G., & Frankenreiter, M. (1977). Quantitative analysis of cochlear structures in the house mouse in relation to mechanisms of acoustical information processing. *Journal of Comparative Physiology, 122,* 65–85.

Ehret, G., & Haack, B. (1982). Ultrasound recognition in house mice: Key-stimulus configuration and recognition mechanism. *Journal of Comparative Physiology, 148,* 245–251.

Ehret, G., Koch, M. Haack, B., & Markl, H. (1987). Sex and parental experience determine the onset of an instinctive behavior in mice. *Naturwissenschaften, 74,* 47–48.

Ehret, G., & Merzenich, M. M. (1985). Auditory midbrain responses parallel spectral integration phenomena. *Science, 227,* 1245–1247.

Ehret, G., & Merzenich, M. M. (1988). Complex sound analysis (frequency resolution, filtering and spectral integration) by single units of the inferior colliculus of the cat. *Brain Research Reviews, 13,* 139-163.

Ehret, G., & Moffat, A. J. M. (1984). Noise masking of tone responses and critical ratios in single units of the mouse cochlear nerve and cochlear nucleus. *Hearing Research, 14,* 45–57.

Eldredge, D. H. (1974). Inner ear-cochlear mechanics and cochlear potentials. In W. D. Keidel & W. D. Neff (Eds.), *Handbook of sensory physiology, Vol. V/1, Auditory system, anatomy, physiology (ear)* (pp. 549–584). Berlin: Springer-Verlag.

Elliott, D. N., & McGee, T. M. (1965). Effect of cochlear lesions upon audiograms and intensity discrimination in cats. *Annals of Otology Rhinology and Laryngology, 74,* 386–408.

Elliott, D. N., Stein, L., & Harrison, M. J. (1960). Determination of absolute-intensity thresholds and frequency-difference thresholds in cats. *Journal of the Acoustical Society of America, 32,* 380–384.

Evans, E. F. (1977). Frequency selectivity at high signal levels of single units in cochlear nerve and nucleus. In E. F. Evans & J. P. Wilson (Eds.), *Psychophysics and physiology of hearing* (pp. 184–192). London: Academic Press.

Feldtkeller, R., & Oetinger, R. (1956). Die Hörbarkeitsgrenzen von Impulsen verschiedener Dauer. *Acustica, 6,* 489–493.

Fleischer, G. (1978). Evolutionary principles of the mammalian middle ear. *Advances in Anatomy Embryology and Cell Biology, 55(5),* 1–67.

Fletcher, H. (1940). Auditory patterns. *Reviews of Modern Physics, 12,* 47–65.

Gibson, D. J., Young, E. D., & Costalupes, J. A. (1985). Similarity of dynamic range adjustment in auditory nerve and cochlear nuclei. *Journal of Neurophysiology, 53,* 940–958.

Glass, I., & Wollberg, Z. (1979). Lability in the responses of cells in the auditory cortex of squirrel monkeys to species-specific vocalizations. *Experimental Brain Research, 34,* 489–498.

Greenwood, D. D. (1961). Critical bandwidth and the frequency coordinates of the basilar membrane. *Journal of the Acoustical Society of America, 33,* 1344–1356.

Haack, B., Markl, H., & Ehret, G. (1983). Sound communication between parents and offspring. In J. F. Willott (Ed.), *The auditory psychobiology of the mouse* (pp. 57–97). Springfield, IL: Charles C. Thomas.

Hack, M. H. (1971). Auditory intensity discrimination in the rat. *Journal of Comparative and Physiological Psychology, 74,* 315–318.

Harris, J. D. (1963). Loudness discrimination. *Journal of Speech and Hearing Disorders Suppl., 11.*

Hawkins, J. E., & Stevens, S. S. (1950). The masking of pure tones and of speech by white noise. *Journal of the Acoustical Society of America, 22,* 6–13.

Heffner, R., Heffner, H., & Masterton, B. (1971). Behavioral measurements of absolute and frequency-difference thresholds in guinea pigs. *Journal of the Acoustical Society of America, 49,* 1888–1895.

Heffner, H., & Masterton, B. (1980). Hearing in glires: Domestic rabbit, cotton rat, feral house mouse, and kangaroo rat. *Journal of the Acoustical Society of America, 68,* 1584–1599.

Henderson, D. (1969). Temporal summation of acoustic signals by the chinchilla. *Journal of the Acoustical Society of America, 46,* 474–475.

Henry, F. M. (1938). Audition in the white rat. *Journal of Comparative Psychology, 26,* 42–62.

Henson, O. W. (1974). Comparative anatomy of the middle ear: In W. D. Keidel & W. D. Neff (Eds.), *Handbook of sensory physiology, Vol. V/1, Auditory system, anatomy physiology (ear)* (pp. 39–110). Berlin: Springer-Verlag.

ISO Recommendation, R. 226 (1961). Normal equal-loudness contours for pure tones and normal threshold of hearing under free field listening conditions. *R 226–1961 (E)*.

Jacobs, D. W. (1972). Auditory frequency discrimination in the atlantic bottlenosed dolphin, *Tursiops truncatus* Montague: A preliminary report. *Journal of the Acoustical Society of America, 52*, 696–698.

Jesteadt, W., Wier, C. C., & Green, D. M. (1977). Intensity discrimination as a function of frequency and sensation level. *Journal of the Acoustical Society of America, 61*, 169–177.

Johnson, C. S. (1968a). Relation between absolute threshold and duration-of-tone pulses in the bottlenosed porpoise. *Journal of the Acoustical Society of America, 43*, 757–763.

Johnson C. S. (1968b). Masked tonal thresholds in the bottlenosed porpoise. *Journal of the Acoustical Society of America, 44*, 965–967.

Khanna, S. M., & Leonard, D. G. B. (1982). Basila membrane tuning in the cat cochlea. *Science, 215*, 305–306.

Khanna, S. M., & Leonard, D. G. B. (1986). Relationship between basilar membrane tuning and hair cell condition. *Hearing Research, 23*, 55–70.

Khanna, S. M., & Tonndorf, J. (1972). Tympanic membrane vibrations in cats studied by time-averaged holography. *Journal of the Acoustical Society of America, 51*, 1904–1920.

Langner, G. (1983). Evidence for neuronal periodicity detection in the auditory system of the guinea fowl: Implications for pitch analysis in the time domain. *Experimental Brain Research, 52*, 333–355.

Liberman, M. C. (1982). Single-neuron labeling in the cat auditory nerve. *Science, 216*, 1239–1240.

Liberman, M. C. (1984). Single-neuron labeling and chronic cochlear pathology. I. Threshold shifts and characteristic frequency shifts. *Hearing Research, 16*, 33–41.

Liberman, M. C., & Beil, D. G. (1979). Hair cell condition and auditory nerve response in normal and noise-damaged cochleas. *Acta Otolaryngology, 88*, 161–176.

Liberman, M. C., & Dodds, L. W. (1984). Single-neuron labeling and chronic cochlear pathology. III. Stereocilia damage and alterations of threshold tuning curves. *Hearing Research, 16*, 55–74.

Long, G. R. (1977). Masked auditory thresholds from the bat, *Rhinolophus ferrumequinum*. *Journal of Comparative Physiology, 116*, 247–255.

Macmillan, N. A., Kaplan, H. L., & Creelman, C. D. (1977). The psychophysics of categorial perception. *Psychological Review, 84*, 452–471.

Maiwald, D. (1967). Ein Funktionsschema des Gehörs zur Beschreibung der Erkennbarkeit kleiner Frequenz- und Amplitudenänderungen. *Acustica, 18*, 81–92.

McGill, W. J., & Goldberg, J. P. (1968a). Pure-tone intensity discrimination and energy detection. *Journal of the Accoustical Society of America, 44*, 576–581.

McGill, W. J., & Goldberg, J. P. (1968b). A study of near-miss involving Weber's law and pure-tone intensity discrimination. *Perception & Psychophysics, 4*, 105–109.

Miller, J. D., Watson, C. S., & Covell, W. P. (1963). Deafening effects of noise on the cat. *Acta Otolaryngology Suppl. 176*, 1–91.

Miyawaki, K., Strange, W., Verbrugge, R., Liberman, A. M., Jenkins, J. J., & Fujimura, O. (1975). An effect of linguistic experience: The discrimination of [r] and [l] by native speakers of Japanese and English. *Perception & Psychophysics, 18*, 331–340.

Møller, A. R. (1981). Coding of complex sounds in the auditory nervous system. In J. Syka & L. Aitkin (Eds.), *Neuronal mechanisms of hearing* (pp. 87–103). New York: Plenum Press.

Moore, B. C. J., & Glasberg, B. R. (1986). The relationship between frequeny selectivity and frequency discrimination for subjects with unilateral and bilateral cochlear impairments. In B. C. J. Moore & R. D. Patterson (Eds.), *Auditory frequency selectivity* (pp. 407–414). New York: Plenum Press.

Nienhuys, T. G. W., & Clark, G. M. (1979). Critical bands following selective destruction of cochlear inner and outer hair cells. *Acta Otolaryngology, 88*, 350–358.

Nordmark, J. O. (1970). Time and frequency analysis. In J. V. Tobias (Ed.), *Foundations of modern auditory theory, Vol. 1* (pp. 57–83). New York: Academic Press.

Palmer, A. R., & Evans, E. F. (1980). Cochlear fibre rate-intensity functions. No evidence for basilar membrane nonlinearities. *Hearing Research, 2,* 319–326.

Pickles, J. O. (1975). Normal critical bands in the cat. *Acta Otolaryngology, 80,* 245–254.

Pickles, J. O. (1982). *An introduction to the physiology of hearing.* London: Academic Press.

Plomp, R., & Bouman, M. A. (1959). Relation between hearing threshold and duration for tone-pulses. *Journal of the Acoustical Society of America, 31,* 749–758.

Raab, D. H., & Ades, H. W. (1946). Cortical and midbrain mediation of a conditioned discrimination of acoustic intensities. *American Journal of Psychology, 59,* 59–83.

Russell, J. J., & Sellick, P. M. (1978). Intracellular studies of hair cells in the mammalian cochlea. *Journal of Physiology, 284,* 261–290.

Ryan, A., & Dallos, P. (1975). Effect of absence of cochlear outer hair cells on behavioral auditory threshold. *Nature, 253,* 44–46.

Ryan, A., Dallos, P., & McGee, T. (1979). Psychophysical tuning curves and auditory thresholds after hair cell damage in the chinchilla. *Journal of the Acoustical Society of America, 66,* 370–378.

Sachs, M. B., & Abbas, P. J. (1974). Rate versus level functions for auditory-nerve fibers in cats: Tone-burst stimuli. *Journal of the Acoustical Society of America, 56,* 1835–1847.

Saunders, J. C., & Garfinkle, T. J. (1983). Peripheral anatomy and physiology I. In J. F. Willott (Ed.), *The auditory psychobiology of the mouse* (pp. 131–168). Springfield, IL: Charles C. Thomas.

Scharf, B. (1970). Critical bands: In J. V. Tobias (Ed.), *Foundations of modern auditory theory, Vol. 1* (pp. 159–202). New York: Academic Press.

Scharf, B., & Meiselman, C. H. (1977). Critical bandwidth at high intensities. In E. F. Evans & J. P. Wilson (Eds.), *Psychophysics and physiology of hearing* (pp. 221–232). London: Academic Press.

Schleidt, W. M., & Kickert-Magg, M. (1979). Hearing thresholds of albino house mouse between 1 and 80 kHz by shuttle box training. *Journal of Auditory Research, 19,* 37–40.

Shaw, A. G. (1974). The external ear: In W. D. Keidel & W. D. Neff (Eds.), *Handbook of sensory physiology, Vol. V/1, Auditory system, anatomy, physiology (ear)* (pp. 455–490). Berlin: Springer-Verlag.

Shower, E. G., & Biddulph, R. (1931). Differential pitch sensitivity of the ear. *Journal of the Acoustical Society of America, 3,* 275–281.

Sinnott, J. M., Sachs, M. B., & Hienz, R. D. (1980). Aspects of frequency discrimination in passerine birds and pigeons. *Journal of Comparative and Physiological Psychology, 94,* 401–415.

Spiegel, M. F., & Watson, C. S. (1981). Factors in the discrimination of tonal patterns. III. Frequency discrimination with components of well-learned patterns. *Journal of the Acoustical Society of America, 69,* 223–230.

Spoendlin, H. (1972). Innervation densities in the cochlea. *Acta Otolaryngology, 73,* 235–248.

Vater, M., & Duifhuis, H. (1986). Ultra-high frequency selectivity in the horseshoe bat: Does the bat use an acoustic interference filter?: In B. C. J. Moore & R. D. Patterson (Eds.), *Auditory frequency selectivity* (pp. 22–30). New York: Plenum Press.

Viemeister, N. F. (1983). Auditory intensity discrimination at high frequencies in the presence of noise. *Science, 221,* 1206–1208.

Watson, C. S. (1963). Masking of tones by noise for the cat. *Journal of the Acoustical Society of America, 35,* 167–172.

Whitney, G., & Nyby, J. (1983). Sound communication among adults. In J. F. Willott (Ed.), *The auditory psychobiology of the mouse* (pp. 98–129). Springfield, IL: Charles C. Thomas.

Wier, C. C., Jesteadt, W., & Green, D. M. (1977). Frequency discrimination as a function of frequency and sensation level. *Journal of the Acoustical Society of America, 61,* 178–184.

Willott, J. F. (Ed.). (1983). *The auditory psychobiology of the mouse.* Springfield, IL: Charles C. Thomas.

Zwicker, E., & Feldtkeller, R. (1967). *Das Ohr als Nachrichtenempfänger.* Stuttgart: Hirzel.

Zwislocki, J. J. (1960). Theory of temporal auditory summation. *Journal of the Acoustical Society of America, 32,* 1046–1060.

Editor's Comments on Saunders and Henry

For some complex sounds such as learned vocal signals, certain species of birds provide the only comparison available for assessing complex acoustic perceptual processes in humans. This volume would be incomplete without consideration of the levels of processing in the avian auditory system.

In this chapter, Saunders and Henry describe what is known about hearing in birds with a special emphasis on the contributions of peripheral processes. As with mammals, the peripheral auditory system exerts a profound influence on the encoding of complex acoustic stimuli. But, as the work of Saunders and colleagues shows, there are dramatic differences in the physiology and anatomy of the peripheral auditory systems of birds and mammals which suggests differences between these two classes of vertebrates in the processing of complex sounds.

The Peripheral Auditory System in Birds: Structural and Functional Contributions to Auditory Perception

James C. Saunders

William J. Henry
University of Pennsylvania

INTRODUCTION

Numerous reviews of the avian peripheral auditory system have recently appeared (e.g., Dooling, 1980; Kühne & Lewis, 1985; Saito, 1980; Smith, 1985) and this presentation will, hopefully, not be redundant of those excellent summaries. In this chapter we examine the structural and functional organization of the auditory periphery from a specific perspective. There are many aspects of hearing and auditory perception in birds that are interesting (Dooling, 1980), and some features of avian auditory behavior can be directly traced to processes found in the peripheral region of the ear. We consider three properties of hearing in which special mechanisms in the periphery appear to play a significant role. These include contributions to the shape of the hearing sensitivity (audibility) curve, frequency resolution, and sound localization. We examine the contribution of the middle and inner ears to each of these by first considering the behavioral evidence and then the associated peripheral process.

I. THE AUDIBILITY CURVE

The audibility curve has been described for 16 different species of birds and each one shows characteristics that are different from their mammalian counterparts. Dooling (1980) has summarized these data and we use his compilation to extract some interesting features. The most sensitive thresholds in his sample of birds occurred between 2.0 and 4.0 kHz and exhibited an average sensitivity of 4.0 dB SPL. The limits of high-frequency hearing, at an arbitrary cutoff of 60 dB SPL averaged 8.5 kHz in comparison to the chincilla and cat whose hearing extends to 35.0 and 65.0 kHz respectively. The rate of decline in sensitivity for frequencies below or above that portion of the hearing curve showing greatest sensitivity averaged 16.8 and 53.9 dB/octave. By comparison the cat shows a low- and high-frequency roll-off of about 13 and 29 dB/octave, while in chinchilla it is around 10 and 20 dB/octave. With the sharper high- and low-frequency cutoffs, and the narrow frequency range of high sensitivity thresholds, the avian audibility curve takes on the appearance of an inverted band-pass filter. The issue here is what mechanisms contribute to this considerable difference between avian and mammalian threshold curves? In this section we argue that the transfer characteristics of the middle ear contribute in an important way to the unique shape of the avian audibility curve.

The middle ear conductive apparatus (the tympanic membrane TM, ossicle(s), suspensory ligaments, and middle-ear muscle(s)) in all vertebrates is designed to improve the efficiency with which sound power is transferred from an air medium to the fluid filled medium of the inner ear (Dear, 1987; Rosowski et al., 1986). The bird accomplishes this "power matching" with a conductive apparatus that is very different from that found in the mammal. It is fascinating to realize that the functional role of the middle ear is the same in the mammal and bird, yet evolution experimented with dramatically different mechanisms to achieve the same goal.

The cavities of the avian middle ear, as well as the general organization of the conductive apparatus, were described in detail during the early decades of this century (Krause, 1901; Pohlman, 1921; Smith, 1904; Stellbogen, 1930; Wada, 1932). More recently Saiff (1974, 1976, 1978, 1981) has provided additional detail on the middle ears of a number of avian orders. Owls have also been examined (Norberg, 1978; Stellbogen, 1930), and Schwartzkopff (1955, 1968) provided quantitative measures of various middle ear dimensions. Saunders (1985) has extended the quantitative data base to five additional species.

The sound conducting parts of the avian middle ear consist of the TM, extra-columella, columella and its footplate, the annular ligament, intrinsic drum ligaments, drum-tubal ligaments, Platner's ligament, and the single middle-ear muscle (the stapedius). All these features can be identified in Figs. 2.1 and 2.2. The most apparent feature of the avian middle ear, when viewed externally, is the convex appearance of the TM. The membrane is supported by the various bones that form the limits of the middle-ear cavity; the sphenoid, occipital, and squamosal bones, as well as the tympanic process of the quadrate bone (Borg, Counter, & Rydquist, 1979; Pohlman, 1921). The membrane is kept taut by a series of ligaments (Fig. 2.2) which also hold the columella system in position. The single middle-ear muscle tenses the extra-columella and TM. The extra-columella is a three legged structure which we label after the description of Pohlman (1921) as the supra-, infra-, and extra-stapedius (Figs. 2.1 and 2.2). The cartilaginous extra-columella and bony columella form a rigid ossicle that

FIG. 2.1. A line drawing of the conductive structures in the parakeet middle ear is presented. The labels are: A_l = annular ligament; C = columella; E_c = extra-columella; E_s = extra-stapedius; I_s = infrastapedius; I_{dt} = inferior drum-tubal ligament; M_{dt} = medial drum-tubal ligament; P_1 = Platner's ligament; S_{dt} = superior drum-tubal ligament; S_s = supra-stapedius; T_m = tympanic membrane. The intrinsic drum ligaments are seen along the lower left-hand rim of the membrane. The middle ear muscle attaches to the inferior stapedius of the extra-columella. As a reference the length of the columella is 1.35 mm. The figure is modified from Saunders (1985).

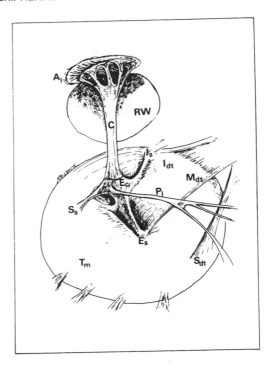

presses into the TM and gives it the convex shape. Saunders (1985) indicated that the membrane is firmly attached along the entire length of the extra-stapedius in the species he examined. The TM consists of three layers. The epidermal layer of the external meatus extends over the surface of the TM and is loosely connected to it (Saiff, 1978; Stellbogen, 1930). The lamina propria is the middle layer and is covered on its inner surface by an extension of the endothelium found in the middle-ear cavity. Across species the surface area of this membrane is quite variable and where measured it extends from 5.87 sq mm in the neonatal chick to 50.6 sq mm in the owl (see for additional details Freye-Zumpfe, 1953; Saunders, 1985; Schwartzkopff, 1955, 1957).

The columella footplate also varies in its form across species (Krause, 1901; Saunders, 1985). In some species like the pigeon or chicken the base of the footplate appears quite solid and massive, while in others (canary and parakeet) it is rather slender with many struts and air spaces that open to a hollow columella (Saunders, 1985; Stellbogen, 1930). It has been suggested that the reduction in mass, without a loss in bending strength may contribute to the ''good hearing abilities'' in species that possess the more slender, lightweight design columella and footplate (Kühne & Lewis, 1985). The footplate is supported in the oval window by the annular ligament. This ligament is broader at its rostral margin and may act as a hinge allowing the footplate to move with a rocking motion (Gaudin, 1968).

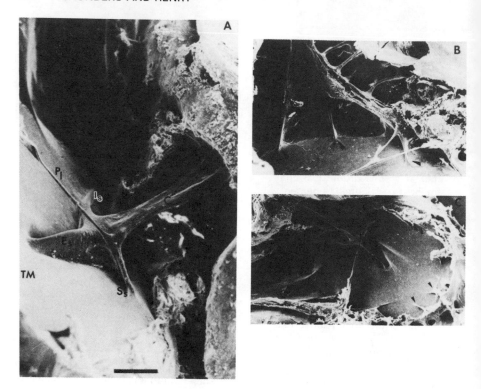

FIG. 2.2. The organization of the extra-columella is seen in panel A
and the labels are the same as in Figure 1. In panels B and C the drum
tubal ligaments (arrows) are seen in detail. The figure is modified from
Saunders (1985).

The ratio between the TM and footplate area is related to the pressure amplification function of the middle-ear system, and has been reported to vary between 11 and 40 across 49 species (Saunders, 1985; Schwartzkopff, 1957). By
comparison the area ratio is 36 in cat, and 30 in chinchilla and mouse (Saunders
& Garfinkle, 1982; Vretakkos, Dear, & Saunders, 1987; Wever & Lawrence,
1954). These areas are important in that pressure is determined by the force-per-
unit area. Thus the same force acting on the TM acts on the footplate, but
because the footplate has a smaller surface, the pressure acting on the membrane
is amplified at the footplate by the area ratio. The TM, however, is attached at its
rim and thus is not free to move over its entire surface. There are arguments over
the "effective" TM area, and because this is not known for the birds, it is
difficult to place any meaning on the differences in area ratios among species at
this time.

An additional pressure advantage in the avian middle ear can be gained from a
levering of the movements between the TM and columella footplate. If the

displacements of the membrane are larger than those of the footplate, then a pressure advantage will be realized. A lever ratio has been directly measured in the dove (Saunders & Johnstone, 1972) and has been modeled on the basis of middle-ear anatomy by Gaudine (1968) and Norberg (1978). The lever advantage is derived from the fact that the extra-columella is off-set on the TM, and this imparts a rocking motion to the columella footplate in the oval window. The estimates of a lever advantage in birds vary between 1.6 to 3.1. By comparison the level advantage in cat is 2.0 (Guinan & Peake, 1967).

The transmission characteristics of the avian middle ear have also been examined (Gummer, Smolders, & Klinke, 1986; Saunders, 1985; Saunders & Johnstone, 1972). This is accomplished by measuring the displacements of the TM or columella footplate at a fixed location, for a number of different frequencies with stimulus intensity held constant. The measurements have been made with Mössbauer or capacitive probe technology which permits detection of mechanical movements to fractions of a micron. In the dove and pigeon the shape of the transfer function at both the TM and footplate was identical. The footplate, however, showed a less sensitive response due to the lever ratio (Gummer et al., 1986; Saunders & Johnstone, 1972). The transfer function of the TM has also been described for the neonatal chick and adult parakeet, and these data are presented in Fig. 2.3. In the left panel of Fig. 2.3 the displacement of the TM was measured at the most convex point of the membrane (at the tip of the extra-columella). The results are presented as membrane displacement when the stimulus applied to the "ear drum" is maintained at 100 dB SPL. These data represent the *best* animal of the many subjects tested in each species. The

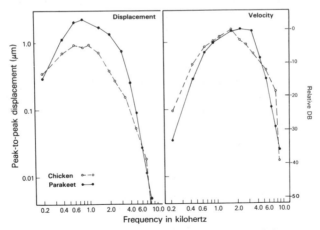

FIG. 2.3. The displacement and velocity response of the tympanic membrane in the chick and parakeet are presented. These data are for the "best" animal tested in each group. The velocity curve shows the typical "band-pass" filter characteristics on the non-mammalian middle ear response. The data are replotted from Saunders (1985).

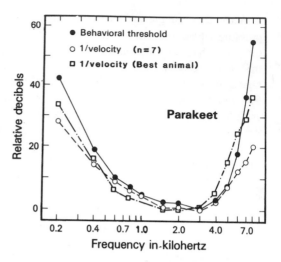

FIG. 2.4. The inverse of the tympanic membrane velocity response is plotted against the behavioral audibility curve of the parakeet obtained by Saunders, Else and Bock (1978). The shape of the middle ear response in the "best" animal closely approximates the shape of the threshold curve. Redrawn from Saunders (1985).

sharpness or selectivity of the transfer curve would be expected to deteriorate as a consequence of surgical trauma, testing time, and other uncontrolled variables. Thus, the *best* preparation provides an indication of what the middle-ear system is capable of performing under the closest approximation to ideal conditions. The displacement data show that a maximum response to the constant stimulus SPL is achieved in the mid-range frequencies, and this most likely corresponds to the resonant frequency of the middle ear. Even though the SPL of the stimulus is held constant at 100 dB, the displacement of air particles will decline at a rate of 6 dB per octave. Thus the TM displacement curves in Fig. 2.3 are not really referenced against a constant input. However, at 100 dB SPL, air particle velocity is constant over frequency, and by replotting the displacement data in terms of velocity (right hand panel of Fig. 2.3) the results are compared against a constant input signal. Moreover, velocity is generally accepted as the essential input signal to the cochlea. The velocity results in Fig. 2.3 reveal that the bird transfer functions exhibit a band-pass characteristic. The high frequency roll-off is about 35 and 32 dB per octave for the parakeet and chick respectively. This characteristic is unlike the high-pass velocity response reported for the TM in mammals (for a summary see Saunders & Tilney, 1982).

In Fig. 2.4 the relation between the behaviorally measured threshold curve for the parakeet (Dooling & Saunders, 1975), plotted as relative dB, is presented along with the inverse velocity function for the TM response. The tympanic membrane response for the average of seven animals (Saunders, 1985) and for the *best* animal are both presented. These results indicate that the shape of the middle-ear response is closely correlated to the shape of the behavioral audiogram. This relation has also been demonstrated in a number of mammalian species (i.e., cat, hamster, mouse; see Khanna & Tonndorf, 1977; Relkin & Saunders, 1980; Saunders & Summers, 1982).

The importance of this observation is that the transfer function of the middle ear sets limits on the parameters of acoustic energy reaching the inner ear. This curve says little about sensitivity, which is largely determined by the transduction properties of the hair cells. However, it does explain why high frequency hearing in birds is so limited. In large measure, the middle ear is incapable of transferring high frequency information to the cochlea. Similarly, the low frequency limitations of the transfer function raise interesting questions about avian infra-sound hearing (Kreithen & Quine, 1979), since the middle ear, at frequencies below 1.0 Hz, is probably incapable of transferring energy to the cochlea.

II. FREQUENCY RESOLUTION

The frequency resolving power of avian hearing is an important perceptual property which takes on added significance when the complexity and diversity of avian vocalizations are considered. Resolving power can be measured at the behavioral level by using conditioning and psychoacoustic methods to determine frequency difference limens, critical bands or ratios, or masking procedures that yield tuning-curve functions. All of these phenomena have been studied in various bird species and they have been interrelated to reveal common principles of frequency analysis in the bird (Dooling & Searcy, 1979, 1980, 1985; Saunders, Rintelman, & Bock, 1979). A number of interesting observations have emerged from this effort, and we consider a few of these below. The most obvious conclusion is that birds exhibit excellent frequency resolution. Indeed, as we will see, frequency selectivity at some frequencies in the parakeet at least, is clearly as good as, if not superior to the best frequency selectivity of many mammals. This would not be so interesting, if the bird inner ear were simply a scaled-down version of the mammalian cochlea; we shall see it is remarkably different in its structural organization. (Saito, 1980; Smith, 1985).

Several examples of frequency resolution in birds are presented in Fig. 2.5. The upper panel illustrates two psychophysical tuning curves obtained in the parakeet using a forward and simultaneous masking paradigm (Kuhn & Saunders, 1980). As expected, the sharpness of tuning changed as a consequence of both test frequency and procedure. Moreover, the tuning curves in this figure appear generally symmetrical on both sides of the center frequency. The observant reader will also note that the trough of the tip region is quite deep, being 60 dB or more for the forward masking conditions. A considerable number of masking procedures have been used with the parakeet and other bird species to examine tuning properties at the behavioral level and they all exhibit more or less symmetrical tuning functions (Dooling & Searcy, 1979, 1980, 1985; Saunders,

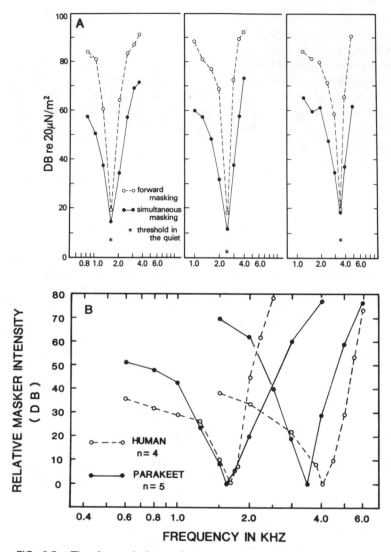

FIG. 2.5. The A panel shows three sets of psychophysical tuning curves obtained by forward and simultaneous masking in the parakeet. The forward masking tuning functions had Q values of 9.2, 13.0, and 14.7 from left to right. The B panel compares parakeet and human psychophysical tuning curves obtained with forward masking. The testing conditions for both species were identical. The data are redrawn from Kühn and Saunders (1980) and Saunders, Rintelman, and Bock (1979).

1976; Saunders, Bock, & Fahrbach, 1978; Saunders, Denny, & Bock, 1978; Saunders & Else, 1976; Saunders & Pallone, 1980).

In Fig. 2.5B simultaneous masking psychophysical tuning curves, at two test frequencies, are related to corresponding tuning curves for human listeners obtained by identical procedures (Saunders, Else, & Bock, 1978; Saunders et al., 1979). The selectivity of these tuning curves can be described by a Q ratio (defined as the center frequency divided by the bandwidth of the tuning function 10 dB above the center frequency), and the higher the value of Q the more sharply tuned or more frequency selective is the auditory filter. The Q ratio for the parakeet and human data of Fig. 2.5B at the low frequency was 2.2. and 4.1 respectively, while at the higher frequencies it was 9.2 and 5.0. At 3.5 kHz the filter characteristics of the parakeet ear were much more selective than the human at 4.0 kHz. As it turns out, human Q ratios for simultaneous masking tuning curves increase from 1.5 to 5.0 between 0.25 and 2.0 kHz. At higher frequencies they remain fairly constant, at least to 8.0 kHz (Saunders et al., 1979). Frequency selectivity in the parakeet, as measured by five different procedures, rises from 1.0 to about 9.0 from 0.3 to 3.5 kHz (Fig. 2.6). At the highest frequencies tested the sharpness of tuning appears to deteriorate (Saunders & Pallone, 1980; Saunders, Pallone, & Rosowski, 1980). A similar curve of frequency selectivity (the Q ratio) across the hearing range of the neonatal chick has been reported by Saunders and Tilney (1979), and is reproduced in Fig. 2.7. A cochlear nucleus

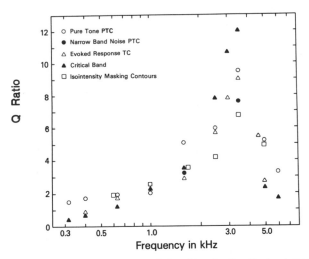

FIG. 2.6.   Frequency selectivity as defined by the Q ratio is plotted for the parakeet as a function of frequency. The parameter in the figure is the procedure for measuring frequency selectivity. With exception of the evoked response procedure, all the data are from behavioral experiments. The figure is replotted from Saunders and Pallone (1980) and Saunders, Pallone, and Rosowski (1980).

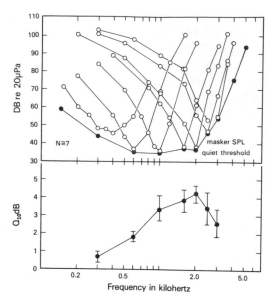

FIG. 2.7. Evoked response tuning curves from the cochlear nuclei of the neonatal chick (7-days-old) are presented (top panel) along with the Q values (lower panel). Each data point is the average of 7 animals. Data from Saunders and Tilney (1979).

evoked response tuning curve procedure employing a simultaneous masking paradigm was used to obtain these data.

It is widely held that the filter properties of the auditory system in mammals are derived from the mechanical properties of the cochlear partition, particularly the interaction between the basilar membrane, hair cell stereocilia, and the tectorial membrane (see for example Khanna, 1983, 1984). Neuroanatomical evidence of orderly projections from the cochlear nerve to the cochlear nuclei (Boord & Rasmussen, 1963), evidence of tonotopic organization of the cells in the cochlear nuclei (Konishi, 1970), indications of orderly frequency selectivity in cochlear ganglion cells and nerve fibers (Gleich, Lappelsack, & Oeckinghaus, 1985; Sachs, Young, & Lewis, 1974), and direct measures of the basilar membrane response (Gummer et al., 1986; von Békésy, 1960) all indicate that frequency analysis also occurs in the bird cochlea. However, as Smith (1985) noted, the intriguing and as yet unanswered question is how the bird ear accomplishes this analysis.

The avian cochlea has been described in ample detail for a number of species (for example, see Smith, 1985; Smith, Konishi, & Schuff, 1985; Takasaka & Smith, 1971; Tanaka & Smith, 1978), and we focus on the receptor epithelium of the inner ear in this presentation. The receptor organ for hearing is called the basilar papilla and is located in the middle chamber of the cochlea. The papilla is covered by the tectorial membrane (Fig. 2.8A) and when this is removed the hair cell field can be seen (Fig. 2.8B). The papilla is relatively short, being on the order of 2.5 to 4.0 mm in most small birds, but as long as 7 mm in the owl (Smith et al., 1985). As Fig. 2.8B shows the papilla has a slight turn to it, and is

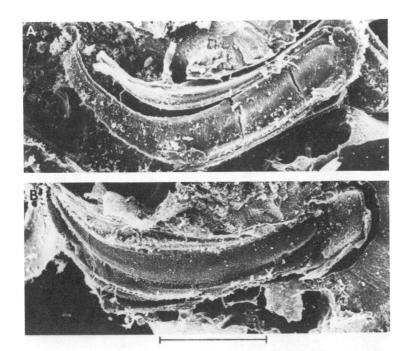

FIG. 2.8.   Two stages of dissecting the chick basilar papilla are seen. In panel A the tectorial membrane is intact. The fibrous nature of this structure can be seen along the inferior edge. In panel B the tectorial membrane has been removed and the dots along the papilla represent the sensory hair tufts on the hair cells. The calibration bar indicates 1.0 mm. These dissections were made from freeze dried ears and the panels are modified from Schneider et al. (1987).

distinctly shaped at its distal (low frequency) and proximal (high frequency) ends. In cross section (Fig. 2.9) the cochlea is seen to have the three chambered organization of the mammal. Scala vestibuli and scala tympani lie above and below the middle chamber (the cochlear duct or scala media). The tegmentum vasculosum forms a boundary between the upper and middle chamber, while the basilar membrane is the boundary between the lower and middle chambers. In a transverse section as many as 40–50 hair cells may lie across the papilla surface (at its widest point). Only a portion of the hair cells are found over the basilar membrane, while the remaining receptor cells are situated on the relatively immobile superior cartilaginous plate.

There are about 10,300 hair cells distributed on this epithelium in the chick (Tilney, Tilney, Saunders, & DeRosien, 1986), and these are organized into three groupings: tall, intermediate, and short hair cells (see Smith, 1985 for a review). The short hair cells are so defined because their cell bodies are relatively

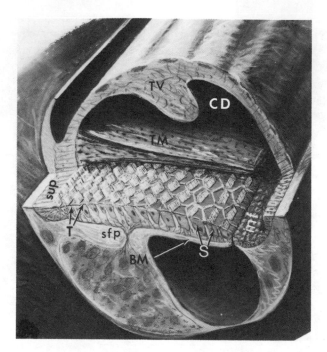

FIG. 2.9. A cross section of the bird cochlea is seen. The labels indicate the following structures: BM = basilar membrane; CD = cochlear duct; inf = inferior edge of the basilar pipilla; S = short hair cells; sfp = superior cartilaginous plate; sup = superior edge of the basilar papilla; T = tall hair cells; TM = tectorial membrane; and TV = tegmentum vasclosum. Tilney and Saunders (1983) redrew this figure from Takasaka and Smith (1971), and this rendering is modified from Tilney and Saunders (1983).

short. They are found over the "free" basilar membrane portion of the cochlea, are innervated by a single afferent synapse, and have large efferent terminals at their basal end (Takasaka & Smith, 1971; Tanaka & Smith, 1978). The tall hair cells have a large columnar appearance, multiple afferent synapses, and relatively few efferent boutons. They are located along the superior edge of the entire papilla above the superior fibrocartilaginous plate (see Fig. 2.9). The vast majority of the fibers from the cochlear nerve innervate the tall hair cells. The intermediate cells occupy a zone between the tall and short hair cells. The tall and short hair cells are often considered as avian analogues of the mammalian inner and outer hair cells.

The important receptive zones for the hair cell is the sensory hair bundle or stereocilia at the apical end. The morphology of the sensory hair tuft changes systematically along the length of the papilla (Tilney & Saunders, 1983; Tilney et al., 1986). These changes from the distal to proximal end, in terms of the number of hairs per cell, the height of the hairs, their diameter, and their orientation on the cell, have been described in detail for the chick, and can be used as signatures to locate specific hair cells on the papilla (Tilney & Saunders, 1983; Tilney et al., 1986; Tilney et al., 1987). Receptor cell transduction occurs when the sensory hairs are deflected (Hudspeth, 1985). It is currently thought that the mechanosensitive transduction channels lie somewhere along the plasma membrane of the sensory hairs. A number of schemes have been proposed to describe how these channels might be activated (see for example, Hudspeth, 1985; Saunders, Schneider, & Dear, 1985). Perhaps the most important is related to the interconnecting "tip" links between stereocilia on adjacent rows in the hair bundle (for review see Hudspeth, 1985). These tip links have been extensively described for hair bundles in the guinea pig cochlea (Furness & Hackney, 1985; Pickles, Comis, & Osborne, 1984). As illustrated in Fig. 2.10, links are also seen interconnecting adjacent rows of sensory hairs on chick hair cells. It is thought that when the sensory hairs are deflected in the excitatory direction the tip links pull on the mechanosensitive transduction channels, thus opening them. This leads to an influx of ionic species (presumably K^+), depolarization of the cell, and the release of neurotransmitter. Deflection in the other direction relaxes the links, which increase the probability that the transduction channel is tightly closed. As a consequence the cell hyperpolarizes.

The underlying processes of frequency analysis in avian hearing are not well understood, however a number of possible mechanisms can be suggested. As already noted the frequency analytic processes in birds, as in mammals, resides in the auditory periphery. The results plotted in Fig. 2.6 showed systematic changes in frequency resolution throughout the audible range of the parakeet. The behaviorally defined functions of frequency selectivity in this figure, such as the psychophysical tuning curves, the critical ratios and bands, and the iso-intensity contours, when normalized by the Q ratio, all had the same degree of selectivity as the evoked response tuning curves obtained from the cochlear nuclei. These data indicate that the behavioral measures were derived from events that originated in the periphery. It appears that little if any additional frequency sharpening occurs in the central auditory pathways of the parakeet.

We have noted that the sensory hair bundles vary in their height from one end of the papilla to the other (Tilney & Saunders, 1983). This gradation is organized so that the tallest hairs are located in the low frequency end of the cochlea (distal tip), whereas the shortest are found at the high frequency end. Sensory hair bundle height is correlated with the distribution of frequency along the receptor organ of six species including a bird (Saunders & Dear, 1983). The stereocilia exhibit resonant properties, and variations in height along the length of the papilla may tune each hair cell to a narrow frequency range (Frischkopf & DeRosier, 1983; Holton & Hudspeth, 1983). In addition, von Békésy (1960) measured stiffness along the basilar membrane in the chicken and concluded that

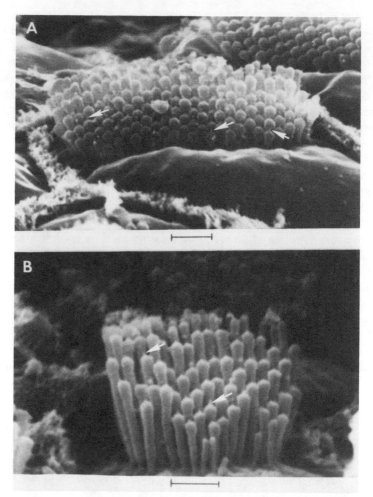

FIG. 2.10. The sensory hair bundles from two cochlear hair cells in the five day old chick are presented. The A panel shows stereocilia from a high frequency cell located at the proximal tip of the cochlea. The B panel is a hair cell from the approximate middle of the papilla. The arrows indicate the tip-links that interconnect adjacent rows of hairs.

this structure could perform frequency analysis. These measures, however, were obtained in cadaver ears, and it is unclear if the same conditions exist in the fresh cochlea. More recently Gummer and his colleagues (Gummer et al., 1986) directly measured the magnitude and phase response of the pigeon basilar membrane in living specimens. Their data also support the hypothesis that the receptor organ is capable of mechanical frequency analysis. The measures of frequency selectivity from cochlear nerve or cochlear ganglion cells provide additional evidence of frequency selective processes on the papilla. In the mammal, the auditory nerve tuning curves are only a reflection of frequency tuning in the receptor cell. Moreover, the receptor cell response appears to be a reflection of the mechanical response of the basilar membrane (Khanna, 1983, 1984). It remains to be seen if the tuning curves of the primary neuron in birds can also be traced to the basilar membrane response. This may be unlikely however, since the tall hair cells lie over the superior cartilaginous plate, and are not influenced directly by the movements of the basilar membrane (see Fig. 2.9). Indeed it is not yet clear how the sensory hair bundles on these cells are stimulated. It is known that the tallest hairs in the bundle of both tall and short hair cells attach to the tectorial membrane (Tanaka & Smith, 1975). Deflections of the basilar membrane, leading to movements of the short hair cells, may pull the tectorial membrane across the receptor surface in such a way that it tugs and pushes on the tall hair-cell stereocilia.

Finally, a general asymmetry is found in all the tuning functions reported for mammalian species. This is seen in the shallow low frequency and steep high frequency slopes of the human psychophysical tuning curves in Fig. 2.5B. The mechanical response of the mammalian basilar membrane, as characterized by the traveling wave, has a long tail and an asymmetric peak response region (see Khanna, 1984). These properties of the traveling wave are thought to contribute directly to the frequency selective processes seen in the mammal. We have suggested that the auditory filters in the avian ear are different, and one feature of this difference is that the high- and low-frequency slopes of the tuning curves are approximately equal. An explanation of this difference may lie in the mechanical action of the basilar membrane response. As the hypothetical data in Fig. 2.11 indicate, it may be that the avian traveling wave has a more symmetric ap-

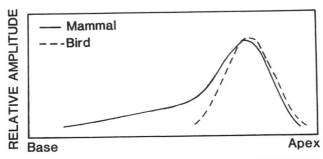

FIG. 2.11. In this hypothetical drawing the envelope of the mammalian traveling wave is shown with its tail and peak region. As suggested in the text the avian traveling wave may lack a tail region and appear more symmetrical on the surface of the papilla.

pearance. This possibility is partially supported by the "V" shaped basilar membrane response data reported by Gummer et al. (1986). Another possibility, recently suggested by Tilney, Tilney, and DeRosier (1987), is that the population of hair cells on the papilla activated by a tone varies considerably with the location of the papilla stimulated. Tilney has demonstrated contours of equal sensory hair bundle height or orientation that lie at an oblique angle to the papilla. If, for example, hair bundles of equal height code for the same frequency (using the assumptions of resonance noted earlier) then the process of frequency analysis in terms of the patterns of activation on the avian papilla is much more complicated than currently appreciated. Tilney et al. (1987) however, did not consider the effects of loading the sensory hairs by the tectorial membrane (Zwislocki, 1986) and this aspect needs to be considered further before iso-height or iso-orientation contours can be considered to have functional importance.

III.   SOUND LOCALIZATION

In this section we consider the contribution of the auditory periphery to the perception of sound in space. Although this treatment is restricted to peripheral processes, the reader should recognize that very important advances have been made in the last decade concerning the central mechanisms in birds that code for auditory space (Knudsen, 1980, 1983). The identification of sound in space appears to be a rather *special* process in the bird, and unlike the situation in the mammal, the mechanisms remain elusive. Nevertheless, a fuller appreciation of this property of avian hearing may be significant for understanding other aspects of complex sound perception in birds.

The minimum audible angle (MAA) provides an indication of the minimum separation between two sounds along the horizontal azimuth that can be detected 50% of the time. The MAA has been measured in great detail for human listeners Mills (1958).   The results indicate that the smallest MAA occurs when the reference position is located near the midline. Across frequency the midline MAA varies from 2 to 4° with the low frequencies showing better resolution. At 30° from the midline the MAA varies from 2 to 12° with resolution deteriorating above 1.5 kHz. At 60° the MAA is even poorer. Egelmann (1928, cited in Erulkar, 1972) made one of the earliest attempts to measure the MAA in a bird. His data for neonatal chicks suggested that they could localize a hen's maternal exodus call to within 4°. Localization data for other birds generally fall far short of this acuity. The early work with the bullfinch concluded that the MAA was between 20° and 25° (Granit, 1941; Schwartzkopff, 1949, 1950). The bobwhite quail, based on the number of correct responses to speakers spaced 180° apart, can discriminate an angle of 25–30° at 2.0 kHz (Gatehouse & Shelton, 1978). Although no MAA data were obtained, Jenkins and Masterton (1979) clearly demonstrated that pigeons could localize sounds. More recent work has attempted to quantify the MAA under conditions of greater control. However, this measure remains elusive both in terms of training the animals, and in controlling the stimulus. Nevertheless, Klump and his associates (Klump, Windt, & Curio, 1986) have shown an MAA of 20° for the great tit. A heart rate conditioning procedure in pigeons revealed a "minimum resoluable angle" between 4 to 6° from 250 to 500 Hz (Lewald, 1987a). In the mid-frequency range (1.0–2.0 kHz) the threshold increased to 25–50°. Park, Okanoya, and Dooling (1987) reported MAA's between 10 and 20° for the canary, zebra finch, and the great tit. More interesting is data from the parakeet in which a spatial resolution of 5° was demonstrated (Park et al., 1987). Remarkably, the barn owl has an acuity of 1 to 2° in both azimuth and elevation, when measured by strike accuracy or head orientation accuracy (Payne, 1971; Knudsen, 1980; Knudsen & Konishi, 1979). On the basis of this literature it is difficult to draw a general conclusion concerning the accuracy of sound localization in birds. The localizing ability of the chick and owl seem unusually acute, and certainly needs to be replicated in the case of the chick. The owl may represent a special case, not only for the biological specializations it posesses in the peripheral ear (Knudsen, 1980; Kühne & Lewis, 1985), but because of its natural tendency to orient or strike at acoustic signals. Indeed, the localizing ability of the owl may be more a reflection of its capacity to provide us with an unambiguous behavioral indication of sound location, rather than with some intrinsic sensory ability unique to this species.

Several cues have been clearly identified as the essential signals for determining the source of a sound (Knudsen, 1980). These include differences at the two tympanic membranes for: (a)   The arrival time of transient sounds;   (b) The ongoing phase of a sustained sound; (c) Sound intensity, and; (d) Sound spectrum distribution. Birds represent a unique evolutionary problem for sound localization, and based on the assumptions that have been applied to localization phenomena in the mammalian system, they should have a poor sense of auditory space. In the following sections we consider why this is so.

Differences in time of arrival, either for transient or continuous stimuli, occur as a consequence of the propagation of a sound disturbance. This disturbance moves away from its source, independent of frequency, at the approximate rate of 344 meters per sec. The wavelength of sound however, is frequency dependent. The time of arrival of a stimulus at the two ears depend on the source of the sound (along the horizontal azimuth), the distance between the two TMs, the orientation of the head, and the speed of sound propagation. Most birds have very small heads and this places severe restraints on their ability to utilize time-of-arrival information. Let us consider a small bird whose intertympanic distance (equal approximately to the diameter of the head) is about 2.0 cm. If a sound source is located 90° to the head along the horizontal axis (0° would be directly in front of the animals beak in the horizontal plane) the difference in time of arrival at the ipsilateral and contralateral ear is given by:

$$TD = (a/c)(\sin \varnothing + \varnothing)$$

where TD is the time delay, a is the radius of the head, c the velocity of sound, and $\varnothing$ is the incident angle of the sound stimulus on the head (Woodworth, 1938). In our example of a bird with an approximate 2.0 cm head diameter, the time of arrival at the two ears (for the best case of sound at 90°) would differ by only 74 usec! By comparison, the human head has a diameter of 17.5 cm, and the interaural time delay for a stimulus at 90° is about 650 usec. In absolute terms as the stimulus is moved from 0° to 90° along the horizontal axis there will be a change of approximately 7.22 usec per degree for the human listener (this value is in slight error as the equation above shows, since the radius of the head must be taken into account). In the case of our hypothetical bird there is a change of about 0.82 usec per degree. Of course, sound localization is not necessarily referenced in absolute terms along the horizontal axis, but may be relative to two points in space. The MAA is smallest for sound sources around the midline and increases rapidly beyond 60° because of complex time delays introduced by the pinna. Nevertheless, as a generalization, the human nervous system can distinguish about a 3° difference between two sounds lying along the horizontal azimuth from 0 to 30° (Mills, 1958). This corresponds to a time difference at the two ears of about 22 usec. Assuming that this difference represents a limit on the detection of synaptic events in the vertebrate nervous system, a bird with the same 22 usec limitation could only discriminate the difference between two sound sources spread apart by about 27°! Alternatively, if the bird could detect a 3° spatial difference, the nervous system would have to successfully distinguish synaptic events occurring with a delay of 2.5 usec. This is roughly three orders of magnitude faster than synaptic transmission time itself (about 1.0 msec)! As far as interaural time differences are concerned, birds are either unable to use this cue or have a remarkable nervous system for detecting time differences. Some recent evidence suggest that the pigeon, between 0.25 and 1.0 kHz can detect ongoing interaural time differences around 10 to 30 microseconds (Lewald, 1987b). This is similar to that found in the mammal.

Differences in sound pressure at the two ears is most effective when the distance between the two TMs (again approximately equal to the diameter of the head) is greater than the stimulus wavelength. An interaural intensity difference occurs because of two phenomena. First, surplus pressure builds up at the ear facing the sound as acoustic energy reflects off the head and interacts with the incident wavefront. Second, the reflected sound does not diffract about the head, and as a consequence there is a loss in sound pressure due to the "head shadow" effect at the contralateral ear (Saunders & Garfinkle, 1982). The interaural intensity difference between the ears of the human head is effective above 2.0 kHz. A bird with an interaural distance of 2.0 cm would exhibit a strong head shadow effect at frequencies above 17.0 kHz! It might be argued that small mammals have overcome this problem by evolving high-frequency hearing. In birds however, the limits of high-frequency hearing rarely exceed 8.0–10.0 kHz (Dooling, 1980). Moreover, the frequencies used in communication tend to lie between 1.0 and 3.5 kHz, and have wavelengths much larger than the head size (e.g., 34.4 to 9.8 cm). Thus, it is difficult to understand how differences in interaural intensity play a role in avian sound localization.

Autrum realized in 1940 that animals with small heads can achieve significant directional sensitivity by using the two ears as a pressure difference detector instead of the mammalian-type pressure detector. An ear designed to operate in this manner must have sound waves strike both the inner and outer surfaces of the TM at the same time. The actual displacement of the eardrum in this situation depends on the net pressure and phase on both sides of the membrane. The phase difference at the membrane depends on the length of the acoustic pathway between the sound source and the outer and inner surfaces. Furthermore, the length of this acoustic path will vary as a function of the sound source direction. The principles behind a differential pressure detector are summarized in Fig. 2.12. If the avian TMs acted as differential pressure detectors, then large pressure differences between the ears might occur without the need to resort to traditional interaural intensity or time difference cues. The problem, of course, is to explain how birds can develop an acoustic signal on the inside of their TMs.

It has long been known that the middle ears of birds are interconnected by air passageways (Coles et al., 1980; Henson, 1974; Hill, Lewis, Hutchings, & Cole, 1980, Payne, 1971; Rosowski, 1979; Rosowski & Saunders, 1980; Schwartz-kopff, 1952; Stellbogen, 1930; Wada, 1923). These air-filled connections result from the joining of the bilateral bony eustachian tubes, and the air spaces at the back of the skull (Kühne & Lewis, 1985; Rosowski, 1979). These interaural pathways are capable of transmitting sound from one middle ear to the other, and provide the necessary delay-line conditions needed for a differential pressure detector (Coles et al., 1980; Hill et al., 1980; Kühne & Lewis, 1985; Lewis, 1983; Rosowski, 1979; Rosowski & Saunders, 1980). Moreover, in some species the intensity of the acoustic stimuli acting on the inside and outside of the TM are not the same. Thus, the differential pressure across the TM needs to be calculated from the complex vector interaction of both magnitude and phase of the internal and external TM signals. In this situation the ears act as *partial* differential pressure detectors.

Rosowski (1979) provided a detailed description of the interaural pathway in the pigeon and it is worthwhile summarizing his observations here. The volume of the skull air spaces connecting the two middle ears was found to be about 1.0 ml. This space included the bony eustachian tube interconnecting the two middle-ear cavities, the middle-ear cavities themselves, and the connected air spaces in the bilayered skull that communicate with the middle ears. The volume of each middle ear was about 0.05 ml, while that of the interconnecting eustachian pathway was 0.5 ml. The remaining 0.4 ml was distributed in the air spaces of the skull. Within the eustachian tube and between the layers of the skull were a

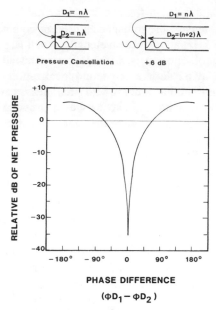

FIG. 2.12.   A general explanation of a differential pressure detector is presented. In the upper panels a tube with a membrane stretched across it is seen. Acoustic stimulation (D_1) on one side of the membrane will cause it to displace because of the pressure variations on its surface. If a second stimulus (D_2), of the same frequency and intensity, but 180° out of phase (upper right panel) is applied to backside of the membrane, the displacement will increase. This is because a pressure condensation (for example) on one side occurs with a pressure rarefaction on the other side. In effect the membrane is "pushed" and "pulled" simultaneously. However, if the two acoustic stimuli are in phase, a positive pressure (for example) on one side of the membrane (upper left panel, D_1) will push against a positive pressure on the other side (D_2) and the net displacement will approach zero. The plot of phase difference across the membrane against net pressure shows this relation. The phase differences at the membrane occur because of the length of the tube and the direction of the sound relative to the tube. This figure was modified and redrawn from Lewis and Coles (1980).

large number of bony struts (trabeculi). Rosowski (1979) noted that the struts in the skull air spaces were sufficiently dense along the midline to prevent a patent pathway between the two middle ears, and he concluded that the eustachian tube was the principal structure of the interaural pathway. The organization of the interaural pathway in pigeon was quite complex. The length, from its opening into the middle ear on either side, averaged 9.4 mm in six skulls. The width of

the path was variable being narrowest at the openings to the middle-ear cavity
(2.7 mm in diameter) and widest at the midline (7.1 mm). The height of the path
also varied along its length being shallowest at the midline (2.0 mm) with a
"tent-like" peak (5.2 mm) occurring between the midline and the opening to the
middle ear. Rosowski (1979) assumed that the length of the interaural pathway
(about 1.1 cm from left to right TMs) was small enough so that the wavelengths
in the pigeon's audible range (below 10 kHz or longer than 3.4 cm) should
minimally influence sound traveling through the path.

Several sources of evidence support the hypothesis that the bird ear acts as a
partial differential pressure detector. Hill and his associates (1980) used probe-
tube microphones to measure acoustic pressure in the outer and middle ear of the
quail. Their data indicated relatively little acoustic loss across the interaural
pathway for mid-range frequencies (2.0–6.0 kHz). Rosowski and Saunders
(1980) made similar measures of sound conduction in the neonatal chick. They
showed 30 dB of attenuation across the TM, but no additional loss in sound
transmission through the pathway itself (Fig. 2.13). These effects, moreover,
were independent of frequency from 100 Hz to 6.0 kHz. Sound transmission
through the pigeon interaural pathway, however, was reported to be frequency

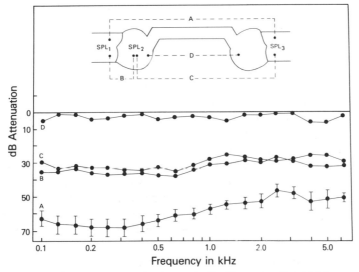

FIG. 2.13. The upper panel schematically illustrates the middle ear
cavities and interaural pathway, the three probe-tube microphone locations from which pressure measures were taken (SPL$_1$, SPL$_2$, SPL$_3$),
and the four measured transmission losses (A, B, C, D). The lower
panel shows the losses observed in the chick. A 30 dB loss occurred
across the TM (B and C), while there was almost no loss through the
interaural pathway (D). The figure is modified from Rosowski and
Saunders (1980).

dependent (Rosowski, 1979). A loss of about 10 dB occurred between 0.15 and 2.0 kHz and this increased to 26 dB at 4.0 kHz. At higher frequencies the loss diminished somewhat and by 10.0 kHz it was only 17 dB. It would thus seem that acoustic measures verify the transmission of sound between the middle-ear cavities of the quail, chick, and pigeon. There appear to be relatively little loss in the quail, whereas in the chick and pigeon loss across the TM and in the pathway itself (pigeon) change the pressure ratios acting on the outer and inner surfaces of the eardrum. Nevertheless, in all species the phase angle of the stimulus on the inner surface was different from that on the outer surface due to the delay line introduced by the interaural pathway.

These acoustic measures are interesting but it is important to empirically verify that the signals reaching the cochlea actually went through a differential pressure detector, and that they show directional sensitivity. There is now ample evidence that this is indeed the case (Coles et al., 1980; Rosowski, 1979; Rosowski and Saunders, 1980). The experimental procedure is relatively simple, and uses the microphonic potential recorded from the round window membrane of the cochlea as an indication of the stimulus energy reaching the inner ear. The potential arises from the inner ear (Dallos, 1973) and its magnitude and phase are a good reflection of the acoustic input to the cochlea.

The presence of a differential pressure detector has been demonstrated in the chick (Rosowski & Saunders, 1980) and the pigeon (Rosowski, 1979). In other species closed-field sound delivery was used to stimulate each ear separately. Differences were noted in stimulus intensity at the TM, for the ipsi- and contralateral stimulation needed to achieve a criterion ipsilateral microphonic response. In addition, bilateral stimulation using these intensities revealed that the microphonic response could be described as the result of a vector addition of individual responses to monaural stimulation. This supported the conclusion that the stimulus on the inner surface of the ipsilateral TM interacted with the stimulus on the external surface to produce the resultant microphonic response. Rosowski and Saunders (1980) mathematically modeled the binaural intensity ratios that might be seen at the chick's ears, based on the microphonic data from binaural stimulation. Fig. 2.14 represents the microphonic binaural intensity ratio as a function of azimuth at four frequencies. These ratios were compared with results from sound diffraction alone using the acoustic model developed by Stewart (1911). As can be seen, a larger binaural intensity difference (shown by a smaller intensity ratio) occurs at all frequencies for the differential pressure model.

Rosowski (1979) also confirmed the presence of a differential pressure detector in the pigeon using the microphonic response. As described earlier, he measured the magnitude and phase of this response during ipsilateral, contralateral, and binaural stimulation. Using a criterion microphonic response the stimuli were adjusted to produce an equal pressure on the inner and outer surfaces of the ipsilateral TM. The phase delays from these monaural conditions were noted. Using the monaural phase data Rosowski (1979) trigonometrically predicted

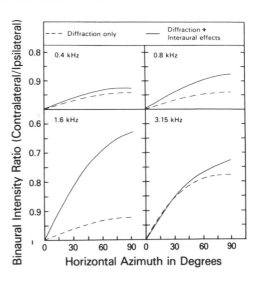

FIG. 2.14. Calculations of the binaural intensity ratio due to sound diffraction alone, and diffraction plus the differential pressure mechanism, are compared using data collected in the chick. At the four representative frequencies the differential pressure model produced larger binaural intensity differences than would be predicted by diffraction alone. This figure redrawn from Rosowski and Saunders (1980).

what the magnitude of the microphonic response would be during binaural stimulation. The resulting microphonic response was then empirically measured during equal intensity binaural stimulation. The empirical and theoretical predictions are plotted in Fig. 2.15 and the results indicate a significant correlation of 0.89. These results as with the chick, confirmed the operation of a differential pressure detector. These closed-field measures of the microphonic response unfortunately, do not directly confirm the contribution of a differential pressure detector to sound localization.

This issue was resolved by Coles et al. (1980). These investigators used the

FIG. 2.15. The measured and predicted microphonic responses are compared for 23 different test conditions. The measured response was determined from closed-field binaural stimulation of the pigeon ears. The stimulus level at each ear was set to produce an equal microphonic response during monaural stimulation. The predicted results were calculated from the phase and magnitude microphonic response during monaural stimulation. The correlation was close to unity and the slope of the line (1.1) was not significantly different from a slope of one. The figure is redrawn from Rosowski (1979).

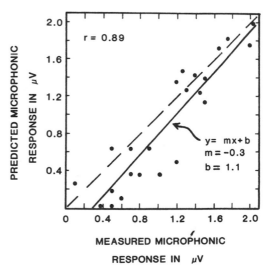

FIG. 2.16. A polar plot of the cochlear microphonic response from the right cochlea is presented during binaural stimulation and during stimulation with the contralateral ear canal blocked. The microphonic response, indicating the input to the right ear is clearly directional with binaural stimulation. If the contralateral ear is blocked, or if the pressure in the right ear canal is measured, there is no indication of stimulus directionality. This figure was modified and redrawn from Coles et al. (1980).

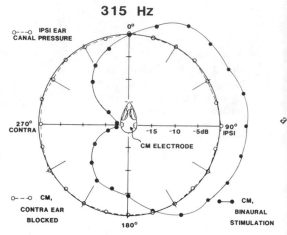

microphonic response to study the directional sensitivity of the quail ear. Anesthetized animals with an electrode placed on the round-window membrane, were mounted in the center of an anechoic chamber. The sound source was moved in an equidistant radius about the animal's head along the horizontal azimuth. A constant frequency and intensity stimulus was used and the microphonic response, at different angles, was referenced to the response when the stimulus was in front of the beak. Ear canal pressure was also measured on the same side as the electrode. The canal pressure was generally constant at all azimuthal positions. The microphonic response, however, showed striking evidence of directional sensitivity, and at 315 Hz, for example, it increased by 7 dB when the stimulus was directly in front of the ipsilateral ear. When the sound source faced the contralateral ear, the ipsilateral microphonic response was attenuated by about 17 dB. Importantly, when the contralateral ear canal was plugged, which in effect blocked the interaural pathway, the directional sensitivity of the microphonic response was lost. These results are summarized in Fig. 2.16. Thus, the input to the ipsilateral cochlea exhibited a 24 dB change from ipsilateral to contralateral stimulation, and this could not be accounted for by acoustic pressure changes in the ipsilateral ear canal.

Rosowski (1979) also described the directional sensitivity of the pigeon ear. Using a fixed speaker in the test environment, he rotated the head (and body) of an anesthetized animal, implanted with a round-window electrode, through the equivalent of 180° of horizontal azimuth. The microphonic response was compared at different angles during binaural stimulation and with the contralateral ear canal occluded. The acoustic testing environment was not anechoic. He found evidence of directional sensitivity with both binaural and monaural stimulation. However, the directionality of the ear was 3 to 5 dB better in every case of binaural stimulation. As with the Coles et al. (1980) experiment, contralateral occlusion removed the interaural pathway from the measurement system. Unlike the quail, where an interaural pressure difference as much as 24 dB emerged, the difference in the pigeon appeared to be considerably less. Similar findings using anchoic test conditions have recently been described for the pigeon (Lewald, personal communication). Thus, there may indeed be species differences in the effectiveness of the interaural pathway.

The above data support the conclusion that (a) the bird ear acts like a differential pressure detector; (b) this mechanism is inherently directional, and; (c) binaural comparisons in this directional sensitivity can provide unambiguous directional cues based on intensity differences at the two receptors. Earlier work with the bullfinch (Schwartzkopff, 1952) recognized the potential importance of the interaural pathway. Binaural studies with this species revealed directional sensitivity in the microphonic response that was much larger than could be predicted on the basis of acoustic diffraction alone. However, no change in the directionality of the microphonic response was found following occlusion of the contralateral ear. This contradictory finding is at odds with the more recent observations and needs to be examined further. In addition the owl appears to be a special case, and sound transmission through the head may be less significant than in other birds (Payne, 1971; Moiseff & Konishi, 1981). Because the issue of localization in the owl is complicated by major structural asymmetries in the outer ear, a head that is larger than most other birds, and a unique behavioral response to sound (Knudsen, 1980), this species will not be considered here. The reader is referred to Knudsen (1980, 1983) and Kühune and Lewis (1985) for further details. Nevertheless, the avian interaural pathway may be an important element in the spatial perception of sound, and hopefully future research will elucidate the function of this pathway in greater detail.

IV. CONCLUSIONS

In this essay we have suggested that certain aspects of the avian peripheral auditory system contributes in a special way to the perception of acoustic signals. The transfer characteristics of the middle ear sets limits on the functional flow of energy to the cochlea, and these limits contribute to the shape of the avian audibility curve. In addition, the mechanism for frequency analysis and resolution in bird hearing is established in the organization and function of the receptor organ. Moreover, since frequency and time resolution are interrelated, it may also be true that the cochlea provides the basis for temporal resolution in birds. Finally, the interaural pathway connecting the middle ear cavities may be important to the process of sound localization. It needs to be clearly recognized, however, that each of the relationships we have tried to establish are somewhat speculative, and further research is needed to tease out the contributions of peripheral and central factors in avian sound perception.

ACKNOWLEDGMENTS

The preparation of this manuscript was supported in part by awards from the Deafness Research Foundation, the Pennsylvania Lions Hearing Research Foundation, the University Research Foundation, and a Biomedical Research Support Grant to the University of Pennsylvania. The authors greatly appreciate the assistance of Ms Miriam Berg.

REFERENCES

Autrum, H. (1940). Das Richtungshören von *Locustra* und Versuch einer Hörtheorie fur Tympanalorgane des Locustidentyps. *Zeitschrift für Vergleischende Physiologie, 28,* 326–352.

Békésy, G. von (1960). *Experiments in hearing.* New York: McGraw Hill.

Borg, E., Counter, S. A., & Rydquist, B. (1979). Contraction properties and functional morphology of the avian stapedius muscle. *Acta Otolaryngology, 88,* 20–26.

Boord, R. L., & Rasmussen, G. L. (1963). Projections of the cochlear and lagenar nerves on the cochlear nuclei of the pigeon. *Journal of Comparative Neurology, 120,* 463–475.

Coles, R. B., Lewis, D. B., Hill, K. G., Hutchings, M. E., & Gower, D. M. (1980). Directional hearing in the japenese quail (*Coturnix coturnix japonica*). II. Cochlear physiology. *Journal of Experimental Biology, 86,* 153–170.

Dear, S. D. (1987). *Impendance and sound transmission in the auditory periphery of the chinchilla.* Doctoral thesis, University of Pennsylvania, Philadelphia, PA.

Dooling, R. J. (1980). Behavior and psychophysics of hearing in birds. In A. N. Popper & R. R. Fay (Eds.), *Comparative studies of hearing in vertebrates* (pp. 261–288). New York: Springer-Verlag.

Dooling, R. J., & Saunders, J. C. (1975). Hearing in the parakeet (*Melopsittacus undulatus*): Absolute thresholds, critical ratios, frequency difference limens, and vocalizations. *Journal of Comparative and Physiological Psychology, 88,* 1–20.

Dooling, R. J., & Searcy, M. H. (1979). The relation among critical ratios, critical bands, and intensity difference limens in the parakeet (*Melopsittacus undulatus*). *Bulletin of the Psychonomic Society, 13,* 300–302.

Dooling, R. J., & Searcy, M. H. (1980). Forward and backward masking in the parakeet (*Melopsittacus undulatus*). *Hearing Research, 3,* 279–284.

Dooling, R. J., & Searcy, M. H. (1985). Nonsimultaneous auditory masking in the budgerigar (*Melopsittacus undulatus*). *Journal of Comparative Psychology, 99,* 226–230.

Erulkar, S. D. (1972). Comparative aspects of spatial localization of sound. *Physiological Reviews, 52,* 237–360.

Freye-Zumpfe, H. (1953). Befunde im Mittelohr der Vögel. *Wissenschaften Martin-Luther Universitäte Halle Wittenberg, 2,* 445–461.

Frischkopf, L. S., & DeRosier, D. J. (1983). Mechanical tuning of freestanding stereociliary bundles and frequency analysis in the alligator lizard cochlea. *Hearing Research, 12,* 393–404.

Furness, D. N., & Hackney, C. M. (1985). Cross-links between stereocilia in the guinea pig cochlea. *Hearing Research, 18,* 177–188.

Gatehouse, R. W., & Shelton, B. R. (1978). Sound localization in bobwhite quail (*Colinus virginianus*). *Behavioral Biology, 22,* 533–540.

Gaudin, E. P. (1968). On the middle ear of birds. *Acta Otolaryngologica, 63,* 316–326.

Granit, O. (1941). Beitrage zur kenntnis des Gehörsinns der Vögel. *Ornis Fennica, 18,* 49–71.

Guinan, J. J., Jr., & Peak, W. T. (1967). Middle-ear characteristics of anesthetized cats. *Journal of the Acoustical Society of America, 41,* 1237–1261.

Gummer, A. W., Smolders, J. W. T., & Klinke, R. (1986). The mechanics of the basilar membrane and middle ear in the pigeon. In J. B. Allen, J. L. Hall, A. Hubbard, S. T. Neely, & A. Tubis (Eds.), *Peripheral auditory mechanisms* (pp. 81–88). New York: Springer-Verlag.

Hensen, O. W. (1974). Comparative anatomy of the middle ear. In W. D. Keidel & W. D. Neff (Eds.), *Handbook of sensory physiology* (pp. 39–110). New York: Springer-Verlag.

Hill, K. G., Lewis, D. B., Hutchings, M. E., & Coles, R. B. (1980). Directional hearing in the japanese quail (*Coturnix coturnix japonica*): I. Acoustic properties of the auditory system. *Journal of Experimental Biology, 86,* 135–145.

Holton, T., & Hudspeth, A. J. (1983). A micromechanical contribution to cochlear tuning and tonotopic organization. *Science, 222,* 508–510.

Hudspeth, A. J. (1985). The cellular basis of hearing: The biophysics of hair cells. *Science, 230,* 745–752.

Jenkins, W. M., & Masterton, R. B. (1979). Sound localization in pigeon (*columbia livia*). *Journal of Comparative and Physiological Psychology, 93,* 403–443.

Khanna, S. M. (1983). Interpretation of the sharply tuned basilar membrane response obtained in the cat cochlea. In R. R. Fay & G. Gourevitch (Eds.), *Hearing and other senses: Presentations in honor of E. G. Wever* (pp. 65–86). Groton, CT: Amphora Press.

Khanna, S. M. (1984). Inner ear function based on the mechanical tuning of the hair cells. In C. I. Berlin (Ed.), *Hearing science* (pp. 213–240). San Diego: College-Hill Press.

Khanna, S. M., & Tonndorf, J. (1977). External and middle ears. The determinants of the auditory threshold curve. *Journal of the Acoustical Society of America, 61,* S4.

Klump, G. M., Windt, W., & Curio, E. (1986). The great tit's (*parus major*) auditory resolution in azimuth. *Journal of Comparative Physiology, A, 158,* (pp. 383–390).

Knudsen, E. I. (1980). Sound localization in birds. In A. N. Popper & R. R. Fay (Eds.), *Comparative studies of hearing in vertebrates* (pp. 289–322). New York: Springer-Verlag.

Knudsen, E. I. (1983). Space coding in the vertebrate auditory system. In D. B. Lewis (Ed.), *Bioacoustics* (pp. 23–44). New York: Academic Press.

Knudsen, E. I., & Konishi, M. (1979). Mechanisms of sound localization in the barn owl (*Tyto alba*). *Journal of Comparative Physiology, 133,* 13–21.

Konishi, M. (1970). Comparative neurophysiological studies of hearing and vocalizations in songbirds. *Zeitschrift für Vergleischende Physiologie, 66,* 257–272.

Krause, G. (1901). *Die Columella der Vögel (Columella Auris Avium). Ihr Bau und dessen Einfluss auf die Feinhörigkeit.* Berlin: Friedländer.

Kreithen, M. L., & Quine, D. B. (1979). Infrasound detection by the homing pigeon: A behavioral audiogram. *Journal of Comparative Physiology, 129,* 1–4.

Kuhn, A., & Saunders, J. C. (1980). Psychophysical tuning curves in the parakeet: A comparison between simultaneous and forward masking procedures. *Journal of the Acoustical Society of America, 68,* 1892–1894.

Kühne, R., & Lewis, B. (1985). External and middle ears. In A. S. King & J. McLelland (Eds.), *Form and function in birds* (pp. 227–271). New York: Academic Press.

Lewald, J. (1987a). The acuity of sound localization in the pigeon (*Columbia livia*). *Naturwissenschaften, 74,* 296–297.

Lewald, J. (1987b). Interaural time and intensity difference thresholds of the pigeon (*Columbia livia*). *Naturwissenschaften, 75,* 151–153.

Lewis, D. B. (1983). Directional cues for auditory localization. In D. B. Lewis (Ed.), *Bioacoustics* (pp. 45–81). New York: Academic Press.

Lewis, D. B., & Coles, R. (1980). Sound localization in birds. *Trends in Neuroscience, 3,* 102–105.

Manley, G. A., Gleich, O., Leppelsack, H.-J., & Oeckinghaus, H. (1985). Activity patterns of cochlear ganglion neurones in the starling. *Journal of Comparative Physiology, A,157,* 161–181.

Mills, A. W. (1958). On the minimum audible angle. *Journal of the Acoustical Society of America, 30,* 237–246.

Moiseff, A., & Konishi, M. (1981). Neuronal and behavioral sensitivity to binaural time differences in the owl. *Journal of Neuroscience, 1*, 409–448.

Norberg, R. A. (1978). Skull asymmetry, ear structure and function, and auditory localization in Tengmalm's owl, *Aegolius funereus* (Linné). *Phil. Trans. Lond. B, 282*, 325–410.

Park, T., Okanoya, K., & Dooling, R. (1987). Sound localization in the budgerigar and the interaural pathway. *Journal of the Acoustical Society of America, 81*, S28.

Payne, R. S. (1971). Acoustic location of prey by barn owls (*Tyto alba*). *Journal of Experimental Biology, 54*, 535–573.

Pickles, J. O., Comis, S. D., & Osborne, M. P. (1984). Cross-links between stereocilia in the guinea pig organ of Corti and their possible relation to sensory transduction. *Hearing Research, 15*, 103–112.

Pohlman, A. G. (1921). The position and functional interpretation of the elastic ligaments in the middle-ear region of the Gallus. *Journal of Morphology, 35*, 229–262.

Relkin, E. M., & Saunders, J. C. (1980). Displacement of the malleus in neonatal golden hamsters. *Acta Otolaryngologica, 90*, 6–15.

Rosowski, J. J. (1979). *The interaural pathway of the pigeon and sound localization: Does the pigeon ear act as a differential pressure transducer?* Doctoral dissertation, University of Pennsylvania, Philadelphia, PA.

Rosowski, J. J., Carney, L. H., Lynch, T. J., & Peake, W. T. (1986). The effectiveness of external and middle ears in coupling acoustic power into the cochlea. In J. B. Allen, A. Hubbard, S. T. Neeley, & A. Tubis (Eds.), *Peripheral auditory mechanisms* (pp. 3–10). New York: Springer-Verlag.

Rosowski, J. J., & Saunders, J. C. (1980). Sound transmission through the avian interaural pathways. *Journal of Comparative Physiology, 136*, 183–190.

Sachs, M. B., Young, E. D., & Lewis, R. H. (1974). Discharge patterns of single fibers in the pigeon auditory nerve. *Brain Research, 70*, 431–447.

Saiff, E. I. (1974). The middle ear of the skull of birds: The Procellariiformes. *Zoological Journal of the Linnean Society, 54*, 213–240.

Saiff, E. I. (1976). Anatomy of the middle ear region of the avian skull: Sphenisciformes. *Auk, 93*, 749–759.

Saiff, E. I. (1978). The middle ear of the skull of birds: Pelecaniformes and Ciconiiformes. *Zoological Journal of the Linnean Society, 63*, 315–370.

Saiff, E. I. (1981). The middle ear of the skull of birds: The ostrich, *Struthio camelus*. *Zoological Journal of the Linnean Society, 73*, 201–212.

Saito, N. (1980). Structure and function of the avian ear. In A. N. Popper & R. R. Fay (Eds.), *Comparative studies of hearing in vertebrates* (pp. 241–260). New York: Springer-Verlag.

Saunders, J. C. (1976). Psychophysical analysis of pure tones masking in the parakeet. In S. K. Hirsh, D. H. Eldrich, I. J. Hirsh, & R. S. Silverman (Eds.), *Hearing and Davis: Essays honoring Hallowell Davis* (pp. 199–212). St. Louis, MO: Washington University Press.

Saunders, J. C. (1985). Auditory structure and function in the bird middle ear: An evaluation by SEM and capacitive probe. *Hearing Research, 18*, 253–268.

Saunders, J. C., Bock, G. R., & Fahrbach, S. E. (1978). Frequency selectivity in the parakeet (*Melopsittacus undulatus*) studied with narrow-band noise masking. *Sensory Processes, 2*, 80–89.

Saunders, J. C., & Dear, S. P. (1983). Comparative morphology of stereocilia. In R. R. Fay & G. Gourevitch (Eds.), *Hearing and other senses: Presentations in honor of E. G. Wever* (pp. 175–197). Groton, CT: Amphora Press.

Saunders, J. C., Denny, R. M., & Bock, G. R. (1978). Critical bands in the parakeet (*melopsittacus undulatus*). *Journal of Comparative Physiology, 125*, 359–365.

Saunders, J. C., & Else, P. V. (1976). Pure tone masking in the parakeet: A preliminary report. *Transactions of the American Academy of Ophthalmology and Otolaryngology, 82*, 356–362.

Saunders, J. C., Else, D. V., & Bock, G. R. (1978). Frequency selectivity in the parakeet (*Melopsittacus undulatus*) studied with psychophysical tuning curves. *Journal of Comparative and Physiological Psychology, 92*, 406–415.

Saunders, J. C., & Garfinkle, T. J. (1982). Peripheral anatomy and physiology I. In J. F. Willott (Ed.), *The auditory psychobiology of the mouse* (pp. 131–168). Springfield, IL: Charles C. Thomas.

Saunders, J. C., & Johnstone, B. M. (1972). A comparative analysis of middle-ear function in nonmammalian vertebrates. *Acta Otolaryngologica, 73*, 353–361.

Saunders, J. C., & Pallone, R. L. (1980). Frequency selectivity in the parakeet studied by isointensity masking contours. *Journal of Experimental Biology, 87*, 331–342.

Saunders, J. C., Pallone, R. L., & Rosowski, J. J. (1980). Frequency selectivity in parakeet hearing: Behavioral and physiological evidence. In R. Nöring (Ed.), *Proceedings of the XVII International Congress of Ornithology* (pp. 615–619). Berlin: Deutsche Ornithologen-Gesellschaft.

Saunders, J. C., Rintelman, W. F., & Bock, G. R. (1979). Frequency selectivity in bird and man: A comparison among critical ratios, critical bands, and psychophysical tuning curves. *Hearing Research, 1*, 303–323.

Saunders, J. C., Schneider, M. E., & Dear, S. P. (1985). The structure and function of actin in hair cells. *Journal of the Acoustical Society of America, 78*, 299–311.

Saunders, J. C., & Summers, R. M. (1982). Auditory structure and function in the mouse middle ear: An analysis by SEM and capacitive probe. *Journal of Comparative Physiology, 146*, 517–525.

Saunders, J. C., & Tilney, L. G. (1979). The relation between frequency selectivity of tuning curves and stereocilia height along the basilar papilla of neonatal chicks. *Abstracts of the Association for Research in Otolaryngology, 2*, 115.

Saunders, T. C., & Tilney, L. G. (1982). Species difference in susceptibility to noise exposure. In R. P. Hamernik, D. Henderson & R. Salvi (Ed.), *New perspectives on noise-induced hearing loss* (pp. 229–248). New York: Raven Press.

Schneider, M. E., Cotanche, D. A., Fambrough, D. M., Saunders, J. C., & Matschinsky, F. M. (1987). Immunocytochemistry and quantitative studies of Na$^+$/K$^+$ ATPase distribution in the chick cochlea. *Hearing Research, 31*, 39–54.

Schwartzkopff, J. (1949). Uber Sitz und Leistung von Gehör und Vibrationssinn bei Vögeln. *Zeitschrift fur Vergleischende Physiologie, 31*, 527–608.

Schwartzkopff, J. (1950). Beitrag zum Problem des Richstungshören bei Vögeln. *Zeitschrift fur Vergleischende Physiologie, 32*, 319–327.

Schwartzkopff, J. (1952). Untersuchungen über die Arbeitweise des Mittelohres und das Richtungshören der Singvögel unter Verwendung von Cochlea-Potentialen. *Zeitschrift für Vergleischende Physiologie, 34*, 46–68.

Schwartzkopff, J. (1955). On the hearing of birds. *Auk, 72*, 340–347.

Schwartzkopff, J. (1957). Die Grössenverhaltnisse von Trommelfell, Columella-Fussplatte und Schnecke bie Vögeln verscheiden Gewichts. *Zeitschrift für Ökologie in Tiere, 45*, 365–378.

Schwartzkopff, J. (1968). Structure and function of the ear and of the auditory brain areas in birds. In A. V. S. de Ruck & J. Knight (Eds.), *Hearing mechanisms in vertebrates* (pp. 41–63). Boston, MA: Little, Brown.

Smith, C. A. (1985). Inner ear. In A. S. King & J. McLelland (Eds), *Form and function in birds. Vol. 3* (pp. 273–310). New York: Academic Press.

Smith, C. A., Konishi, M., & Schuff, N. (1985). Structure of the barn owl's (*Tyto alba*) inner ear. *Hearing Research, 17*, 237–247.

Smith, G. (1904). The middle ear and columella in birds. *Quarterly Journal of Microscopic Science, 48*, 11–22.

Stellbogen, E. (1930). Über das äussere und mittlere Ohr des Waldkauzes. *Zeitschrift für Morphologie und Ökologie in Tiere, 19*, 686–731.

Stewart, G. W. (1911). The acoustic shadow of a rigid sphere, with certain applications in architectural acoustics and audition. *Physics Review, 33*, 467–479.

Takasaka, T., & Smith, C. A. (1971). The structure and innervation of the pigeon's basilar papilla. *Journal of Ultrastructure Research, 35,* 20–65.

Tanaka, K., & Smith, C. A. (1975). Structure of avian tectorial membrane. *Annals of Oto-Rhino-Laryngology, 84,* 287–296.

Tanaka, K., & Smith, C. A. (1978). Structure of the chicken's inner ear: SEM and TEM study. *American Journal of Anatomy, 153,* 251–272.

Tilney, L. G., & Saunders, J. C. (1983). Actin filaments, stereocilia, and hair cells of the bird cochlea. I. The length, number, width and distribution of stereocilia of each hair cell are related to the position of the hair cell on the cochlea. *Journal of Cell Biology, 96,* 807–821.

Tilney, M. S., Tilney, L. G., & DeRosier, D. J. (1987). The distribution of hair cell bundle lengths and orientations suggests an unexpected pattern of hair cell stimulation in the chick cochlea. *Hearing Research, 25,* 141–151.

Tilney, L. G., Tilney, M. S., Saunders, J. C., & DeRosier, D. J. (1986). Actin filaments, stereocilia, and hair cells of the bird cochlea. III. The development and differentiation of hair cells and stereocilia. *Developmental Biology, 116,* 100–118.

Vrettakos, P. A., Dear, S. D., & Saunders, J. C. (1988). Middle ear structure in the chinchilla: A quantitative study. *American Journal of Otolaryngology, 9,* 58–67.

Wada, Y. (1923). Beiträge zur vergleichenden Physiologie des Gehörogane. *Pflügers Archives, 202,* 46–69.

Wever, E. G., & Lawrence, M. (1954). *Physiological acoustics.* New Jersey: Princeton University Press.

Woodworth, R. S. (1938). *Experimental psychology.* New York: Henry Holt.

Zwislocki, J. J. (1986). Analysis of cochlear mechanics. *Hearing Research, 22,* 155–169.

Editorial Comments on Espinoza-Varas and Charles Watson

With this chapter, we find pattern perception defined explicitly as a central process—as distinguished from a peripheral sensory mechanism. Complex patterns are characterized by their temporal or spectral characteristics and there is great emphasis on the role of gestalt mechanisms in pattern perception. At the same time, the authors developed the idea that patterns can be actively heard so as to analyze their detail. Complex acoustic perception represents an interplay between these two perceptual modes.

These ideas emerge in many ways. For example, there is Bregman's work on grouping and streaming. For another, there is research on the effect of stimulus uncertainty and the processes through which this variable modulates the perceptual process. And there are studies of the factors controlling perception when decisions must be made about the characteristics of tones that are imbedded in complex auditory patterns. Throughout, a strong case emerges for the proposition that people construct perceptual patterns with experience. Although they may hear few details in a complex pattern when they first begin listening to it, for example, they begin to hear more and more as experience accumulates.

Finally, in addressing the bearing of their work on a comparative approach to acoustic perception, the authors stress that species share many commonalities in their peripheral auditory system. They propose, quite reasonably, that where species differ, they do so primarily because there are vast differences in the way that acoustic information is processed at high levels of organization.

3 Perception of Complex Auditory Patterns by Humans

Blas Espinoza-Varas
Charles S. Watson
Indiana University

INTRODUCTION

The psychophysical study of human listeners' abilities to discriminate and identify complex auditory patterns is a relatively recent endeavor, dating back less than 20 years (except, of course, for those special classes of complex patterns which are perceived as speech or music). Major handbooks or review articles on hearing published between 1950 and 1980, with but a few exceptions (e.g., Jones, 1978), include little or nothing on listeners' abilities to perceive complex patterns.[1] This is partly because the study of complex patterns requires control of a large number of stimulus parameters, and the required technology became widely available only within the past 15–20 years. However, it is also a reflection of prevailing theories of audition.

Prior to 1960 the dominant view of the auditory system was that first developed by Helmholtz (1863), and elaborated by Fletcher (1940), at Bell Laboratories. The ear was modeled as a bank of band-pass filters, each with specific bandwidths and integration times. The functional properties of the auditory system were studied with the simplest possible stimuli such as noise or tone bursts, and the results were interpreted as reflecting stable, "hardwired" characteristics of the system. Hearing was conceived as a process that took place primarily in the "ear" (i.e., the cochlea). The transduction of pressure waves into auditory sensations was seen as a relatively fixed, invariant process. Auditory information

---

[1]Our review included the handbooks edited by Stevens (1951), Tobias (1970, 1972), Keidel and Neff (1975), and the recent Handbooks on Hearing and on Perceptual Coding edited by Carterette and Friedman (1978).

was thought to be directly and immediately available on the receptor surface (Neisser & Hirst, 1974). Recent evidence suggests that, although expanded versions of this "filter-bank" view of hearing can successfully predict listeners' abilities to process simple sounds (single tones, noise bursts, clicks), it is not adequate to deal with the hearing of complex sounds. Experiments with complex sounds (Yost & Watson, 1987) suggest that the experience of hearing involves a multiplicity of internal levels of processing. The representation of a sound in the peripheral auditory system is just one of several that are available to listeners. Rather than being "hardwired" to the output of the peripheral receptor, the auditory sensations (or perceptions) exhibit considerable plasticity, and depend strongly on experience, attention, and learning. What we hear depends strongly on the immediate form of central processing, which is largely influenced by the listener's cognitive strategy. In sum, this view suggests that *hearing* is something that takes place, to a good extent, in the brain rather than in the ear. Sensory information is not directly available to listeners, but rather it must be actively extracted, and this process of information extraction depends on skill, experience, learning, memory, and other variables generally called "central factors" in perception.

This chapter reviews recent research with complex auditory patterns that emphasizes the involvement of central processes in the process of hearing. In the phylogenetic scale, *Homo Sapiens* exhibit the most elaborated, *or at least the most well-documented,* abilities to process complex auditory patterns.[2] Abilities comparable to those of humans to process the auditory patterns of connected speech and melodic phrases have not been demonstrated in other species. A central tenet of this chapter is that the remarkable processing abilities of human listeners cannot be accounted for by special characteristics of the peripheral auditory system. Instead, it is suggested that those abilities are a manifestation of enhanced cognitive and information-processing capabilities. At present it is difficult to decide whether differences in position processing abilities between human and infrahuman species are simply quantitative, or in some sense are qualitative in nature. We have avoided taking a posture on this matter because considerable research is still needed. The message in this chapter is rather that, whatever the nature of the differences, they probably reflect properties of central information processing mechanisms (e.g., ability to selectively attend, or capacity of long-term memory), rather than differences in the anatomy or physiology of the auditory periphery.

This chapter is devoted primarily to a review of experimental evidence which demonstrates the fundamental roles of memory, attention, learning, and top-down analysis in the processing of complex auditory patterns. The performance-

---

[2]Although simple forms of music and speech perception have been demonstrated in infrahuman species, the vast repertoire and complexity of music and speech sounds that humans routinely process is unparalleled.

oriented approach taken here reflects, in our opinion, the inability of any existing theoretical framework to account for certain systematic limits on the discrimination and identification of complex sounds. The discussion is restricted to complex patterns that are neither musical or phonemic. Perception of music and of phonemic patterns is discussed in the chapters by Carterette and by Pisoni, respectively.

I. GENERAL PRINCIPLES

Temporal and Spectral Ranges of Auditory Patterns

Perception of auditory patterns is associated with sounds that are either spectrally and/or temporally complex. If the spectral complexity of a sinusoid is increased by addition of harmonics, a simple timbre (spectral pattern) is perceived. Similarly, the temporal complexity may be increased by presenting the sinusoid as a component of a three-tone sequence, to create a pattern that may vary both in pitch and in rhythm. It has been argued that, to induce the perception of an auditory pattern, temporal complexity, or variation over time, is more effective than spectral complexity (Hirsh, 1974; Jones, 1978). For example, a spectrally complex tone that is invariant over time (e.g., a hum), is perceived as a background sound rather than as a distinct auditory pattern. The perception of temporal patterns depends very strongly on the rate of presentation of the elements. Most authors (Hirsh, 1959; Kelly & Watson, 1986; Warren, 1974) agree that very different results can be obtained and that conclusions based on one rate do not apply to a different rate. At very fast rates of presentation (less than 5–15 ms per element or component), listeners cannot resolve the elements of multicomponent sequences in the time domain (Hirsh, 1959). Such brief elements are perceptually fused, and the entire ensemble of sounds is heard as a unitary spectrally rich sound. These brief patterns are usually discriminated on the basis of the overall spectral properties of the ensemble. At intermediate presentation rates (25–100 ms per component or element) the individual elements are temporally resolved by the auditory system, and the perceptual impression is that of a single pattern comprised of a succession of elements (Hirsh, 1974; Warren, 1974). At these intermediate rates, there are significant temporal interactions between the elements such as informational or temporal masking (Leshowitz & Cudahy, 1973; Ronken, 1972), and it is not possible to accurately report the temporal order of the elements with verbal labels. At still slower presentation rates (> 150 ms/element), listeners report a sequence of discrete events that can be accurately labeled, if the sounds have familiar names (Warren, 1974). Most of the following discussion of the perception of *temporal* patterns concentrates on the intermediate and slow presentation rates, since they encompass the sounds of music and speech. In music, the rate of presentation of notes ranges from about 50–

1500 ms per note, i.e., 0.5–20 elements/sec (Winckel, 1967). In conversational English, the average rate is 80–100 ms per phoneme (Warren, 1983), with 30–40 ms as the limit on the most rapid intelligible speech (Foulke & Sticht, 1969). The fast presentation rate also plays a significant role in speech and music but, as mentioned above, sounds with these rates are not perceived as temporal patterns. For example, the sequence of spectral changes occurring in the first 20 ms of the syllable /ba/ has an important role in the identification of the syllable (Stevens & Blumstein, 1978), but such a sequence of spectra is perceived as a temporally compact spectral pattern rather than as a temporal sequence.

In the frequency domain, the counterpart of presentation rate is the spectral range or bandwidth covered by the elements of a temporal pattern. Patterns with 1.0-Hz bandwidths (or less) are of course simple sinusoids. Increasing the spectral bandwidth of the elements to a value slightly larger than the JND for frequency, causes the perception of frequency modulation (Shower & Biddulph, 1931); that is, a single sound is perceived with a pitch that fluctuates over time. Spectral bandwidths greater than a critical band are perceived as two or more different pitches, which may still form a strongly unitary pattern (Miller & Heise, 1950). If the elements span a bandwidth that includes several critical bands, the listener not only reports several pitches, but they tend to be perceived as unrelated. The previous generalizations apply to patterns with both medium and slow presentation rates. Several other perceptual effects are determined by the rate of presentation and spectral bandwidth. In general, faster presentation rates tend to weaken the coherence or perceptual grouping of elements into unitary patterns (Bregman, 1978; van Noorden, 1975). Another important variable is whether the frequency transition from one element of the pattern to another is abrupt or gradual. Gradual transitions increase the coherence of the pattern (Bregman & Dannenbring, 1973; Nabelek, Nabelek, & Hirsh, 1973).

Perceptual Correlates of Auditory Patterns

On the perceptual side, by auditory *patterns,* we mean sounds characterized by a perceptual impression that is global, and that commonly is elicited by the overall spectral or temporal form of a sound rather than by the sensations associated with its individual components. In other words, many acoustic patterns tend to be perceived as a Gestalt, which possesses a specific form or figure. This global property, Gestalt, or figure, is defined not by the properties of individual components of the pattern, but rather, by the relations among the elements that comprise the pattern. For example, a rapid sequence consisting of a repeating series of three brief pure tones, 1000, 1200, 1400 Hz, gives rise to a very strong "staircase" pitch pattern (Divenyi & Hirsh, 1974). This staircase pattern is not a property of any of the component tones. Rather, it is a global property of the entire tonal sequence, that is derived from the spectral relations between the individual tones. Similarly, by adjusting the duration of the individual tones, a "gallop" rhythm pattern may be induced. Again, the gallop rhythm is a property of the tonal sequence, which is derived from the temporal relations between the tones. Similarly, in the spectral domain, a timbre pattern may be defined by the amplitude relations between the harmonics of a complex tone. The acoustic parameters of the components of a pattern often can be changed in a way that does not alter the *relations* between the components. For example, the pitches of a series of tones can be transposed or the durations increased proportionally (Divenyi & Hirsh, 1978). Such manipulations, over considerable ranges, typically leave the auditory patterns unchanged, suggesting very clearly that the relations between components are the essential factors in the perception of Gestalt properties of auditory patterns.

When an auditory pattern is perceived, the overall properties of the pattern (i.e., the figure or Gestalt) often are more salient than those of the components of the pattern. However selective attention may also allow the listener to successfully focus on either "holistic" pattern properties or on one or more discrete elements within the pattern. Thus, in the previous example, it is possible to learn to ignore the staircase pitch pattern, focus attention on the pitches of the individual components, and discriminate them very accurately. Considerable training is often required to learn to ignore whatever property of an acoustic complex tends to initially dominate perception. An important consequence of the dominance of a Gestalt over the perceptual properties of individual components, is that patterns are often perceived as single, perceptually integrated sounds, rather than as a collection of elemental sounds. For instance, musical phrases, or spoken words are perceived as single, strongly unitary sounds, rather than as collections or sequences of notes or of phonemes. In summary, under appropriate conditions auditory patterns can be perceived in two fundamentally different ways: holistically, in which case we focus on the figure or Gestalt of the entire pattern; or analytically, in which case we focus on details of specific components of the pattern.

II. AREAS OF RESEARCH ON PATTERN PERCEPTION

Two classes of experimental questions have guided much of the research on auditory patterns. One general class of questions concerns the factors that determine the perceptual organization or grouping of elements in the pattern (e.g., Bregman, 1978). Which physical relations between the dimensions or parameters of the pattern elements are most effective in inducing the perception of overall relational properties, or *Gestalten*? For example, what determines that an alternation of two pitches be perceived as a single moving pitch rather than as two unrelated pitches? The second general class of questions is in a sense the complement of the previous one. Namely, given that two or more components are perceived as an auditory pattern, how accurately can the individual components be heard? (e.g., Watson, Wroton, Kelly, & Benbasset, 1975). Associated with each class of experimental questions are different experimental methods and characterizations of the auditory system. Research on the perception of Gestalt or pattern figures usually reveals aspects of auditory processing related to a synthetic mode of listening, which typically demonstrates coarse resolution. Research aimed at the ability to hear specific details, on the other hand, tends to tap an analytic mode of listening, which is characterized by relatively precise resolution. Research and theories about analytic listening often appear to be at odds with conclusions derived from the Gestalt approaches, and vice versa. We have attempted, in the following sections, to show how such disagreements are mainly the result of differences in fundamental assumptions, methodology, or research goals.

Auditory Figures and Perceptual Organization

A series of studies carried out by Bregman and his collaborators illustrate the kind of results that are obtained when listeners are instructed to listen to sounds in a synthetic mode; that is, to listen to the ways in which the components of patterns are *related,* rather than to the acoustic details of individual components. For example, in one of the early studies (Bregman & Campbell, 1971), subjects listened to a recycling sequence of six pure tones, 100 ms each. All tones had different frequencies. Three of them were in a high frequency range, and the other three in a low frequency range. Subjects were asked to report the temporal order of the tones in the sequence. This task required, of course, that the listener monitor all tones in the sequence. However, because the frequency differences between tones were large, the fine detail of the individual tones was not relevant to the task. The results showed that at high rates of presentation, subjects perceived two separate trains or streams of tones (high and low frequency), and correct report of the temporal order of the tones was possible only within streams but not across streams. The interpretation was that pitch similarity is a strong determinant of perceptual grouping. Many variations of this basic experiment have been undertaken over the past 15 years (see Bregman, Abramson, Doehring, & Darwing, 1985, for a recent review). For example, the frequency difference or the rate of presentation of the tones can be varied, or the transition from one tone to the other made gradual rather than abrupt. The pure tones can be replaced by complex tones which overlap in frequency by various amounts, and have similar or different periodicity pitches. Stimulation may be monotic or dichotic. In general, the results have been consistent with the layman's intuition, and with well-established rules of musical composition. Two or more successive tones are more likely to be perceived as a group or Gestalt if their pitches are not too different (e.g., both pitches within the same critical band), or if they are arranged to form simple auditory figures (e.g., ascending pitch movement), or if the transition from one tone to another is gradual. The exact pitch differences within which these effects are observed depend on the presentation rate (Bregman & Dannebring, 1973).

An alternation of two pure tones can be perceived as a single pitch pattern, depending on the frequency separation and repetition rate of the tones. Van Noorden (1975) alternated two 40-ms pure tones, with repetition rates ranging from 50–400 ms. He measured the maximum frequency separation at which the tones ceased to be perceived as a single pattern, and *split* into two perceptually discrete pitches. It was found that at very small frequency separations (less than 0.5 semitones) the tones are perceived as a single pattern for rates ranging from 50–400 ms. This is probably related to the limited frequency discrimination ability of the auditory system (Kelly & Watson, 1986). As the frequency separation is increased, a point is reached at which the two tones are no longer perceived as a single pattern. At very fast rates (50 ms/tone) a frequency separation of 2–3 semitones is sufficient to split the single pattern, whereas at slow rates (250 ms/tone) frequency separations as large as 15 semitones are required. The grouping of the two tones can be strengthened by means of frequency transitions that physically *connect* the frequencies of the two tones (Bregman & Dannenbring, 1973). Thus, other stimulus properties being equal, a greater frequency separation is required to disrupt the holistic pattern percept, when the tones are physically connected by frequency glides. The tonal grouping has also been shown to depend on the relative loudnesses of the tones (Van Noorden, 1975). Sounds that are very different in loudness tend not to be grouped together to form a single pattern. The grouping of sounds is also facilitated by similarity of spectral structure or timbre (McAdams & Bregman, 1979).

Central Factors in Perceptual Organization

Several results suggest that the grouping or perceptual organization of sounds is strongly influenced by central processing. First, many of these effects are obtained primarily, if not exclusively, when listeners are presented with recycling patterns, that is patterns presented as an endless loop. The listener is explicitly instructed to make judgments of the *relations* of the tones in the set (e.g., the relative order of occurrence), rather that of the details of the individual tones. Strong Gestalt effects are reported with patterns comprised of fairly long elements (100–200 ms) when subjects are instructed to listen synthetically or holistically. In contrast, studies of discrimination of tonal sequences (Espinoza-Varas & Watson, 1986; Watson et al., 1975; Watson, Kelly, & Wroton, 1976) show that at these same durations, listeners can also adopt an analytic strategy; in this case, the listener can focus attention on specific components (especially if the pattern is repeated over and over) and *ignore* (i.e., be unaffected by) all of the other elements in the pattern (Spiegel & Watson, 1981). The diversity of perceptual effects illustrates what we believe to be one of the primary characteristics of the auditory processing of complex sounds: the same acoustic stimulus can often elicit a broad range of perceptual experiences, and there is a good deal of flexibility in terms of which specific percept a given pattern will elicit.

The perceptual organization of a specific pattern is often developed only after a significant amount of formal or informal training. The perceptual effects of a particular stimulus, or class of stimuli, following prolonged experience may differ greatly from that which was originally elicited, or it may be very similar. Some listeners never manage to achieve the perceptual organizations reported in the literature; individual differences in pattern processing are significantly larger than those reported for simpler stimuli (Johnson, Watson, & Jensen, 1987). All of the above implies that the perceptual organization of a complex pattern is in no way *hardwired* to the output of the peripheral receptor.

It should be noted that generalizations based on studies of perceptual grouping are necessarily limited because of the common use of *recycling* sequences, in which the subject listens to repetitions of the same sounds over and over. Many of the reported perceptual effects weaken or disappear altogether if the same stimulus is presented in a nonrecycling format (Bregman, personal communication). This of course seriously limits the applicability of the results to the perception of many patterns that do not recycle such as those of speech and music. As noted earlier, these effects are also strongly dependent on the strategy adopted by the listener, his or her experience with the sounds, and focus of attention.

Knowledge, Predictability and Uncertainty

The majority of complex sounds that (normal-hearing) humans routinely identify by the time they reach adulthood represent frequently occurring classes of acoustic wave-forms. By this time, speech, music, and many environmental sounds are all quite familiar. The relevance of knowledge to the manner in which we hear can be appreciated when we listen to a foreign language in which we are not fluent. Frequently that feeling is one of being unable to resolve the discrete sounds of the language, and of being overwhelmed by the rapidity with which the sounds are produced. The process of learning the new language seems to be associated with a remarkable slowing of its phoneme rate, and corresponding increase in the clarity with which individual phonetic sounds are perceived. A general conclusion based on studies of complex patterns carried out over the past 15 years, is that the listener's knowledge and experience with the patterns has a very strong effect on perception. Until recently, the variables of *knowledge* or *predictability* had not been systematically manipulated in studies of the perception of complex auditory patterns, although different research orientations had dictated a wide variety of amounts of practice and knowledge (stimulus certainty or predictability). Studies grouped under the headings of "auditory psychophysics" or "psychoacoustics" have generally been addressed to questions about asymptotic performance, that is, the performance achieved when subjects have become thoroughly familiar with the stimuli, and when no further effects of training are observed. Researchers on perceptual organization and speech perception, on the other hand, generally do not train listeners for very extended periods of time, often on the grounds that their concern is with "naive perception." For the case of speech, it is often assumed that, since these are sounds with which the listeners are fluent, listeners' previous experience makes them quite practiced at processing any speech sound of their mother tongues. It is clear, from many studies, that even the highly experienced speaker of a language can process it more accurately if he or she knows the properties of the subset of speech sounds from which stimuli are drawn on a given trial (e.g., Miller, Heise, & Lichten, 1951).

The most effective way of studying the impact of knowledge on listening is by manipulating the level of *stimulus uncertainty* in the experimental paradigm. Stimulus uncertainty denotes the extent to which the stimulus parameters vary from trial to trial, and therefore the extent to which the values of such parameters can be predicted. Very high levels of trial-to-trial variability of stimulus parameters make predictions nearly impossible, and listeners, performance under such conditions may reflect their most unbiased, or "open-mode" style of listening. High stimulus uncertainty and variability also necessarily imply that the stimulus sets are very large, and no single stimulus has a high a priori probability of occurring. With complex auditory patterns, there are many ways in which the stimulus uncertainty can be increased. For example, in a sequential pattern consisting of three pure tones, uncertainty can be introduced in the frequency, intensity, and duration of the tones and in the pattern of intertone intervals. Several levels per dimension can thus generate extremely large stimulus sets.

In terms of cognitive processing, stimulus uncertainty means that the listener cannot usefully refer to a *long-term* memory representation (or internal standard) of the stimulus expected on a given trial, as a template to either identify the pattern with a label, or as a reference against which to detect changes in individual pattern components. As a result, under high levels of stimulus uncertainty, very accurate detection or discrimination judgments arc possible only if an external standard is provided to the listener (by "very accurate" we mean performance predictable from the resolving power of the auditory system, as demonstrated with single tonal stimuli). This external standard must be presented in close temporal proximity ($< 100–200$ ms) to the target stimulus (Braida et al., 1984). In this way, the representation of the external standard held in *short-term* memory (STM) apparently can be compared with the target stimulus. Obviously, this STM standard could only be provided for the case of brief, fairly simple patterns that do not overload STM. From the above, it follows that it would be practically impossible to obtain very accurate resolution in identification tasks under high uncertainty, since by definition *identification* tasks provide no external standard.

Another effect of high levels of stimulus uncertainty (or lack of knowledge about where or what to listen for) on cognitive processing of complex patterns appears to be that listeners use a synthetic rather than an analytic mode of listening (Espinoza-Varas & Watson, 1986). For the case of detection and/or discrimination of changes in individual pattern components, this appears to result because the subject does not know in which spectral-temporal region the signal (a change in one component of a complex pattern) will occur. Consequently, he or she attempts to keep "all options open." That is, a multiple channel strategy is used. Such a listening strategy might improve the *average* rate of correct detection or discrimination over a catalog of potential signals. However, is is also typically associated with a deterioration in the detection accuracy for individual signals, implying a limit in the total information processing capacity.

Hearing Single Components of Temporal Patterns.   Earlier, it was mentioned that sequential patterns are often perceived holistically, and that the individual components tend to lose their separate identity. An interesting question is how the components are actually heard when the prominent feature is the Gestalt. This question is particularly relevant to sequential patterns with intermediate or slow rates of component presentation. At high rates (i.e., individual components as short as 2–6 msec), the ability to resolve individual elements in the pattern is greatly degraded or altogether absent (Green, 1971).

Direct measurements of the detectability of changes in individual components of temporal patterns have been reported by Watson et al. (1975, 1976), Spiegel and Watson (1981), and by Espinoza-Varas and Watson (1986). The patterns in each of these studies were tonal sequences, 450 ms in duration, comprised of ten 40-ms tones, with 5-ms intertone intervals. All tones in the sequence had different frequencies (separated by a critical bandwidth or more) generally sampled from the range from 300 to 3000 Hz, and presented at 75 dB SPL. Temporally, the duration of the components is similar to that of the briefer phonemes, while the total duration of the sequence approaches that of average polysyllabic words. A typical procedure consists of presenting a standard pattern followed by a comparison pattern, after a 0.5-sec interval. On half of the trials the comparison pattern is identical to the standard. In the remaining half, a single component of the comparison pattern is changed by a small amount in either the frequency, intensity, or the duration (relative to the corresponding components in the standard pattern). Listeners are instructed to decide whether the comparison pattern is in any respect different from the standard. Figure 3.1 illustrates the case of discrimination of increments in the duration of components. The precision of the discrimination, indexed in terms of thresholds or Weber fractions, along various dimensions, gives a direct measure of the precision with which listeners hear individual pattern components. It is assumed that if the listener can hear a component presented in a pattern as precisely as when it is presented in isolation, then its discrimination threshold should be identical under the two conditions. If the discrimination thresholds are larger for components embedded in patterns, in some manner the context (nonsignal) components are limiting the listener's

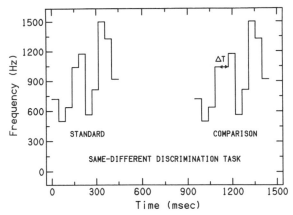

FIG. 3.1.   Structure of a "same-different" trial for the case of discrimination of increments of individual components (ΔT) of ten-tone sequences.

ability to resolve the acoustic signal. Typical results of discrimination of increments in duration of single components are shown in Fig. 3.2. In these experiments, the increment in duration, ΔT, sometimes occurred in sequential components 1, 4, 7, or 10. The frequencies of each of the test components could be either 565, 721, 920, 1175, or 1500 Hz, so that 20 combinations of test-component frequency and temporal position were investigated. Three levels of stimulus uncertainty were:

a. *high uncertainty:* for any of the 20 test tones, the context was a random sample from the set of 9! different sequences that result from permutation of the temporal positions of the nine components forming the context;

b. *medium uncertainty:* only ten different sequences served as contexts for any of the 20 test components; and

c. *minimal uncertainty:* a single sequence was used as context and only one of the 20 test components was used as a signal within that context.

Subjects were given about 2 months of daily training on each condition to insure that asymptotic performance had been approached, before moving to the next level of uncertainty. Figure 3.2 shows the magnitude of the increment in component duration that was needed for listeners to achieve threshold-level discrimination performance ($d' = 1.5$), as a function of number of trials. The results shown in Fig. 3.2 are for the four (out of 20) test conditions studied under all three levels of uncertainty. The expected threshold of about 6.0 ms for duration increments in 40-ms tones presented in isolation is shown by the dotted horizontal line. It can be seen that at the beginning of training, and under high levels of

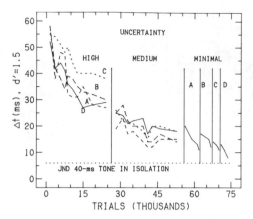

FIG. 3.2. Discrimination thresholds for increments in component duration obtained under high, medium, and minimal levels of stimulus uncertainty, after various amounts of training. Results from four selected target conditions are shown. The temporal position and frequency of the targets in these conditions were: (A): 4/1175 Hz; (B): 7/565 Hz; (C): 4/565 Hz; and (D): 7/1175 Hz. The dotted horizontal line shows the threshold for 40-ms tones presented in isolation. Adapted from Espinoza-Varas and Watson (1986) and Creelman (1962).

uncertainty, component increments of about 50–60 ms were required to obtain d' = 1.5 discrimination performance. That is, discrimination is about an order of magnitude poorer than that for the same component presented in isolation. After about 25,000 trials, performance under high uncertainty approached an asymptote of about 30 ms. The shift to a medium level of stimuli uncertainty was followed by a further reduction of the threshold to about 15 ms, after 20,000–25,000 additional trials. Finally, under minimal uncertainty, the thresholds reflect temporal resolution almost as accurate as that for 40-ms components presented in isolation. Results very similar to these have been reported by Watson et al., (1975, 1976), Spiegel and Watson (1981), and Watson and Kelly (1981), for the cases of discrimination of increments in frequency and intensity of components of patterns. These results show very clearly that the ability to hear individual components of patterns depends quite strongly on knowledge about where to listen, and on being able to predict the spectral-temporal characteristics of the signal. Under high uncertainty and with limited practice the listener does not know "what to listen for and where," and the ability to hear the details of components is severely degraded. Under minimal uncertainty, and with sufficient practice, that knowledge is available and the listener can discriminate details of components nearly as accurately as if those components were presented in isolation.

The interpretation of the above results hinges on the fact that, physically, the stimuli and structure of individual trials were *identical for all three levels of stimulus uncertainty and, of course, across the training period.* Given this fact, the following conclusions are justified:

a. the representation of the patterns in the *auditory periphery* is equally precise for all levels of uncertainty, even though discrimination performance is grossly different;

b. degraded performance under high uncertainty must be caused by inability to extract and process information that is available in the peripheral auditory system; and

c. the amount of information listeners can extract from complex sounds is not limited by "hardwired" constraints of the auditory system.

On the contrary, listeners exhibit an impressive plasticity in terms of their ability to learn to extract selected information from complex patterns. Whether the *total information* listeners can extract from complex patterns is constant, or varies under these levels of stimulus uncertainty cannot be determined from data like those shown in Fig. 3.2.

The results of studies of the effects of stimulus uncertainty also indicate that under high uncertainty listeners tend to employ holistic, or possibly synthetic listening strategies. That is, strategies aimed at detecting gross changes in overall features of patterns, with correspondingly poor sensitivity for details of individual components. For example, they appear to detect changes in frequency or duration of components whenever the changes alter the spectral or temporal bounds of the pattern. Another conclusion suggested by these results is that under minimal- and possibly medium- uncertainty conditions listeners may have multiple representations of the patterns available to them. The effects of stimulus uncertainty demonstrated with tonal patterns are reminiscent of those observed in studies of judgments of multidimensional stimuli (Garner, 1962; Miller, 1956). It is known that subjects are able to monitor multiple stimulus dimensions to identify and discriminate complex displays (Pollack, 1953; Pollack & Ficks, 1954; Espinoza-Varas, 1983). However, evidence from many of these studies suggests that multi-dimensional distribution of processing capacity is associated with a loss of detail in the individual dimensions. This result is particularly important in understanding the processing of speech patterns. As a rule, there are multiple acoustic cues that differentiate phonemes, which are distributed in time and in frequency. More information could theoretically be extracted if the listener monitored all the cues simultaneously. However, attempts at multi-dimensional discrimination have been invariably associated, in experimental studies, with degradation of resolution in each of the individual dimensions (Garner, 1962).

Channel Capacity Limits in the Processing of Complex Patterns.   One of the principal factors determining the amount of information contained in complex auditory patterns is of course the number of components of which the patterns are comprised. Early studies on auditory channel capacity (Pollack, 1953; Pollack & Ficks, 1954), made it clear that a very effective way of increasing the stimulus information listeners could process in patterns was by generating sequences of sounds, with each component varying along two or more dimensions. For example, consider sequential patterns of five components, in which each component can be varied along four dimensions, with two levels per dimension. This seemingly small set can generate 8^5 or 32,768 different sequences. It therefore is important to determine how auditory pattern processing is influenced by this very powerful stimulus variable. A fundamental question in this context concerns the maximum number of pattern components that can be accurately processed, and how the (presumably) finite information capacity is allocated to each component.

Watson and Foyle (1985), have recently conducted experiments to determine information-capacity limits for processing components of tonal sequences. In these experiments subjects had to discriminate patterns with total durations, t, ranging from 62.5–2000 ms. The number of components in the pattern, n, was varied from 1 to 34, with individual component durations always equal to t/n. The frequencies of the components were randomly sampled from a 300–3000 Hz range, with the restriction that the frequency difference between two successive components could not be less than 1/3 oct. Thus the stimulus uncertainty in these experiments was very large, as subjects listened to patterns of different durations, number of components, and frequencies. The number of alternative patterns than can be generated in this case is so large that subjects probably never listened twice to any single pattern.

In the "same-different" paradigm of these experiments, the subject's task was to detect large changes in the frequency (20% or greater) of one or more pattern components, or to detect silent gaps created by deleting a component. The detectability of these changes was studied as a function of the number of components in the patterns. The main results are shown in Fig. 3.3 in which the maximum number of components that yields d' = 1.0 is shown as a function of the total duration of the pattern. The interesting result in this Figure is that, compared to the 32-fold range of pattern durations (62.5 to 2000 ms), the maximum number of components for which frequency changes are detected at d' = 1.0 was relatively constant, usually within the range of 5–8 components. Detectability of frequency changes was thus only weakly related to the duration of the components in the pattern or to the duration of the total pattern. These results suggest that in this condition of very high uncertainty, the channel capacity *for pattern discrimination* resembles the well-known 7 ± 2 limit (Miller, 1956) that has been previously shown to describe performance in identification tasks.

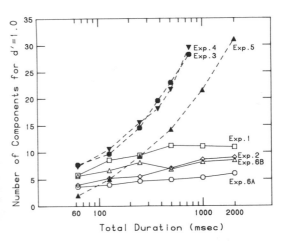

FIG. 3.3. Maximum number of components yielding d′ = 1.0 performance for detection of either 20 percent increments of component frequency (open symbols), or detection of gaps (solid symbols). The Figure shows results from three experiments on detection of gaps (Exp. 3, 4, 5), and from four experiments on detection of ΔF (Exp. 1, 2, 6A, 6B). Adapted from Watson & Foyle (1985).

Figure 3.3 also shows that in the conditions in which the presence or positions of temporal gaps were to be detected, performance appeared to be determined mainly by the duration (rather than by the number) of individual components. Subsequent studies have shown that the difference between the condition involving detection of a gap and that involving detection of changes in component frequency has a simple interpretation. Subtle changes of specific properties in a pattern can be detected, under high stimulus uncertainty, only if those changes are along physical dimensions on which less than the system's informational capacity is encoded. In other words, in a pattern of fixed-level, variable-frequency components, a small change in the level of one component might be readily detected, while a similarly small change in the frequency of a component (in terms of peripherally determined resolving power) would be missed. Like many important generalizations this one seems obvious, perhaps even trivial, but it can account for a great many facts of auditory pattern processing. In summary, an important limitation on the processing of complex patterns appears to be the finite channel capacity of the auditory processor. Details of patterns whose information content exceeds the channel capacity, are not processed very accurately, although the exact limit is to some extent dimension specific.

Discrimination of Single Components of Spectral Patterns: Profile Analysis

In the frequency domain, a complement of the temporal pattern studies is the case of discrimination of details of individual frequency components of multicomponent complexes. Resolving power for sinusoidal components embedded in a variety of complex spectra has been studied for many years as instances of "masking." Most of the previous studies have dealt with the detectability of individual components rather than with discrimination of subtle changes in components that are otherwise clearly detectable. Relevant to the aims of the present chapter are recent results on discrimination of changes in the intensity of components of spectral complexes which show such discrimination ability to be dependent, in some cases, on central factors such as stimulus uncertainty and learning.

Spiegel, Picardi, and Green (1981) studied discrimination of increments in the intensity of individual sinusoidal components presented in a spectral complex consisting of m components. The number of components in the complex, m, ranged from 1–20. Three conditions were studied:

a. masker uncertainty: the signal was always an increment in the intensity of a specific component, but the frequency of the other m-1 components was randomly varied from trial to trial;

b. signal uncertainty: the frequency of nonsignal components of the complex was fixed, but the frequency of the component to which the intensity increment was added was varied from trial to trial; and

c. no stimulus uncertainty: the frequencies of the signal and of the nonsignal components were both fixed from trial to trial.

Typical results are shown in Fig. 3.4. As observed in the case of temporal patterns, uncertainty about the masker, the signal frequency, or both, lead to degradation in performance, i.e., to higher discrimination thresholds. Masker uncertainty was found to be more effective in increasing the thresholds than was signal uncertainty. In another condition, Spiegel et al. (1981) found that uncertainty in the overall level of the complex did not increase the thresholds as much as uncertainty in the component frequencies. Trial-to-trial variability in the overall

FIG. 3.4. Intensity discrimination thresholds as a function of the range of variation in masker level. Four conditions of stimulus uncertainty are shown: signal and masker uncertainty (diamonds); masker uncertainty (squares): signal uncertainty (open circles); and no uncertainty in either the signal or masker (open triangles). The ordinate shows the threshold intensity increment expressed as a proportion of the level of the masker component to which the increment is added. Adapted from Spiegel, Picardi, and Green (1981).

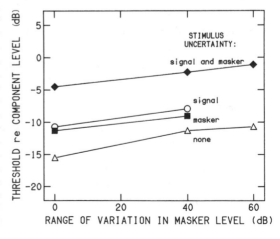

level, over ranges as large as 60 dB, caused increases of no more than 5–6 dB in the intensity discrimination threshold. According to Green (1983), discrimination in these tasks is accomplished through a simultaneous comparison of the output of the critical band containing the target component, against the output of the critical bands containing the remaining nontarget components. This process of simultaneous comparisons across critical-band outputs was termed "profile analysis." In subsequent experiments, Kidd, Mason, & Green (1986) have also demonstrated strong learning effects for intensity discrimination of components of multitone complexes. They observed improvements of up to 10 dB in the intensity discrimination thresholds in the first 3000 trials, and after many additional thousands of trials still greater improvements are found, approaching 15 dB. These results led the authors to conclude that "the peripheral critical-band levels representing the spectrum of a sound are compared with a similar set of stored values reflecting the relative critical-band levels of the reference stimulus" (cf. Kidd et al., 1986). That is, an operation of matching the output of the peripheral receptor to a long-term memory template is involved in profile analysis, similar to that hypothesized earlier for the discrimination of components of temporal patterns.

In the profile-analysis experiments, stimulus uncertainty seems to cause only moderate loss of accuracy in the discrimination of spectral shapes. On the other hand, in the tonal-sequence studies of Watson and collaborators, uncertainty is more often associated with severe degradation in performance. This diversity of effects of uncertainty may be explained on the basis of whether or not the dimension along with uncertainty is introduced is that which must be monitored to detect or discriminate the signals. The foregoing explanation is consistent with the results of experiments on information capacity (Watson & Foyle, 1985) discussed earlier. In those experiments uncertainty was created by varying, from trial to trial, the frequency, the duration, and the number of components, as well as the total duration of the patterns. There was no uncertainty in the durations of the intertone intervals or in the level of the components. The results showed that the detection of frequency increments was limited primarily by the number of components in the pattern, whereas that the detection of gaps was limited primarily by the duration of the components rather than by the number.

Perceptual Construction of Auditory Patterns

Studies of the perception of simple sinusoidal tones in isolation seem to suggest that hearing is an immediate and fairly stable consequence of the arrival of an acoustic stimulus in the ear canal. This is indicated, for example, by the fact that discrimination of the details of isolated tones does not improve significantly with prolonged training. Whatever resolving power is available, is manifested almost from the very beginning of testing. In contrast, discrimination of the same tones embedded in complex auditory patterns improves significantly with training over periods of at least 20–30 hrs (Watson, 1980). This suggests that in the first few trials of listening to a complex pattern, very little of the details of the components may be resolved, and that, in a sense, the pattern must be constructed perceptually as training proceeds. The hearing of complex patterns appears then as a very plastic, evolving process. For a number of years, cognitive psychologists within the contructivist approach (Gibson, 1969; Neisser, 1967) have maintained that perception of complex patterns is not an immediate process. Their argument that perception relies on prior knowledge implies a gradual development of the percepts. Until recently, the main evidence to support construction processes in the perception of complex patterns derived from studies of the effects of training on pattern perception. For example, Neisser and Hirst (1974) studied effects of training on the perception of temporal order in tonal sequences. They observed that the component duration required for correct order identification decreased from 200 to 20 ms after prolonged training.

Another approach to the question of auditory perceptual learning was taken by Leek and Watson (1984). Using a single 10-tone sequence, similar to that shown in Fig. 3.1, they measured the *detection threshold* for each of the ten components of the sequence. On each trial, subjects listened to three renditions of the ten-tone sequence, separated by 500-ms intervals. In the first rendition (and with equal probability, in either the second or the third), an individual target component was deleted and replaced by a silent gap of equal duration. In the remaining rendition (either the second or the third) the same target component was presented at an intensity level specified by an adaptive threshold track. Using the first rendition as "standard," listeners were asked to decide whether the second or the third rendition differed from the standard. With this procedure, the detection thresholds were measured for each of the 10 tones comprising the sequence. The results, in Fig. 3.5, show the average amount of masking (i.e., the difference in

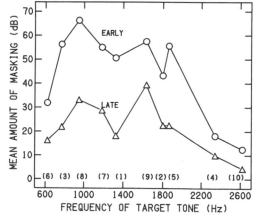

FIG. 3.5. Average amount of masking (four listeners) for each pattern component. The circles represent masking during the first 200 trials for each tone (function labeled "Early"); the triangles show masking over trials 600–800 (labeled "Late"). Numbers in parentheses indicate the temporal location of each tonal frequency within the pattern. Adapted from Leek and Watson (1984).

the detection thresholds of targets when presented in patterns and when presented in isolation) as a function of the frequency of the test component. The figure shows a set of thresholds obtained at the beginning of training (early), and after prolongued experience in the task (late). The major results are, first, that in all cases the detection thresholds for tones embedded in patterns are clearly greater than the same thresholds for tones presented in isolation. Second, the results show that there are significant reductions in the thresholds for targets in patterns after prolonged training (i.e., *the effective sensation level of the components increases*). This latter finding clearly supports a process of perceptual construction. In the earlier presentations of a pattern, listeners literally hear few of its details. However, with sufficient training they are often able to construct a very detailed representation of the same pattern.

Capabilities, Proclivities, and Perceptual Learning

Elsewhere one of us (CSW) has distinguished between the measurement of *sensory capabilities* and *response proclivities* (Watson, 1973). The first of these two goals of psychophysical measurement refers to hypothetical properties of a sensory system or, more properly, of an entire functioning organism endowed with such a system. Those properties include, at least, sensitivity and resolving power, but also must reflect the limits of selective attention, memory capacity and constraints on retrieval from memory. In psychophysical research, sensitivity and resolving power are inferred from performance in *detection and discrimination tasks*. Limits of attention or memory, are more often estimated from performance in *identification tasks*. A great deal of research effort has been focussed on the measurement of sensitivity and resolving power, much of it intended to establish the behavioral correlates of the functions of the peripheral auditory system. We suspect that, in contrast to this "peripheral psycho-acoustics," the next couple of decades will see an increasing number of studies of identification tasks, as part of a general effort to cstimate central limits on sensory information processing, those imposed by the capacities of directed attention, learning and memory. In terms of the operations of measurement, those "central" properties are as fundamental as sensitivity or resolving power. As the sounds to be processed become more complex, and particularly when they include so many (potentially resolvable) details that a listener cannot attend to all of them at once, central factors may become relatively more important determinants of psychophysical performance than are the properties of the peripheral sensory channels (Watson & Foyle, 1985).

Sometimes sensory studies are not conducted to estimate the sensory capabilities of a person or animal, but instead to establish the characteristic responses elicited by some specific stimuli. It is those characteristic stimulus-response relations for which we have used the term "response proclivities." This term was intended to be as neutral as possible, implying no presuppositions about the origins of characteristic responses, either in experience or in innate properties of the nervous system. We have been concerned, in recent years, with the choice of ways in which response proclivities and sensory capabilities might best be measured (Robinson & Watson, 1972; Watson, 1973). The differences between those two goals of psychophysical research provide reasonably clear guidelines for the selection of methods. If the goal is to estimate sensitivity, for example, the psychophysical method should allow a subject to demonstrate the lowest sound pressure level at which he or she can reliably detect the stimulus. Sufficient practice, with feedback, should be provided so that it is reasonable to assume that performance has approached a lower asymptote, and the trial-to-trial stimulus uncertainty should be set to a level below which no lowering of the threshold results. Different rules, however, apply to the measurement of response proclivities. The reason is fairly clear in the definition of response proclivities as psychophysically measured *tendencies to respond to specific stimuli with specific responses.*[3] If the goal of an experiment is to determine the responses that are characteristically elicited by a particular stimulus, then clearly it would be self-defeating to attempt to train the listener to give some other response to that stimulus. Similarly, if we are attempting to learn what a listener calls a given sound, when left to *label* it without interference, there is obviously no basis by which to provide right-wrong feedback. In other words, if one wishes to determine what phonemic label a particular speech sound elicits, it would seem reasonable to present that sound to each of several subjects and ask them to write down what they heard. They might agree, as demonstrated in innumerable experiments, that plosive noise bursts followed immediately by voicing (e.g., the /a/ vowel) sound like the consonant-vowel /ba/, while those with voicing delayed by 25 msec or more results in their labeling the sounds as /pa/ (Abramson & Lisker, 1970). Only with such a nonjudgemental approach to the psychophysical process can an investigator be certain that the stimulus-response relation that has been observed is a characteristic (a proclivity) that the subject brought to the experiment.

The difficult part of the study of proclivities is, of course, to determine their *origin,* once their existence has been demonstrated. In the case mentioned above, for example, some early investigators seemed to believe that the categorical

---

[3]If we were not making a modest effort to avoid mentalistic language, the easiest way to explain this issue would be to say that when we measure proclivities we are determining the way people *perceive* stimuli. The effort to avoid retreating to that subjective terminology results, as usual, in a good deal of circumlocution. Nevertheless, we really don't know how anyone perceives anything, other than ourselves, and we *do not* equate the study of response proclivities with that of perception. We do believe, however, that the determination of proclivities is as close as one can come to that goal (of measuring perception, or personal experience) in the framework of objective science. Historically, similar conclusions have been reached by Stevens (1951), who proposed sensational scaling as the method of choice; and by Brunswick (1956) and Gibson (1969) who emphasized the need to measure proclivity-like aspects of sense-based behavior in ecologically valid settings.

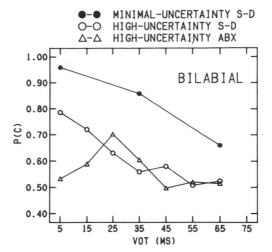

●-● MINIMAL-UNCERTAINTY S-D
○-○ HIGH-UNCERTAINTY S-D
△-△ HIGH-UNCERTAINTY ABX

FIG. 3.6. Discriminability of differences in voice-onset time, of a /ba-pa/ continuum, obtained whith three psychophysical methods: high uncertainty ABX; high uncertainty same-different (S-D); and minimal-uncertainty same-different. Adapted from Kewley-Port et al. (1988).

boundary (the tendency to employ different labels depending on whether the delay of voicing is smaller or greater than the category boundary) was a hard-wired property of the listener, and also that it was employed only when the sound to be judged was perceived as human speech. But the experiments conducted, while appropriate for the determination of proclivities, were not suited to the measurement of sensory capabilities which, presumably, were implicated if the proclivity was based in a "property of the sensory system." Training was inadequate to demonstrate that asymptotic performance levels had been approached, and the levels of stimulus uncertainty were generally high enough that it appeared likely that their reduction might result in improved performance. Figure 3.6, from a recent study by Kewley-Port, Watson, and Foyle (1988), shows how performance on this task changes when various psychophysical methods are used to measure the discriminability of stimuli along the voice-onset-time (VOT) continuum. When the high-uncertainty, ABX method is used, with very little training, the characteristic peak in performance signifying the categorical /b-p/ boundary is demonstrated. When a minimal-uncertainty, same-different method is used, not only is performance significantly improved for all stimuli, but the nonmonotonic discrimination function is eliminated. Under this last condition, discrimination of a fixed increment in VOT is found to improve monotonically, as the standard value of VOT is reduced toward zero. Thus, the *proclivity* of categorical perception of the voicing feature (a) does not reflect an invariant property of the auditory system's capability to resolve temporal details of complex sounds, and (b) may be most parsimoniously intepreted as an acquired tendency to focus available resolving power on a particular spectral-temporal region within a complex waveform. Abilities to learn to hear specific high-information-carrying details of familiar waveforms have been studied in several of our tonal-pattern experiments (e.g., Leek & Watson, 1984, Spiegel & Watson, 1981). In general, it has been found that the time-course of learning to hear details of a pattern is significantly longer than that required to learn to hear similar details of simpler sounds. Learning times also are longer as more information is processed in the learned task; identification requires more training to reach asymptote than discrimination, and discrimination requires more training than detection (Watson, 1980).

Proclivities and Capabilities in Animal Research.   It is reasonably easy to explain to a human subject that the goal of a psychophysical experiment is to learn to attend to some subtle detail of an acoustically complex stimulus, even though that detail was formerly of little or no interest to the subject. Verbal mediation is very effective in directing a listener's attention to a specific spectral-temporal region of a complex sound, and the explanation of a new psychophysical task can also be facilitated by use of graphic representations of the stimuli. But despite such efforts to speed task acquisition, it often takes from a few hundred to several thousand trials for the human subject to approach asymptotic performance. Such lengthy training, especially under minimal-stimulus-uncertainty conditions, has been shown to reduce thresholds for the detection of single components of a complex pattern by 40–50 dB, and to have similarly large effects on discrimination performance for changes in the frequency, intensity, and duration of the same components (Watson & Kelly, 1981). It seems possible that the difference between human and animal auditory processing abilities may be more a matter of the degree of difficulty in teaching subjects to attend to specific properties of stimuli, especially in cases in which some other aspect of the sound was previously important to the subject (as reflected in proclivity experiments). The recent history of animal psychophysics, like similar work with human infants (e.g., Kuhl & Miller, 1975), seems to support this hypothesis. Each time a more sensitive psychophysical procedure is invented, babies, birds, chinchillas, bats, etc., appear to become more sensitive to all sorts of stimuli and to various differences between stimuli. What the cautious investigator can do about this problem is not clear, other than to devise psychophysical methods appropriate to a species' cognitive and motor capacities and common behavioral repertoire, and then to continue training until performance has clearly approached asymptotic levels. Despite this sort of effort, it is still difficult to interpret poor discrimination for cues unimportant to a species as clear evidence of a *sensory* deficit. The basic problem is that the results of a psychophysical measurement never define precisely the level of performance a subject *can* achieve on a sensory task, but only demonstrate that the subject can process the stimuli *at least as well as* is demonstrated by that performance. This doesn't mean that either human or animal psychophysics are fruitless occupations. But it certainly does suggest some danger in theorizing that prematurely invokes either anatomical or ethological considerations to account for apparent limitations on performance, or for differences in performance between species.

III. INTEGRATION OF REMOTE FREQUENCY REGIONS

This section discusses a somewhat different set of experimental evidence that has begun to limit the general applicability of the critical bandwidth concept. Fletcher (1940) proposed that for detection of a sinusoidal signal in broadband noise, only a narrow band of frequencies around the signal causes effective masking; namely the frequencies within the critical bandwidth centered at the signal frequency. This has been a dominant concept in auditory theory for almost 5 decades, however, recent evidence has cast doubt on its general validity. In a number of situations energy remote from the critical band centered at the signal frequency has been shown to be effective in influencing the detectability of the signal.

The first line of evidence derives from work on intensity discrimination for single components of multitone complexes, or *profile analysis*. Green, Kidd, and Picardi (1983) studied this case of intensity discrimination as a function of the number and frequency spacing of the components in multitone complexes. In different experimental conditions, the number of components was varied from 3 to 21, and in each case the component spacing ranged from values smaller. to values considerably larger than the critical bandwidth. Two very surprising results were obtained: first, detectability *improved* with increases in both the number and the spacing of the components; second, this improvement was obtained even if components were added at frequencies well outside the signal's critical band.

A second source of evidence that is consistent with the critical bandwidth interpretation is the phenomenon of comodulation masking release, CMR, first described by Hall, Haggard, and Fernandez (1984). In CMR, the detection of a sinusoidal signal is measured under two conditions. In one, the signal is masked by a narrow band of noise, amplitude modulated at low frequencies. Detection in this condition is compared to a condition in which a second narrow-band noise is added, also amplitude modulated in-phase with the first band, but with a different center frequency. Differences in detectability between these two conditions are studied as a function of differences in modulation and in the center frequencies of the noise bands. The first surprising result is that the detectability of the sinusoidal frequency *improves* (up to 10–12 dB) with *addition of the second noise band,* provided that its amplitude modulation (and therefore its temporal envelope) is correlated with that of the first band (hence called "comodulation masking release"). No masking release is observed if the amplitude modulation of the noise bands is uncorrelated. The second surprising result is that comodulation masking release is obtained even if the second noise band is added at frequency regions considerably removed from the critical band centered at the signal frequency.

The third source of evidence derives from experiments on fusion and separation of spectral components of complexes, by means of frequency modulation

(McAdams, 1984). These experiments typically employ multitone complexes consisting of 6–12 harmonics, the frequencies of which are modulated sinusoidally at 2–4 Hz, and with modulation extent of less than 5 percent. An interesting result is obtained when the modulation functions applied to different harmonics of the complex are made to differ slightly by, for example, introducing phase differences between the modulating functions. In this situation, the components that share identical modulation functions are grouped together and perceived as separate or different from the remaining components with different modulations functions. This grouping of spectral components in terms of communality of frequency modulation is observed even with components that are widely separated in frequency.

IV. SUMMARY AND CONCLUSIONS

The main goal of this chapter was to review several lines of evidence which demonstrate the relatively greater involvement of central, rather than peripheral mechanisms, in the processing of complex patterns by humans. One line of evidence showed that the perceptual organization of complex auditory patterns is not determined by the output of the auditory receptor. The same complex pattern can elicit a variety of perceptual organizations, for the same listener. Which organization is constructed depends on attention, listening strategy, and task demands. Other evidence shows that the ability to hear details of individual components of either temporal or spectral patterns is strongly determined by knowledge about "what to listen for and where." Acquisition of such knowledge depends in turn on the level of stimulus uncertainty, and the experience of the listeners with the patterns. Low stimulus uncertainty and prolonged experience allow the development of highly detailed representations of the patterns, which the listener can use as perceptual references. Similarly precise memory references cannot be developed under high uncertainty or without training.

Another central limitation in the processing of complex patterns is the finite channel capacity of the auditory processor. If the information content of a pattern exceeds the channel capacity, degradation in resolution occurs. The information content is strongly determined by the *number* of discrete components which comprise the pattern. Finally, perception of complex patterns does not seem to be an immediate, stable process. The sensations elicited by complex patterns appear, instead, to be an evolving, very plastic result of perceptual construction. Prolonged practice seems required to achieve *fully developed* perceptual representations of patterns.

What is the main implication of the previous discussion for the comparative psychoacoustician? The single most important implication is perhaps that in the processing of complex patterns by animals, the limitations may not be imposed primarily by the peripheral receptor, but instead, by more central processes such as attention, learning, and the capacity of memory. Consistent with this possibility are, for example, the results of studies on speech perception in the chinchilla (Kuhl & Miller, 1978). These studies have shown that, after prolonged training, chinchillas can exhibit human-like categorical perception for synthetic syllables. Where are the differences between animal and human speech perception to be found? Because chinchilla and human auditory systems share a number of structural and psychoacoustic similarities, it is likely that the peripheral representation of the speech sounds is also similar in the two species. Generalizing to other mammals, it may be proposed that the chinchilla, cat, monkey, man, and other mammals probably *hear* speech sounds in much the same way. In fact, this is what studies of representation of speech sounds in the auditory nerve have begun to show (e.g., Sachs, Voight, & Young, 1983; Sinex & Geisler, 1983). Strong differences between mammals would emerge when more central processes intervene in the auditory-perceptual representation of sounds. The previous conclusion has an additional implication for research in the comparative psychoacoustics of complex pattern processing. In our opinion, little will be learned if investigators focus exclusively on species differences in *peripheral* auditory processing, using tasks that minimize the role of central processes. We believe that more prominent and interesting differences emerge as central mechanisms are allowed to influence performance. Specifically, tasks which place demands on attention and memory may be particularly informative. This can be achieved, for example, by manipulating the level of stimulus uncertainty, introducing distracting stimuli, or overloading the animal's channel capacity using multidimensional stimuli. Most of what we currently know about pattern processing abilities of infrahuman species, seems to derive from experimental situations in which the involvement of central processing is greatly minimized.

ACKNOWLEDGMENTS

Preparation of this chapter was supported by grants from the National Institutes of Health, and the Air Force Office of Scientific Research awarded to Indiana University.

REFERENCES

Abramson, A. S., & Lisker, L. (1970). Discriminability along the voicing continuum: Cross-language tests. *Proceedings of the 6th International Congress of Phonetic Sciences.* Czechoslovak Academy of Sciences, Academia, Prague.

Braida, L. D., Lim, J. S., Berliner, J. E., Durlach, N. I., Rabinowitz, W. M., & Purks, S. R. (1984). Intensity perception. XIII. Perceptual anchor model of context coding. *Journal of the Acoustical Society of America, 76,* 722–731.

Bregman, A. S., Abramson, J., Doehring, P., & Darwing, C. J. (1985). Spectral integration based on common amplitude modulation. *Perception and Psychophysics, 37,* 483–493.

Bregman, A. S. (1978). The formation of auditory streams. In J. Requin (Ed.) *Attention and Performance VII.* Hillsdale, NJ: Lawrence Erlbaum Associates.

Bregman, A. S., & Campbell, J. (1971). Primary auditory stream segregation and the perception of order in rapid sequences of tones. *Journal of Experimental Psychology, 89,* 244–249.

Bregman, A. S. & Dannenbring, G. L. (1973). The effect of continuity on auditory stream segregation. *Perception and Psychophysics, 13,* 308–312.

Brunswick, E. (1956). *Perception and the Representative design of Psychological Experiments.* Berkeley: University of California Press.

Carterette, E. C., & Friedman, M. P. (1978). *Handbook of perception: Hearing.* New York: Academic Press.

Carterette, E. C., & Friedman, M. P. (1978). *Handbook of perception: Perceptual Coding,* New York: Academic Press.

Creelman, C. D. (1962). Human discrimination of auditory duration. *Journal of the Acoustical Society of America, 34,* 582–593.

Divenyi, P. L., & Hirsh, I. J. (1974). Identification of temporal order in three-tone sequences. *Journal of the Acoustical Society of America, 56,* 144–151.

Divenyi, P. L., & Hirsh, I. J. (1978). Some figural properties of auditory patterns. *Journal of the Acoustical Society of America, 64,* 1369–1385.

Espinoza-Varas, B., & Watson, C. S. (1986). Temporal discrimination for single components of nonspeech auditory patterns. *Journal of the Acoustical Society of America, 80,* 1685–1694.

Espinoza-Varas, B. (1983). Integration of spectral and temporal cues in discrimination of nonspeech sounds: a psychoacoustic analysis. *Journal of the Acoustical Society of America, 74,* 1687–1694.

Fletcher, H. (1940). Auditory patterns. *Review of Modern Physics, 12,* 47–65.

Foulke, E., & Sticht, T. G. (1969). Review of research on the intelligibility and comprehension of accelerated speech. *Psychological Bulletin, 72,* 50–62.

Garner, W. R. (1962). *Uncertainty and structure as psychological concepts.* New York: Wiley.

Gibson, E. J. (1969). *Principles of perceptual learning and development.* New York: Appleton-Century-Crofts.

Green, D. M. (1971). Temporal auditory acuity. *Psychological Review, 78,* 540–551.

Green, D. M. (1983). Profile analysis: A different view of auditory intensity discrimination. *American Psychologist, 38,* 133–142.

Green, D. M., Kidd, G., Jr., & Picardi, M. C. (1983). Successive versus simultaneous comparisons in auditory intensity discrimination. *Journal of the Acoustical Society of America, 73,* 639–643.

Hall, J. W., Haggard, M. P., & Fernandez, M. A. (1984). Detection in noise by spectro-temporal pattern analysis. *Journal of the Acoustical Society of America, 76,* 50–56.

Helmholtz, H. (1954). *On the sensations of tone as a physiological basis for the theory of music.* New York: Dover. (Originally published, 1863.)

Hirsh, I. J. (1959). Auditory perception of temporal order. *Journal of the Acoustical Society in America, 31,* 759–767.

Hirsh, I. J. (1974). Temporal order and auditory perception. In: H. R. Moskowitz et al. (Eds.), *Sensation and Measurement.* Dordrecht-Holland: Reidel.

Johnson, D. M., Watson, C. S., & Jensen, J. K. (1987). Individual differences in auditory capabilities. I. *Journal of the Acoustical Society of America, 81,* 427–438.

Jones, M. R. (1978). Auditory patterns: studies in the perception of structure. In: E. C. Carterette and M. P. Friedman, *Handbook of perception, Vol. VIII, Perceptual Coding.* New York: Academic Press.

Keidel, W. D., & Neff, W. D. (1975). *Handbook of sensory physiology: Auditory system.* Berlin: Springer-Verlag.

Kelly, W. J., & Watson, C. S. (1986). Stimulus-based limitations on the discrimination between different temporal orders of tones. *Journal of the Acoustical Society of America, 79,* 1934–1938.

Kewley-Port, D., Watson, C. S., & Foyle, D. (1988). Auditory temporal acuity in relation to category boundaries: speech and nonspeech stimuli. *Journal of the Acoustical Society of America, 83*, 1133–1145.

Kidd, G., Mason, C. R., & Green, D. M. (1986). Auditory profile analysis of irregular sound spectra. *Journal of the Acoustical Society of America, 79*, 1045–1053.

Kuhl, P. K., & Miller, J. D. (1975). Speech perception in early infancy: Discrimination of speech sound categories. *Journal of the Acoustical Society of America, 58*, S56.

Kuhl, P. K., & Miller, J. D. (1978). Speech perception by the chinchilla: Identification functions for synthetic VOT stimuli. *Journal of the Acoustical Society of America, 63*, 905–917.

Leek, M. R., & Watson, C. S. (1984). Learning to detect auditory pattern components. *Journal of the Acoustical Society of America, 76*, 1037–1044.

Leshowitz, B., & Cudahy, E. (1973). Frequency discrimination in the presence of another tone. *Journal of the Acoustical Society of America, 54*, 882–887.

McAdams, S. (1984). Spectral fusion, spectral parsing, and the formation of auditory images. Unpublished Ph.D. Dissertation, Stanford University.

McAdams, S., & Bregman, A. (1979). Hearing musical streams. *Computer Music Journal, 3*, 26–44.

Miller, G. A., Heise, G., & Lichten, W. (1951). The intelligibility of speech as a function of the context of the test materials. *Journal of Experimental Psychology, 41*, 329–335.

Miller, G. A. (1956). The magical number seven, plus minus two. *Psychological Review, 63*, 81–97.

Miller, G. A., & Heise, G. A. (1950). The trill threshold. *Journal of the Acoustical Society of America, 22*, 637–638.

Nabelek, I. V., Nabelek, A. K., & Hirsh, I. J. (1973). Pitch of sound bursts with continuous and discontinuous change of frequency. *Journal of the Acoustical Society of America, 53*, 1305–1312.

Neisser, U. (1967). *Cognitive psychology.* New York: Appleton-Century-Crofts.

Neisser, U., & Hirst, W. (1974). Effect of practice on the identification of auditory sequences. *Perception and Psychophysics, 15*, 391–398.

Pollack, I. (1953). The information of elementary auditory displays: II. *Journal of the Acoustical Society of America, 25*, 765–769.

Pollack, I., & Ficks, L. (1954). Information of elementary multidimensional auditory displays. *Journal of the Acoustical Society of America, 26*, 155–158.

Robinson, D. E., & Watson, C. S. (1972). Psychophysical methods in modern psychophysics. In: J. V. Tobias (Ed.) *Foundations of Modern Auditory Theory, Vol. II*, New York: Academic Press.

Ronken, D. A. (1972). Changes in frequency discrimination caused by leading and trailing tones. *Journal of the Acoustical Society of America, 51*, 1947–1950.

Sachs, M. B., Voight, H. F., & Young, E. D. (1983). Auditory nerve representation of vowels in background noise. *Journal of Neurophysiology, 50*, 27–45.

Shower, E. G., & Biddulph, R. (1931). Differential pitch sensitivity of the ear. *Journal of the Acoustical Society of America, 3*, 275–287.

Sinex, D. G., & Geisler, C. D. (1983). Responses of auditory-nerve fibers to consonant-vowel syllables. *Journal of the Acoustical Society of America, 73*, 602–615.

Spiegel, M. F., Picardi, M. C., & Green, D. M. (1981). Signal and masker uncertainty in intensity discrimination. *Journal of the Acoustical Society of America, 70*, 1015–1019.

Spiegel, M. F., & Watson, C. S. (1981). Factors in the discrimination of tonal patterns. III. Frequency discrimination with components of well learned patterns. *Journal of the Acoustical Society of America, 69*, 223–230.

Stevens, K. N., & Blumstein, S. (1978). Invariant cues for place of articulation in stop consonants. *Journal of the Acoustical Society of America, 64*, 1358–1368.

Stevens, S. S. (1951). *Handbook of experimental psychology.* New York: Wiley.

Tobias, J. V. (1970). *Foundations of modern auditory theory.* Vol. I. New York: Academic Press.

Tobias, J. V. (1972). *Foundations of modern auditory theory*. Vol. II. New York: Academic Press.

van Noorden, L. P. A. S. (1975). Temporal coherence in the perception of tone sequences. *The Institute of Perception Research*, Eindhoven, The Netherlands.

Warren, R. M. (1974). Auditory temporal discrimination by trained listeners. *Cognitive Psychology, 6*, 237–256.

Warren, R. M. (1983). Multiple meanings of "phoneme" (articulatory, acoustic, perceptual, graphemic) and their confusions. In: N. J. Lass (Ed.) *Speech and Language: Advances in research and practice, Vol. 9*. New York: Academic Press.

Watson, C. S., & Foyle, D. C. (1985). Central factors in the discrimination and identification of complex sounds. *Journal of the Acoustical Society of America, 78*, 375–380.

Watson, C. S. (1973). Psychophysics. In B. B. Wolman (Ed.), *Handbook of General Psychology*. New York: Prentice-Hall.

Watson, C. S., & Kelly, W. J. (1981). The role of stimulus uncertainty in the discrimination of auditory patterns. In D. J. Getty and J. H. Howard, Jr. (Eds.) *Auditory and visual pattern recognition*. Hillsdale, NJ: Lawrence Erlbaum Associates.

Watson, C. S., Wroton, H. W., Kelly, W. J., & Benbasset, C. A. (1975). Factors in the discrimination of tonal patterns. I. Component frequency, temporal position, and silent intervals. *Journal of the Acoustical Society of America, 57*, 1175–1185.

Watson, C. S., Kelly, W. J., & Wroton, H. W. (1976). Factors in the discrimination of tonal patterns. II. Selective attention and learning under various levels of stimulus uncertainty. *Journal of the Acoustical Society of America, 60*, 1176–1186.

Watson, C. S. (1980). Time course of auditory perceptual learning. *The Annals of Otology, Rhinology and Laryngology*. Suppl. 74, 96–102.

Winckel, F. (1967). *Music, sound, and sensation*. New York: Dover.

Yost, W. A., & Watson, C. S. (1987). *Auditory processing of complex sounds*. Hillsdale, NJ: Lawrence Erlbaum Associates.

Editor's Comments on Mullennix and Pisoni

Decades of research on the perception of speech sounds has winnowed this area of complex auditory perception down to several critical focal issues around which much of modern research on speech perception is organized. These issues are linearity, acoustic invariance, and segmentation. The failure of basic psychoacoustics to adequately account for these phenomena point to the necessity of invoking higher order, "top-down" influences on perception. The efficiency with which speech is processed by the human auditory system has led to the notion that a special "speech mode" is involved.

In this chapter, Mullennix and Pisoni describe the major problems in speech perception today providing a plethora of evidence that higher-level sources of information interact with the auditory encoding process in humans listening to speech. These authors rally support most eloquently for the notion that speech perception processes in humans may operate in a qualitatively different manner than analogous complex perceptual processes in animals but that the evidence does not yet support ". . . a specialized phonetic processor organized as an autonomous phonetic module. . . ."

4 Speech Perception: Analysis of Biologically Significant Signals

John W. Mullennix
David B. Pisoni
Indiana University

INTRODUCTION

Over the last 35 years, the study of speech perception has been largely concerned with describing the acoustic parameters which are important to phonetic distinctions in speech. Although a large amount of research has been conducted in this area, the evidence which has accumulated to date has not resolved a number of critical issues central to the understanding of the perception of speech sounds. One such issue is concerned with describing the nature and origin of the perceptual processes which transform the acoustic waveform into a speech percept. It has been suggested by some researchers that specialized, speech-specific biological mechanisms may exist in the human which are devoted to processing speech sounds (e.g., Liberman, 1982; Liberman & Mattingly, 1985). These mechanisms are hypothetically instantiated in a modular subsystem characterized by a specialized neural architecture for perceiving acoustic (speech) signals (Liberman & Mattingly, 1985). This idea was originally based on evidence from various experimental paradigms suggesting that the human perceptual system responds differently to speech input than to other auditory input (e.g., Liberman, Harris, Kinney, & Lane, 1961, Mattingly, Liberman, Syrdal, & Halwes, 1971). When this observation is compared to observations in the animal world that responses to species-specific vocalizations critical for survival are ''special'' (e.g., in treefrogs, birds, etc.), then the hypothesis can be advanced that the processes involved in speech perception may be specialized for perceiving speech much as mechanisms in nonhumans are specialized for perception of species-specific vocalizations. In order to resolve an issue of this type, it is useful to compare the processing of complex acoustic sounds across species. Although these comparisons provide valuable information about the nonhuman species themselves, this work can function directly to elucidate the nature of speech perception processes in the human. In particular, by examining nonhuman perceptual responses to speech stimuli, evidence can be obtained that can guide construction of hypotheses considering whether certain speech processes are specific to the human being or not. When this evidence is related to the biological commonalities and differences in the auditory systems of humans and nonhumans, a cohesive description of the processes and mechanisms by which humans perceive speech may begin to emerge.

Although much research has been conducted in examining and comparing the complex acoustic perception of different species (e.g., this volume), the focus in this chapter is mainly on issues and research that are pertinent to human speech perception. The human being is decidedly adept in his or her ability to quickly and efficiently decode the speech waveform. Despite variations in the physical waveform resulting from such factors as surrounding phonetic context, individual speaker differences, smearing of phonetic information across speech segments, differences in rate, loudness, pitch, etc., speech is readily perceived and understood. There are a number of basic issues and problems of research in speech perception that bear on the question of whether perception of speech signals by the human is "unique" when compared to other species. Among these are the lack of acoustic-phonetic invariance, the linearity problem, segmentation and units of encoding, and perceptual normalization. There is also evidence that higher-level sources of information (i.e., phonological, lexical, syntactic, and semantic) are available to interact with and substantially affect lower-level speech perception processes. Use of information in this manner may also be unique. In this chapter, we first briefly describe some of the basic issues concerning perceptual constancy in speech perception, and later, present evidence concerning the involvement of top-down knowledge in speech perception. Then, we consider the notion that perception of speech may involve specialized, speech-specific biological mechanisms. There have been a number of claims suggesting that speech is "special" (Liberman, 1970a), and that a specialized speech processor or perceptual mechanism is needed to process speech sounds. A body of experimental evidence has recently accumulated relevant to this subject which will be described under the rubric of perception in the speech mode.

Finally, we briefly compare and contrast perception of speech by humans (infants and adults) across languages and across species. Similarities and differences across languages in the perception of phonetic contrasts have important implications concerning the development of perceptual processes in the infant. The comparison of humans to nonhumans in processing speech provides valuable evidence concerning the nature of the mechanisms utilized in human speech perception.

I. BASIC ISSUES: VARIABILITY AND PERCEPTUAL CONSTANCY

One of the most fundamental characteristics of speech is its inherent physical variability. The tremendous variability in the speech waveform ultimately reflects the consequences of a wide range of possible articulatory configurations used when producing speech. Such factors as rate of speech, voice, pitch, loudness, and accent all dictate the form that the acoustic waveform will take. The coarticulation of adjacent acoustic segments and the effects of phonetic context also affect how the acoustic waveform will appear. The observation that these sources of variation are transparent to the listener with regard to perceiving speech has led to a number of basic questions and problems concerning speech perception.

Linearity, Invariance, and Segmentation

The complex manner with which linguistic information is encoded into the speech waveform is exemplified by the failure of speech to meet the conditions of linearity and invariance (Chomsky & Miller, 1963). The condition of linearity requires that each phoneme in the utterance must have associated with it a particular stretch of sound. In other words, if phoneme A precedes phoneme B in the phonemic representation of the utterance, then the stretch of sound corresponding to phoneme A must precede the stretch of sound corresponding to phoneme B in the physical acoustic waveform. This condition has not been met because of the context-conditioned variability of speech due to coarticulation and the effects of immediate and distant phonetic context. As a speech sound is being articulated, the exact articulatory configuration will depend on the phones uttered before and after the present phone (see Fig. 4.1).

As an example, in the word *bat* the lips remain unrounded during articulation of the word. However, in the word *boot,* which has an identical initial phoneme, the lips are rounded before and during articulation. Although the initial consonants are identical, the difference in articulation as a function of the following vowel context manifests itself in the acoustic waveform, i.e., the portion of the waveform corresponding to the /b/ in *bat* is different than the portion of the waveform corresponding to the /b/ in *boot.* Thus, information about the following vowel is carried in the acoustic segment corresponding to /b/. This situation is quite typical when examining fluent speech. Identical phonemes are often represented in the acoustic waveform in substantially different ways (e.g., Liberman, Delattre, Cooper, & Gerstman, 1954). For example, in Fig. 4.2 the acoustic segments corresponding to the phoneme /t/ vary widely as a function of context.

More importantly, a "smearing" of acoustic information often occurs such

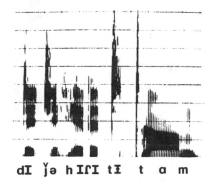

dI Ĭə h IʃI tI   t   ɑ   m

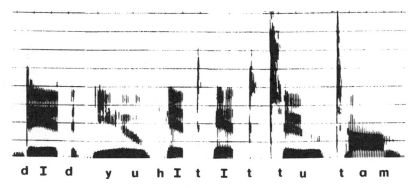

d I   d   y u h I t   I   t   t u   t ɑ m

FIG. 4.1. Two spectrograms of the utterance "Did you hit it to Tom?".
The upper panel shows the utterance produced in a normal sentence
context, the lower panel shows the same words produced in isolation.
Adapted from Luce and Pisoni (1987).

that each stretch of the waveform may contain acoustic information about adjacent and even nonadjacent phonemes (Liberman, 1970b). The failure to meet the linearity condition reflects the nonlinear and complex nature of the encoding of speech.

Closely related to linearity is what has been termed the ''lack of invariance'' in speech. Simply put, the requirement for invariance in speech perception is that a set of criterial acoustic attributes or features exists which is present when a phoneme or its allophone is present, and is absent when the phoneme is absent. As mentioned earlier, there exists evidence that different acoustic representations exist for identical phonemes. Identical acoustic cues for particular phonemes can also give rise to different percepts as a function of context (e.g., Liberman, Delattre, & Cooper, 1952). As a result of these contextual effects, it has been difficult to isolate acoustic attributes or features that satisfy the invariance condition. This problem has generated a great deal of research devoted to searching for invariant cues to phonemes, particularly with stop-consonants (e.g., see Blum-

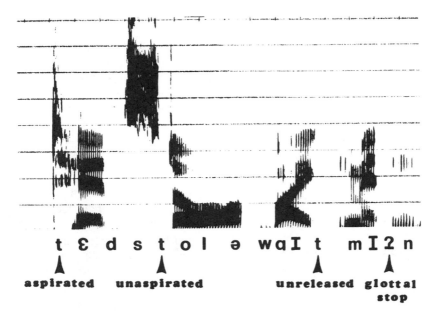

t ɛ d s t o l ə waɪ t m ɪ 2 n

aspirated unaspirated unreleased glottal stop

FIG. 4.2. Spectrogram of the utterance "Ted stole the white mitten". /t/ is shown as aspirated, unaspirated, unreleased, and as a glottal stop. Adapted from Luce and Pisoni (1987).

stein, 1986; Kewley-Port & Luce, 1984; Stevens & Blumstein, 1978, 1981). To date, a simple invariant mapping between acoustic attributes and phonemes has yet to be found.

As a result of the lack of invariance and the linearity problems in speech, an additional problem arises which deals with the segmentation of the acoustic waveform into phonemes, syllables, words, and sentences. As previously noted, a given segment of the acoustic waveform does not contain information solely corresponding to one linguistic unit, and furthermore, the acoustic manifestation of a particular linguistic unit differs as a function of context. When you add to these observations the fact that the speech signal varies continuously and does not contain breaks or silent intervals corresponding to word boundaries, it appears as though there is no simple way of mapping the acoustic waveform onto discrete linguistic units. Consequently, it has been difficult to pinpoint at what level segmentation takes place. In fact, evidence has been presented at one time or another to suggest that the primary perceptual units are features, phonemes, syllables, context-sensitive allophones, context-sensitive spectra, words, and sentence clauses. Regardless of the outcome of this continuing debate over units, it is clear that there is no simple one-to-one relationship between the acoustic segments of the speech waveform and units of perception.

Perceptual Normalization

Another source of variability present in the speech waveform results from intra-talker and intertalker differences. Intratalker differences from utterance to utterance occur as a function of changes in pitch, loudness, speaking rate, stress, rhythm, and affect. Intertalker differences occur as a result of these factors plus variability due to individual differences in articulatory and vocal tract configurations, accent, dialect, etc. In perceiving speech, the listener must not only deal with variability due to lack of invariance and linearity, but he or she must also adjust (normalize), in some way, for intra- and intertalker variability in extracting speech information.

There is some evidence that suggests that intratalker variation due to rate changes, stress, timing and rhythm, and prosody (pitch contour changes over the utterance) are instantiated in the waveform in similar ways across talkers. For example, research in production and perception has documented the effects of speaking rate on the durations of vowels and consonants, syllables, words, and silent intervals (e.g., see Grosjean & Lane, 1981; Miller, 1981). Durational changes of speech segments due to rate changes appear to be fairly regular and rule-based, with changes occurring both within and across talkers.

On the other hand, intertalker variation due to vocal tract shape and configuration, voice, affect, accent, and dialect are much less quantifiable. The effects of talker voice characteristics have been documented in studies examining vowel perception (e.g., Nearey, 1978; Strange, Verbrugge, Shankweiler, & Edman, 1976; Summerfield, 1975; Summerfield & Haggard, 1973; Verbrugge, Strange, Shankweiler, & Edman, 1976) and word perception (Allard & Henderson, 1976; Cole, Coltheart, & Allard, 1974; Craik & Kirsner, 1974; Mattingly, Studdert-Kennedy, & Magen, 1983; Mullennix, Pisoni, & Martin, in press). It is clear that differences between talkers have consequences for perceptual processing of the utterance. However, the acoustic parameters which underly differences among talkers have not been adequately identified (but, see Carrell, 1984, for a recent review; see also O'Shaughnessy, 1986). It may turn out that intertalker differences can be described by a set of parameters or rules which can predict perceptual performance, but further investigation is needed.

Given that we can quickly and easily understand speech despite intra- and intertalker variability, it can be hypothesized that there are perceptual processes or mechanisms which *normalize* the speech input. The manner in which such a hypothetical normalization might occur is not clear, but a transformation of the acoustic waveform into a normalized form that can be operated on by processes for further analysis seems warranted.

Conclusion

As briefly outlined, a number of basic issues in speech perception remain unresolved. These issues have been rather intractable because of the complex nature of the context-conditioned and talker-conditioned variability of speech. Phenomenally, this complexity seems to be of little consequence: spoken language is quickly and readily processed. The likelihood is very strong that the human possesses sophisticated processes and mechanisms that are suited to preserving perceptual constancy in speech. If similar processes are at all present in non-humans, they may be considerably less complex.

II. PERCEPTION IN THE SPEECH MODE

For a number of years a debate has occurred concerning the idea that speech is perceived directly as a result of specialized, speech-specific processes and/or mechanisms. At one level, the idea that special systems exist for language processing probably cannot be disputed as suggested by the use of syntactic and semantic knowledge in comprehending fluent speech. However, the specific issue of whether the perceptual encoding of phonetic information is performed by specialized speech-specific neural mechanisms is controversial. One rationale for postulating such a mechanism follows from observations with animals. Given that animals respond to species-specific vocalizations differently than they do for extraneous auditory signals, it is tempting to make the analogy that humans respond to speech signals in a similar species-specific fashion (Mattingly, 1972; Pisoni, 1979). Any evidence gathered which shows that humans respond differently to speech than to nonspeech signals would support this hypotheses. It is possible that the perceptual mechanisms involved in coding phonetic information in speech are instantiated in a specialized, dedicated neural system functioning as a modular speech processor (Liberman & Mattingly, 1985; Mattingly & Liberman, 1986).

Further evidence suggesting a mechanism of this sort follows from observing the phenomenon of perceptual constancy. If a mechanism exists which is particularly suited to extracting intended phonetic information from the highly variable acoustic signal, the temptation is strong to attribute this extraction process to a specialized mechanism of some sort. Existence of a mechanism of this type has predominantly been advocated in the form of theories which posit a relationship between perception and articulation (i.e., motor theory, Liberman, 1970b, Liberman, 1982; Liberman, Cooper, Shankweiler, & Studdert-Kennedy, 1967; Repp, 1982; Studdert-Kennedy, Liberman, Harris, & Cooper, 1970). More recently, a modified version of motor theory postulating a specialized ''module'' which detects the intended articulatory gestures of the talker has also been proposed (Liberman & Mattingly, 1985; Mattingly & Liberman, 1986). Alternatives to this view have also been proposed suggesting either that a specialized mechanism of this sort is not needed (Cutting, 1978; Pastore, 1981; Schouten, 1980), with perception proceeding by the use of general auditory coding mechanisms. Also, theories have been advocated incorporating both auditory and phonetic coding processes (Pisoni & Sawusch, 1975; Sawusch, 1986).

A great deal of research involving phenomena such as categorical perception (e.g., Fry, Abramson, Eimas, & Liberman, 1962; Liberman, Harris, Hoffman, & Griffith, 1957; Mattingly et al., 1971), lateralization (Studdert-Kennedy & Shankweiler, 1970), cross-modal integration (MacDonald & McGurk, 1978; McGurk & MacDonald, 1976), trading relations (see Repp, 1982, for a review), and duplex perception (Liberman, Isenberg, & Rakerd, 1981; Repp, 1984; Repp, Milburn, & Ashkenas, 1983; but see Nusbaum, 1984; Nusbaum, Schwab, & Sawusch, 1983) has been cited in favor of a specialized, speech-specific processing mechanism based on some form of motor mediation (Liberman et al., 1967; Liberman & Mattingly, 1985). Within this theoretical framework, perception of speech is accomplished by a biologically distinct, specialized speech processing subsystem which recovers the phonetic information via intimate links between production and perception. As this work has been extensively reviewed elsewhere (Liberman, 1982; Liberman & Mattingly, 1985; Repp, 1982) we will not elaborate on it here. However, a number of studies recently conducted using nonspeech stimuli are of direct importance to the issue of whether a specialized mechanism of this particular sort exists. This evidence is briefly reviewed in the next sections.

Nonspeech Studies

Categorical perception of speech is a robust phenomenon. Numerous studies using identification and discrimination procedures (e.g., Liberman et al., 1957) have shown that consonants differing along a phonetic contrast are perceived in a discontinuous fashion, while vowels and certain nonspeech sounds are perceived in a continuous fashion (Fry et al., 1962; Mattingly et al., 1971). Categorical perception has been used to argue for a motor theory explanation of speech perception. It is hypothesized that since consonants are perceived and produced in a discontinuous fashion (i.e., categorically) and vowels are perceived and produced in a continuous fashion, a link between perception and production must exist. Therefore, a specialized processor which utilizes knowledge about articulation operates on the acoustic input to produce a speech percept.

One of the critical assumptions on which this theory is based is that nonspeech sounds which are not processed as speech are not perceived in a categorical manner. This assumption has been challenged by the work of Miller, Wier, Pastore, Kelley, and Dooling (1976) and Pisoni (1977) in which certain nonspeech continua containing parameters mimicking important dimensions in speech were perceived categorically. For example, Miller et al. (1976) constructed a stimulus continuum composed of noise-buzz sequences. The stimuli resembled speech in that the aperiodic noise bursts were similar to noise bursts found in stop consonants, with the buzz portion of the stimulus corresponding to voicing. The stimuli across the continuum also varied in the lead-time of the burst to the buzz portion of the stimulus (emulating VOT in natural speech).

Miller et al. (1976) obtained identification and ABX discrimination functions that were similar to those found with synthetic speech VOT continua. Hence, the nonspeech continuum was perceived categorically, even though the stimuli were not perceived as speech.

Pisoni (1977) investigated VOT timing relations in a somewhat more abstract manner. He constructed a nonspeech two-tone stimulus continuum where the onset of the lower tone either preceded, was identical with, or followed the onset of the higher tone. This continuum preserved the timing information found in VOT continua in speech (where the first formant onset varies in relation to the second formant onset depending on whether the stimulus is prevoiced, voiced, or voiceless). The results showed that the nonspeech continuum was perceived categorically, and moreover, that the category boundaries corresponded closely to the VOT boundaries found in speech (Lisker & Abramson, 1970). Pisoni (1977) concluded that the discriminability of temporal order differences of component dimensions was an important attribute determining voicing perception of word initial stops. Again, this study illustrated the fact that a stimulus continuum containing information pertinent to perception of speech which was not heard as speech was perceived categorically.

Categorical perception has also been shown to occur in the visual domain as well (see Pastore et al., 1977). As this shows that categorical perception is not just peculiar to the processing of speech, the argument using categorical perception as evidence for a specialized processing mechanism is weakened further. As discussed below, categorical-like perception has also been observed with animals (e.g., Kuhl & Miller, 1975, 1978; Kuhl & Padden, 1982, 1983). Thus, it appears as though categorical perception cannot be used to support a motor-theory-based explanation of speech perception.

Additional evidence that nonspeech signals are processed in a speech-like manner was shown by the finding that context effects occurring in speech can be found with nonspeech stimuli. For example, temporal order identification thresholds for tones with asynchronous onsets are dependent on stimulus duration (Pastore, Harris, & Kaplan, 1982) much as category boundaries for consonants with asynchronous formant onsets are dependent on duration (Summerfield, 1981). Analogous findings have also been found with labeling of tonal analogs to the F1-cutback voicing cue in speech (Pastore, Morris, & Layer, 1985). It has been shown that shifts in the category boundary of a stop-glide speech continuum as a function of overall syllable duration (Miller & Liberman, 1979) are also found with nonspeech tonal analogs of the stimuli (Pisoni, Carrell, & Gans, 1983). Trading relations between VOT and formant transitions in perception of voicing (e.g., Lisker et al., 1977) can be emulated with nonspeech sinewave stimuli (Hillenbrand, 1984), and trading relations between low-frequency glottal pulsing and closure duration have been found with nonspeech square-wave stimuli (Parker, Diehl, & Kleunder, 1986).

Context effects of the kinds reviewed above found with speech (e.g., speaking rate, trading relations) have been used to argue for the existence of a specialized speech processor (Liberman, 1982; Liberman & Mattingly, 1985; Repp, 1982). But, the fact that similar context effects can be found with nonspeech tonal analog stimuli eliminates the need to suppose that these effects are simply due to a specialized mechanism of this sort. Hence, this line of evidence cannot be used to support the idea of a special speech processor of the type advocated by Liberman and colleagues (see also Repp, 1983).

Manipulation of Speech/Nonspeech Modes

A line of research has emerged directly investigating perception of speech as a function of the perceptual mode that the listener is engaged in. In these studies, nonspeech sinewave tonal analogs of speech which preserve pattern information (see Cutting, 1974) are used. The critical manipulation concerns whether the subjects hear these stimuli as speech or nonspeech (Bailey, Summerfield, & Dorman, 1977; Best, Morrongiello, & Robson, 1981; Grunke & Pisoni, 1982; Ralston, 1986; Ralston & Sawusch, 1984, 1986; Remez, Rubin, Pisoni, & Carrell, 1981; Schwab, 1982; Tomiak, Mullennix, & Sawusch, 1987; Williams, 1986). An assumption that is critical in interpreting data obtained from these experiments is that when the listener hears the sinewave analog stimuli as nonspeech, he or she is engaged in a nonspeech perceptual mode, and when the listener hears the sinewave analog stimuli as speech, he or she is engaged in a speech perceptual mode. Given this assumption, if qualitative differences in performance exist as a function of the perceptual mode the subject is engaged in when processing acoustically identical stimuli, then this suggests that operations or computations are invoked which are peculiar to a speech mode of processing.

Performance differences of this sort have been exhibited in experiments examining categorical perception (Bailey et al., 1977; Ralston, 1986; Ralston & Sawusch, 1984, 1986), phonetic labeling (Grunke & Pisoni, 1982; Schwab, 1982), trading relations (Best et al., 1981), sentence perception (Remez et al., 1981), and integral processing of speech (Tomiak et al., 1987). Remez et al. (1981) provided a convincing demonstration that sinewave analogs can be processed as speech even though they do not contain the traditional acoustic cues found in phonetic segments. Remez et al. used time-varying sinusoidal patterns which followed the changing center formant frequencies of naturally produced sentences. Subjects who were not told anything about the stimuli spontaneously reported them as sounding like "science fiction sounds," "computer bleeps," "bird sounds," etc. However, subjects who were linguistically primed (i.e., were told they were listening to a sentence and had to transcribe it) were able to identify the phonetic segments of the stimulus. Remez et al. (1981) concluded that, "The linguistically primed listeners were capable, for the most part, of directing their attention to the phonetic properties of the sinusoidal signal, merely by virtue of the instruction to listen in the speech mode of perception" (p. 949).

Thus, even though the stimulus information was identical in both conditions, performance differed simply as a function of instructions which primed subjects to listen in a "speech mode."

Differences in categorical perception of place of articulation continua have been reported as a function of speech and nonspeech modes of perception. Bailey et al. (1977) found shifts in category boundaries between "b" and "d" when subjects heard the sinewave analogs as speech as opposed to nonspeech. A more detailed investigation of categorical perception of place was conducted in a recent series of experiments by Ralston and Sawusch (1984, 1986; Ralston, 1986). In brief, identification and discrimination procedures were used in conjunction with speech/nonspeech instructional manipulations for one and three-component sinewave analogs. Evidence was found supporting the idea that both speech and nonspeech continua were perceived categorically. In addition, some differences were exhibited between speech and nonspeech groups in category labeling. Thus, evidence existed refuting the idea that categorical perception is only found with speech stimuli, and evidence also existed suggesting that processing in the speech mode affects the categorization of speech stimuli.

Given that performance differs as a function of the perceptual mode (speech or nonspeech) the subject engages, the question arises as how to characterize this "speech mode" of processing. Schwab (1982) examined auditory and phonetic processing of place information in syllable-initial and syllable-final positions using sinewave analogs and speech/nonspeech instructions. Using a signal detection analysis, she found that differences in labeling between speech and nonspeech groups were the result of systematic changes in perceptual sensitivity rather than a criterion shift. This suggests that the engagement of a "speech mode" may have something to do with changes in the perceptual processes themselves, as opposed to judgmental or decision processes.

One attempt at characterizing processing in the speech mode is concerned with the dependency relations existing between adjacent phones within syllables (Tomiak et al., 1987). Tomiak ct al. (1987) constructed noise-tone analogs of fricative-vowel syllables (i.e., /fae/, /shae/, /fu/, and /shu/). They used a selective attention procedure incorporating a two-choice speeded classification task (see Garner, 1974) where the stimulus dimensions were ordered into single-dimension, orthogonal, and correlated sets. By observing the pattern of latencies across the stimulus set conditions, the presence or absence of dependency relations (i.e., whether the stimulus dimensions were processed in an integral or separable fashion) between the dimensions of noise and tone (nonspeech condition) and fricative and vowel (speech condition) was able to be assessed. Although the stimuli were acoustically identical in both conditions, the results obtained showed that when subjects heard the syllables as nonspeech, they processed the noise and tone as separable entities. However, when the noise-tone analogs were heard as speech, the syllables were processed in an integral fashion. This latter result was also exhibited with naturally produced speech. These results were taken by Tomiak et al. (1987) as evidence that a speech mode exists which incorporates knowledge of the acoustic consequences of coarticulation. As the stimulus dimensions in their study were specified independently of one another, the integrality found between adjacent phones within a syllable was simply a function of the processing mode engaged. Whether or not coarticulatory information was actually present in the signal was irrelevant.

These results can also be related to the idea of "emergent features" (Pomerantz, Sager, & Stoever, 1977; Sawusch & Nochajski, 1982). As stated by Pomerantz et al. (1977), ". . . wholes are perceived by their emergent features which are not the parts themselves but rather stem from the interaction of these parts" (p. 434). Thus, it is possible that the engagement of a "speech mode" results in a merging and interaction of acoustic components in the stimulus which are then extracted as a wholistic entity or pattern.

Conclusion

The issue with which we began in this section, i.e., whether the perceptual coding of phonetic information is a result of specialized, speech-specific neural mechanisms, has not been settled. Recently, criticisms have been leveled against the use of data from nonspeech studies to argue against the concept of specialized, speech-specific mechanisms (see Kuhl, 1986a, 1986b, this volume). Kuhl claims that confusion arises as a result of the interchangeable use of the terms "speech-specific" and "specially evolved for speech" (Kuhl, 1986a). As stated by Kuhl (1986a), "The implication here is that mechanisms could have evolved 'especially for speech' without being 'speech-specific.' What I am suggesting, then, is the possibility that if feature-detecting or other "dedicated" mechanisms exist, they may not be so narrowly tuned that nonspeech sounds mimicking the critical features in speech are excluded. In other words, nonspeech sounds may 'fool' them" (p. 240). So, in this view, effects that have been obtained with humans using nonspeech continua emulating critical acoustic cues in speech are only useful in determining the underlying tuning of the mechanisms underlying speech perception. Furthermore, convergent performance of speech and nonspeech only proves that the two signals are tied to a common mechanism.

This viewpoint suggests that one cannot discriminate between accounts proposing that general auditory processing is responsible for nonspeech results or whether a mechanism specially evolved for speech is responsible. However, this argument is largely based on the hypothesis that nonspeech signals "fool" the processing mechanism. Although it is possible that this occurs, there is little evidence currently available to support such a conjecture. If a mechanism which has evolved especially for the perception of speech also processes certain nonspeech sounds, then by definition the mechanism is not strictly dedicated to perception of speech signals. Furthermore, it is difficult to explain the results of speech/nonspeech manipulations where identical acoustic information produces different patterns of performance with a mechanism of the sort which Kuhl (1986a, 1986b, this volume) suggests. If a "dedicated" mechanism of this sort exists which is instantiated in the neural hardware, it would seem that a "processing mode" adopted by the listener would have little consequence, as the mechanism should supposedly operate only as a function of the acoustic input. However, a wide variety of studies have shown that the perception of speech is substantially affected by cognitive factors as well as factors related to the acoustic input.

Perhaps the most well-developed account proposing that speech perception is "special" depends on postulating links between perception and production (Liberman, 1982; Liberman et al., 1967; Liberman & Mattingly, 1985; Repp, 1982). This account, however, fails to explain the results obtained from the manipulation of speech/nonspeech instructions. With a motor-theory type of account, the stimulus information drives the specialized processes translating the input into terms of articulatory gestures in a deterministic manner. Indeed, Liberman and Mattingly (1985), in adopting Fodor's (1983) idea of modularity, suggest that the operation of a specialized speech perception module is "mandatory" and "informationally encapsulated." Given that this module is instantiated in a rigid, specialized neural architecture, it is difficult again to reconcile the finding that processing of sinewave analogs is different when the listener *engages* a speech mode with the idea of a deterministic, modularized mechanism. It would seem that the acoustic input should trigger the *specialized* processes without cognitive mediation. These findings suggest that a speech mode of processing must have the involvement of some type of cognitive component, as performance differences with identical stimuli are exhibited simply on the basis of the listener's expectations.

III. EFFECTS OF HIGHER-LEVEL INFORMATION

If speech is viewed as a form of species-specific vocalization, another aspect of the processing of speech which may be unique, or at the very least is much more highly developed and sophisticated in the human being is access to and use of higher-level knowledge sources. In the course of perceiving normal fluent speech, utterances are processed under a variety of different constraints including phonological, lexical, syntactic, and semantic. In the following sections, the effect of these knowledge sources on perception of speech is described.

Phonological Constraints

Knowledge of phonological rules and permissible phonological sequences (i.e., phonotactics) of a language appears to affect lower-level perceptual processes.

Some of the psychological evidence supporting this assertion comes from experimental work on misperceptions (Bond & Garnes, 1980; Bond & Robey, 1983) and perceptual identification (Brown & Hildum, 1956; Massaro & Cohen, 1983). For example, Bond and Garnes (1980) collected instances of errors in the perception of a number of spoken utterances by comparing the actual utterance with the misperceived utterance. Among the misperceptions ("slips of the ear") they examined were errors that seemed attributable to the misapplication of phonological rules. For instance, certain errors resulted from the deletion or insertion of entire phonetic segments or syllables by listeners (e.g., perceiving "test" instead of "text" and perceiving "amples" instead of "apples"). Deletions were interpreted by Bond and Garnes (1980) as resulting from a listener's failure to recover a segment or syllable which had been reduced in production by application of a simplification rule, whereas for insertions the listener wrongly assumed that the phonological rule for reduction was applied. These results suggest that perceptual processes involved in speech perception are affected by the listener's knowledge of particular phonological rules (see also Oshika, Zue, Weeks, Nue, & Aurbach, 1975).

Evidence also exists to suggest that knowledge of permissible phonological sequences affects perception. Brown and Hildum (1956) presented CVC (consonant-vowel-consonant) syllables to subjects with the CVC's being either words, phonologically admissible pseudowords, or phonologically inadmissible nonwords (e.g., /glib/, /spib/, and /tlib/). The VC portion of the syllable was always the same, with phonological variation manipulated in the initial consonant cluster. They found that listeners were worst in identifying the sequences which were phonologically inadmissible, and were best in identifying words. This finding suggests that subjects used phonological constraints in the form of knowledge of sequential contingencies in perceptual processing of the items. In a somewhat more detailed exploration of this context effect, Massaro and Cohen (1983) constructed a synthetic /ri/-/li/ continuum. These sounds were placed after four different consonants (/s/, /t/, /p/, and /v/) in order to vary the phonological context. By examining the effect on labeling of the continua, the effect of phonological sequence permissibility could be examined. The results for the /sri/-/sli/ continuum showed that more "l" responses were produced than "r" responses; and for the /tri/-/tli/ continuum, more "r" responses were exhibited than "l" responses. Identification functions for the /pri/-/pli/ and /vri/-/vli/ continua were not biased in either direction, because in one case both endpoint stimuli were permissible, and in the other case, both endpoints were not permissible. The results obtained by Massaro and Cohen (1983) suggested that phonological context biased listener's labeling judgments of the continua. Furthermore, the effect of context was greatest where there was ambiguous stimulus information (i.e., for items near the category boundary). Overall, these results support the idea that the permissibility of phonological sequences constrains and affects perceptual processing of the stimuli, as listeners were biased towards perceiving a phonologically permissible item. Massaro and Cohen (1983) hypothesized that these context effects were independent of low-level, sensory feature extraction processes. However, their results can still be interpreted as affecting some level of perceptual processing involved in phonetic labeling.

Effects of Lexical Context

There is also recent evidence suggesting that lexicality directly affects speech perception processes. Ganong (1980) conducted a study that investigated the effects of lexical status on the perception of word-initial stop consonants. Two series of tokens were created varying in VOT. One endpoint was a word item and the other endpoint was a nonword item (e.g., /dash/-/tash/ and /dask/-/task/). When subjects were asked to identify the initial stop, the results demonstrated that perception of the ambiguous items in the middle of the stimulus continuum was influenced by the lexicality of the endpoint stimuli. In other words, more /d/ responses were obtained in the /dash/-/tash/series, while more /t/ responses were obtained in the /dask/-/task/ series. Ganong (1980) interpreted these results in terms of an interactive criterion-shift model. In this model, he hypothesized that higher-level lexical information was used to change the criterion used to compare VOT information for categorization. Ganong suggested that since the effects of lexicality were primarily exhibited with ambiguous items near the phoneme boundary, a postcategorical type of correction process was not tenable (as a model of this type would predict that the endpoint stimulus would also be affected). The results suggested that lexical information directly affected some aspect of the phonetic categorization process itself.

The effects of lexicality on phoneme boundaries found by Ganong (1980) have been replicated using somewhat similar procedures (see Connine & Clifton, 1987; Fox, 1984). However, the additional manipulation of reaction-time measurement in these later studies led to different interpretations of the mechanism by which the lexical level affects perceptual processing. Fox (1984) measured latencies along with identification responses, and divided latencies into three categories: slow, medium, and fast. Fox (1984) found that there were more word responses for slow and medium reaction times compared to the fast reaction times. Fox argued that if lexical context directly affected phonetic categorization processes, then more word responses should have been found in each reaction time range. Hence, he hypothesized that the effect of lexical context may be separate and independent from phonetic categorization processes. However, as pointed out by Connine and Clifton (1987), Fox's argument is based on the idea that an interactive mechanism in which lexical knowledge is present does not accrue the lexical information over time. It may be the case that the contribution of lexical information increases over time, in which case the pattern of results Fox (1984) found is not unexpected. In two experiments, Connine and Clifton (1987) also compared reaction times for words and nonwords at the phoneme boundary and at the endpoints of the continua. In one condition, a monetary payoff was instantiated to induce bias, while in the other condition this was not present. They demonstrated that reaction times were faster for bias-consistent responses only with the endpoint stimuli for the payoff condition, while reaction times were faster only for responses to ambiguous items near the boundary when the payoff was not present. The difference in reaction times as a function of the different types of bias was taken as evidence for the operation of two different mechanisms. In one mechanism, the effect of lexicality is interactive and directly affects phonetic categorization processes. In the second mechanism, factors such as response bias induced by payoff operate postperceptually in a more hierarchical manner. Thus, these results support the idea that lexical knowledge may be directly involved in phonetic coding operations.

A different series of experiments examining lexical context effects involves what is called the "phonemic restoration" illusion (Warren, 1970). Warren (1970) first reported this phenomenon in an experiment in which the first /s/ phoneme in the word "legislatures" was removed and replaced either by a cough or a 1000-Hz tone. When this word was presented within a sentence context, subjects were unaware that the /s/ phoneme had been removed and, in effect, perceptually restored the missing phoneme. In later studies, Samuel (1981a, 1981b) investigated this phenomenon as a function of different types of context (phonetic, lexical, and sentential) in parceling out the contributions of higher-level information to perceptual processes involved in the restoration effect. Among the results Samuel (1981a) obtained, he found that a greater amount of restoration existed when word length was increased, greater restoration was found for words versus pronounceable nonwords, and high-frequency items produced greater restoration than low-frequency items. Although bottom-up acoustic information also played a role in performance, these results suggested that a top-down flow of expectancies from the lexical level of processing directly affected the perceptual processes involved in the restoration effect. As a result, Samuel (1986) has proposed an interactive model of auditory word recognition where the lexicon directly influences and constrains perceptual processing at lower levels.

Sentence-level Constraints

The effect of sentential context on the perception of fluent speech has been documented using a number of experimental techniques. These include perception of speech in noise (Miller, Heise, & Lichten, 1951; Miller & Isard, 1963), perception of words excised from sentence context (Lieberman, 1963; Pollack & Pickett, 1963), detection of mispronunciations (Cole & Jakimik, 1978, 1980), gating (Cotton & Grosjean, 1984; Grosjean, 1980; Salasoo & Pisoni, 1985; Tyler, 1984), monitoring tasks (Marslen-Wilson & Tyler, 1980; Marslen-Wilson & Welsh, 1978), phonemic restoration (Samuel, 1981a), and perceptual labeling (Garnes & Bond, 1976; Miller, Green, & Schermer, 1984). Overall, these studies and others have shown that the context of the sentence affects perception of speech at some processing level, whether this be perceptual or postperceptual.

Early studies examining perception and intelligibility of speech in noise (Miller et al., 1951; Miller & Isard, 1963) found that words in sentence context were identified better than words in isolation. This was corroborated by work showing that words excised from fluent speech context were identified very poorly (e.g., Pollack & Pickett, 1963). Further investigations around this time period suggested that syntactic and semantic variables may have been responsible for these context effects. Miller and Isard (1963) compared intelligibility of words in noise for normal sentences, semantically anomalous sentences, and ungrammatical strings. They found that words in normal sentences were identified most accurately, words in ungrammatical sentences were identified least accurately, and performance for words in semantically anomalous but syntactically correct sentences fell in between the other two conditions. It was suggested that both syntactic and semantic constraints were used in the perception of speech (see also Lieberman, 1963).

More recent work has attempted to focus on the nature of the knowledge sources which have been subsumed under the generic label of sentential context. Experiments conducted which have used the gating paradigm (Cotton & Grosjean, 1984; Grosjean, 1980; Salasoo & Pisoni, 1985) have shown that less acoustic-phonetic information is needed to identify items within sentence context than in isolation. In the study by Salasoo and Pisoni (1985), the target word in the sentence was first replaced entirely by noise. Then, on successive trials, selected increments of the original segments of the word replaced the noise segments of the stimulus with the increments accumulating in interactive fashion until the entire waveform is finally presented. The point at which subjects recognize the word is measured (gate duration), and in this way the amount of acoustic-phonetic information needed to recognize a word can be estimated. Salasoo and Pisoni (1985) used this paradigm to present sentences that were either normal or semantically anomalous. Fifty-msec increments of the original waveform replaced the envelope-shaped noise portions of the target word on each trial. The gating direction of the words started from the beginning or end of the word. Among their results, they found that performance in normal sentences was better than both in the semantically anomalous sentences and isolated words (i.e., less gate duration was needed for recognition), while performance differed between the anomalous condition and the isolated word condition. This can be interpreted as evidence that a tradeoff existed between an acoustic-phonetic source of knowledge and higher-level semantic and syntactic sources of knowledge, with less acoustic-phonetic information needed as higher-level constraints were utilized.

Other research has shown that sentential context can bias perception of ambiguous acoustic-phonetic information. Garnes and Bond (1976) constructed a continuum of 16 stimulus words varying in place of articulation ("bait" to "date" to "gate"). They presented these words embedded within various sentence contexts which were semantically constrained for a particular word (e.g., "Here's the fishing gear and the _____" for "bait"), and in an isolated control condition. They discovered that when the acoustic-phonetic information in the word was unambiguous, the word was reported regardless of the sentence context. However, when the word was ambiguous (i.e., the continuum stimulus word fell in between the boundaries of "b" and "d" or "d" and "g") the subjects' judgments of the word were biased towards the semantically appropriate item (compared to the item in isolation). Thus, categorization of the stimulus word was influenced by the semantic content of the sentence *only* when the acoustic-phonetic information was ambiguous. This result has been replicated more recently using a similar procedure by Miller et al. (1984) for categorization of a stimulus word continuum varying in voicing (but, see Connine, 1986).

Given that sentential context influences categorization of speech continua, the question arises as to whether the knowledge sources subsumed under sentential context *directly* or *indirectly* affect lower-level perceptual processes. Miller et al. (1984) argued that semantic context effects are not obligatory, because they found that context effects were only present when the subject was explicitly required to attend to the sentence context. Because semantic context only affected the identification of ambiguous stimuli near the category boundary, they suggested that, ". . . the context effect was not due to a late decision process that operated on the discrete, categorical outcome of an earlier process responsible for the analysis/interpretation of the acoustic input. . ." (p.334). If a late decision process had been operating, they postulated that the influence of context would have been seen across all the items of the continuum. Connine (1986) followed up on the results of Miller et al. (1984) by using a similar procedure while collecting response times in addition to identification responses. Connine (1986) replicated the identification results of Miller et al. (1984), however, reaction times for ambiguous items at the category boundary did not show an advantage for responses consistent with semantic context, while an advantage *was* exhibited with unambiguous items at the endpoint for context-consistent responses. Connine (1986) interpreted these results as support for an effect of semantic context on the postperceptual mechanisms (see also Connine & Clifton, 1987). Additional evidence for this hypothesis has been provided by Samuel (1981a), who found that sentential context predicting a target word resulted in greater perceptual restoration. Using the results of a signal detection analysis, he argued that the effect of the sentence context was due to a bias effect and suggested that information from the higher syntactic/semantic levels was not passed down to the lower phonetic-phonological level. Instead, context operated at a postperceptual decision-making stage.

Thus, conflicting explanations exist in the current literature regarding the exact locus of sentential context effects. However, it is clear that higher-level knowledge sources (syntactic, semantic, etc.) do affect some aspect of the processing and labeling of speech.

Conclusion

Overall, the idea that perceptual processes are influenced by higher-level constraints is fairly well-supported. Knowledge of phonological rules and sequential contingencies, lexicality, and higher-order semantic/syntactic information all affect the perception of the acoustic-phonetic input in the speech signal. The processing locus during perception at which each of these knowledge sources has its effect is still a matter of some debate. Studies where the effects of phonological and lexical constraints are exhibited on categorization of speech have shown that changes occur only for items which are ambiguous in acoustic-phonetic terms (Connine & Clifton, 1987; Fox, 1984; Ganong, 1980; Garnes & Bond, 1976; Massaro & Cohen, 1983). This suggests that higher-level information sources are directly interacting with categorization processes, and therefore acoustic-phonetic coding processes in a top-down manner. Categorization changes of this type have also been shown for semantic/syntactic constraints (Connine, 1986; Miller et al., 1984). However, it is not clear whether this information directly affects categorization or whether it operates on the output of categorization processes (see also Samuel, 1981a). In addition to evidence for categorization, work with the gating paradigm has shown that less acoustic-phonetic input is needed for perception when semantic/syntactic constraints are present (Cotton & Grosjean, 1984; Grosjean, 1980; Salasoo & Pisoni, 1985). This suggests that bottom-up acoustic-phonetic coding processes and top-down contextual constraints interact and cooperate to support recognition of the intended message. These findings provide support for interactive theories of speech perception (e.g., Elman & McClelland, 1986) and blackboard models of speech recognition (Reddy, 1980; Reddy & Newell, 1974).

In short, perception of speech by human listeners involves complex interactions with higher-order knowledge concerning the linguistic structure of language, as well as interactions with long-term memory representations of several different linguistic entities. The nature of these interactions suggests a number of important differences in perceptual processing between humans and nonhumans. Current evidence suggests that a specialized mechanism for perceiving species-specific vocalizations (speech) in the human may not be informationally encapsulated and isolated from higher-level cognitive processes and structural representations.

IV. DEVELOPMENTAL ISSUES AND CROSS-LANGUAGE COMPARISONS

The question of whether speech perception processes (at the level of phonetic coding) are speech-specific and/or specialized can also be elucidated by examining the perceptual performance of human infants and by comparing similarities and differences between infants and adults across languages (for a review, see Aslin, Pisoni, & Jusczyk, 1983). While there is evidence that speech is perceived and categorized differently by adults from language to language, there is also evidence that infants from different language cultures discriminate and perceive speech sounds in a fashion similar to one another.

Much of the adult cross-language research has dealt with identification and discrimination of selected phonetic contrasts. For instance, Lisker and Abramson (1970; Abramson & Lisker, 1970) obtained categorization data for English, Spanish, and Thai listeners for voicing judgments. Their results showed that VOT boundaries were placed at different points on the voicing continuum for each respective language. This was replicated for VOT perception for Spanish and English speakers (Williams, 1977). Also, identification and discrimination of the /r/-/l/ contrast has been shown to differ between English and Japanese listeners (Miyawaki et al., 1975). Differences in the processing of phonetic information in consonants exist simply as a function of how the phonetic contrast is used within the language. Although this implies that perceptual strategies develop during the course of learning a particular language, these strategies can be changed by specific laboratory training (e.g., Pisoni, Aslin, Perey, & Hennessy, 1982).

Perceptual differences across language could be construed as support for the existence of a specialized processing mechanism which is linked to the articulatory representations peculiar to a particular language. That is, listeners do not perceive certain contrasts if they do not normally produce them. This claim is weakened somewhat by the finding that a new perceptual contrast can be induced by training (see Pisoni et al., 1982), but one must look to data obtained from infants to further substantiate this hypothesis.

In 1971, Eimas, Siqueland, Jusczyk, and Vigorito conducted a seminal experiment which investigated infants' discrimination for a /b/-/p/ voicing continuum. Using a high-amplitude sucking technique, they found that infants were able to discriminate between pairs of VOT stimuli when they were drawn from different categories, however, they were unable to discriminate between pairs of stimuli drawn from the same phonetic category. Thus, evidence was obtained that categorical-like perception was present very early in the infant (at 2 weeks old), suggesting at the time that specialized mechanisms for speech perception existed and were innate. This pattern of results with infants has also been replicated with a wide variety of other phonetic contrasts for consonants and vowels (Aslin et al., 1983). It appears that the infant possesses the ability to discriminate a widely variant assortment of phonetic cues which are pertinent to speech perception (see Aslin et al., 1983).

The similarity of the categorical discrimination performance of infants to adults becomes even more interesting when comparisons of infants are made across languages. A number of studies have shown that infants from different cultures process speech in remarkably similar ways. Lasky, Syrdal-Lasky, and

Klein (1975) found that VOT discrimination for infants from Spanish-speaking homes was similar to discrimination performance for the infants in the Eimas et al. (1971) study; this was also found for infants from a Kikuyu-speaking environment (Streeter, 1976). Trehub (1976) found that 1- to 4-month-old infants from English-speaking homes can discriminate phonetic contrasts which occur in Czech and Polish, but not English. More recently, Werker and colleagues (Werker, Gilbert, Humphrey, & Tees, 1981; Werker & Tees, 1983, 1984) have conducted a series of experiments explicitly comparing performance for infants and adults from the same and different language environments on selected phonemic contrasts. Among their results, they found that infants from English-speaking environments could discriminate pairs of Hindi (nonnative) speech contrasts as well as Hindi-speaking adults, while English-speaking adults apparently could not; identical results were found with an American Indian language (Thompson). Furthermore, they found evidence that this ability begins to significantly decline as early as 8- to 10-months-of-age. Thus, infants initially possess the ability to make a large variety of discriminations of phonetic contrasts, but as experience is gained with the infant's native language, this ability is modified and shows some alignment or tuning with the categories used by adults (see Aslin & Pisoni, 1980).

Returning to the question of whether specialized speech processes exist in the infant and adult, an argument could be made for some type of specialized mechanism based on infants' categorical discrimination performance. However, the evidence that exists for categorical perception of nonspeech continua (e.g., Miller et al., 1976; Pisoni, 1977) suggests that this proposal should be viewed with some caution. There are three criteria that must be met in order to postulate a phonetic mode of analysis in the infant: (1) the infant's perceptual performance must be unique to speech (i.e., not shown with nonspeech, (2) performance must be unique to the human phonological system (i.e., not shown in nonhumans), and (3) performance must conform to the phonetic distinctions within the native language. With regard to the third criterion, as discussed above, infants can indeed discriminate phonetic distinctions that are both native and nonnative to their environment. With regard to the first criterion, it has been shown that infants also show categorical discrimination of nonspeech continua emulating speech contrasts. Jusczyk, Pisoni, Walley, and Murray (1980) conducted a study using tone-onset stimuli that were identical to those used by Pisoni (1977) in his adult study. They presented these stimuli to 2-month-old infants and found that they discriminated them categorically, although the category boundaries differed somewhat from those of adults. This particular result suggests that the postulation of a specialized phonetic processing mechanism may be unwarranted. An explanation for categorical discrimination by infants of phonetic contrasts can be offered in terms of general auditory processing without recourse to phonetic coding.

Further evidence supporting this proposal comes from a finding by Eimas and

Miller (1980) indicating that syllable duration affected placement of a formant transition boundary in infants (as found by Miller & Liberman, 1979, with adults). Jusczyk, Pisoni, Reed, Fernald, and Myers (1983) conducted a similar experiment, with the exception that they used analogous nonspeech tonal stimuli. They obtained identical results with the nonspeech stimuli as Eimas and Miller (1980) had found with speech stimuli, suggesting that the effect of speaking rate on infants could be due to a more general auditory level of processing.

The second criterion delineated above concerns whether performance obtained with infants using speech stimuli is also observed with nonhuman species. Simply put, if similar performance is obtained with nonhumans, then the fact that nonhumans do not possess access to a phonetic/phonological system suggests that specialized mechanisms incorporating phonetic-level processes are not necessary to produce categorical perception. A brief discussion of this area of research follows (for a more comprehensive review, see Kuhl, this volume). However, it has been demonstrated that categorical-like performance with speech stimuli can be observed in chinchillas (e.g., Kuhl & Miller, 1975, 1978) and monkeys (e.g., Kuhl & Padden, 1982, 1983). Hence, the second criterion also fails for postulating a specific phonetic mode of analysis in human infants.

The debate about whether some type of specialized processes or mechanisms exist in infants is far from over, however. Some evidence has been obtained that shows that infants exhibit forms of perceptual constancy for speech sounds. Kuhl (1979a) found that infants are capable of perceiving speech sounds regardless of differences in spectral composition that result from talker variability and changes in pitch contour (see also Carrell, Smith, & Pisoni, 1981). In addition, infants were able to perceive similarities between phonetic tokens, even though they could discriminate between them (Kuhl, 1983). These findings suggest that a specialized mechanism of some sort exists producing these patterns of responses. However, it has been shown that species such as the dog (Baru, 1975) and the chinchilla (Burdick & Miller, 1975; Kuhl & Miller, 1975) exhibit a very similar pattern of generalization responses suggesting that they can adjust to variation in voice and contour. Hence, the perceptual constancy displayed by infants and/or adults could possibly be due to characteristics inherent in the general mammalian auditory system and/or general perceptual processes that are not necessarily unique to speech perception.

To briefly summarize, differences in perceptual resolution for certain speech contrasts differ across languages. However, infants appear to possess the ability to categorically discriminate a plethora of speech contrasts which are found in many languages other then their native one. A specialized mechanism of the sort producing categorical-like perception may be ruled out, because infants display categorical discrimination with nonspeech continua. There are instances where perceptual constancy appears to be operating, however, some of these behaviors may also be shown with nonhuman species. Examining the three criteria put forth to postulate a phonetic mode of analysis in the infant, two of the three criteria failed. Although it is possible that a specialized capacity for perceptual processing of speech of some sort may be present in the infant, the nature of this putative mechanism is not clear at the present time.

V. HUMAN/NONHUMAN COMPARISONS

The comparison of perceptual performance between humans and other animals provides valuable data concerning two separate but related issues. The first issue deals with testing the notion of a specialized, speech-specific processor in the human. The second issue is concerned with examining similarities and differences between humans and nonhumans in how the perceptual system responds to vocal signals that are biologically important to each species. Here, we are primarily concerned with the first issue. Because much of the relevant research has been reviewed in detail elsewhere (see Kuhl, 1979b, 1986a, this volume), we briefly highlight a few of the major findings of direct relevance and try to draw several general conclusions.

A number of well-known studies have examined the perception of human speech signals in chinchillas (Kuhl, 1981; Kuhl & Miller, 1975, 1978) and monkeys (Kuhl & Padden, 1982, 1983; Morse and Snowden, 1975; Sinnott, Beecher, Moody, & Stebbins, 1976; Waters & Wilson, 1976). These investigations obtained identification and discrimination data for synthetic speech continua varying either in VOT or place of articulation. Kuhl and colleagues have conducted the most extensive series of studies to date of speech perception in nonhumans, namely in the chinchilla and the macaque (Kuhl, 1981; Kuhl & Miller, 1975, 1978; Kuhl & Padden, 1982, 1983).

Using avoidance training and generalization procedures with the chinchilla, Kuhl and Miller found that category boundary functions for a /da/-/ta/ voicing continuum were essentially identical as those obtained for adult humans. This result was replicated for a labial /ba/-/pa/ series and for a velar /ga/-/ka/ series. In a later study, discrimination performance for the same /da/-/ta/ voicing continuum revealed that the animals were sensitive to changes near the category boundary and insensitive to changes near the centers of the categories. Thus, the identification and discrimination data suggested that chinchillas perceive VOT contrasts categorically much like humans. In further work, discrimination of voicing and place continua were also assessed for another species, the Japanese macaque (Kuhl & Padden, 1982, 1983). The discrimination performance peaked at the phonetic boundaries for three voicing continua and one place continuum. This "phoneme boundary" effect suggested that primates perceived these speech distinctions in roughly the same manner as do humans and chinchillas, with all species sharing similar mammalian auditory systems.

In addition to categorical perception, the phenomena of perceptual constancy has been shown to occur with animals. Burdick and Miller (1975) demonstrated that not only can chinchillas differentiate between the vowels /a/ and /i/, but that their performance generalizes to phonetically similar but spectrally different vowel tokens from different talkers. This result was replicated with dogs for similar vowels (Baru, 1975). Kuhl and Miller (1975) showed that chinchillas can categorize /b/ and /d/ regardless of talker voice and vowel context. This result is particularly interesting, because it suggests that the mechanisms involved in perception in chinchillas may be performing computations that adjust or "normalize" for types of variations in the speech signal. Thus, perceptual adjustments leading to perceptual constancy for phonetic categories may also be present in nonhumans.

The significance of the finding that nonhuman species appear to perceive speech continua categorically is directly relevant to the arguments surrounding the postulation of a specialized speech processor in humans. Previously, categorical perception had been taken as strong evidence for a specialized mechanism, although this was later disputed with the findings of categorical perception of nonspeech. Since this phenomenon is displayed in nonhuman species that do not possess the capability to phonetically process speech, this suggests that categorical perception in humans is due to general processing characteristics of the mammalian auditory system. Any putative speech-specific specialized mechanism therefore could not be supported by the existence of categorical perception. In addition, the fact that speech stimuli may be perceived by nonhumans in the same manner regardless of voice and pitch contour suggests that if a mechanism exists in humans for perceptual normalization, this may also ultimately be explained in terms of general auditory processing principles as well and may not be a "specialized" mechanism.

Recently, Kuhl (1986a, 1986b, this volume) has argued that the results obtained in testing speech with nonhumans do not rule out the existence of specially evolved mechanisms for perceiving speech in the human. Rather, she suggests that these kinds of results should be viewed as "existence proofs" simply demonstrating that these phenomena can indeed exist in the absence of special mechanisms. Hence, the only thing that can be proved by these findings is that specially evolved mechanisms are not *necessary* to obtain the phenomenon. So, one can entertain the notion that these types of effects with humans are due to general auditory processing, but it remains to be seen whether this is, in fact, the case. However, the contribution of comparative animal studies to resolving the issue must be closely linked with other data to form a coherent view of whether speech-specific specialized perceptual processes exist.

VI.   GENERAL CONCLUSIONS

We have described some of the major problems in speech perception and presented a brief summary of recent research which is related to two important issues regarding the nature of speech perception processes. The first issue is concerned with ascertaining the degree to which human speech perception is "unique" when compared to the perception of complex acoustic sounds by animals. As shown by the inherent physical variability of speech and the problems of perceptual constancy and perceptual normalization, the processing and encoding of speech appears to be extremely complex. In animals, even if an analogous amount of variability in vocal signals was shown within various species, it remains to be seen whether perceptual mechanisms of the complexity utilized by humans exist which process the species-specific vocalizations. The complexity and variability of vocal signals and the processes devoted to perceiving the signal constitutes one important difference between human and animals in perceiving complex acoustic signals.

A second factor is the access to and use of higher-level knowledge sources in the perception of speech signals. In animals, the existence of higher-level sources of information which interact with auditory encoding processes in a like manner is purely a matter of speculation at this time. However, the existence of interactions between higher-level knowledge sources (phonology, morphology, syntax, and semantics) and perceptual processes in human listeners supports the idea that speech perception processes operate in a qualitatively different manner than complex acoustic perceptual processes in animals. We believe this is true because of the duality of patterning in human language and the complex encoding of the linguistic message in the speech waveform.

The second issue that we were concerned with deals with the specialization of mechanisms for perceiving species-specific vocalizations. Research showing that categorical perception and context effects are obtained with nonspeech analogs of speech and with nonhumans as well raises the possibility that general mammalian auditory coding mechanisms are responsible for producing these phenomena. Further evidence obtained from manipulating speech/nonspeech modes and effects due to higher-level knowledge sources does not provide support for the proposal that a biologically specialized speech processor is instantiated in an informationally encapsulated, modularized neural system. The proposal of a specialized phonetic processor organized as an autonomous phonetic module must be treated with some caution at this time.

One possible explanation of phonetic processing which may be ultimately explained in terms of a "specialized" mechanism incorporates both perceptual and cognitive components. We suggest that it is possible that the integration of acoustic cues may produce "emergent features" or wholistic entities which correspond to phonetic percepts. Here, phonetic information is perceived as a result of a cognitive processing component "activating" the output of auditory coding processes to produce the final phonetic representation. The mechanism which produces the final phonetic output could loosely be described as "specialized." Indeed, it seems possible that a *capacity* for processing speech may have evolved which is specific to the human being (Lieberman, 1984). Although the current models proposing that phonetic processing is specialized presently have mixed support (e.g., Liberman & Mattingly, 1985), the proposal is one that should not be prematurely discarded until further research concerning this issue has been conducted.

Much research needs to be conducted with both human and animal observers in order to address the question of whether specialized, species-specific perceptual mechanisms exist. Studies examining contextual variability, perceptual constancy, and higher-level information, among other issues, will provide us with valuable information on the processes involved in perception of complex acoustic sounds by various animals species, and will serve to test several important assumptions regarding processes employed in human speech perception. As more research evidence accumulates, the similarities and differences in perceptual processing of complex sounds between humans and animals should become much clearer.

ACKNOWLEDGMENTS

This research has been supported in part, by NIH Research Grant NS-12179, and in part, by NIH Training Grant NS-07134 to Indiana University in Bloomington, IN.

REFERENCES

Abramson, A. S., & Lisker, L. (1970). Discriminability along the voicing continuum: Cross-language tests. *Proceedings of the 6th international congress of phonetic sciences* (pp. 569–573). Prague: Academia.

Allard, F., & Henderson, L. (1976). Physical and name codes in auditory memory: The pursuit of an analogy. *Quarterly Journal of Experimental Psychology, 28,* 475–482.

Aslin, R. N., & Pisoni, D. B. (1980). Some developmental processes in speech perception. In G. Yeni-Komshian, J. F. Kavanagh, & C. A. Ferguson (Eds.), *Child phonology: Perception and production* (pp. 67–96). New York: Academic Press.

Aslin, R. N., Pisoni, D. B., & Jusczyk, P. W. (1983). Auditory development and speech perception in infancy. In P. Mussen (Ed.), *Carmichael's manual of child psychology, 4th ed., volume II: Infancy and the biology of development,* M. M. Haith & J. J. Canpor (Vol. Eds.). (pp. 573–687). New York: Wiley.

Bailey, P. J., Summerfield, Q., & Dorman, M. (1977). On the identification of sine-wave analogues of certain speech sounds. *Haskins laboratories status report on speech research SR–51/52* (pp. 1–25). New Haven, CT: Haskins Laboratories.

Baru, A. V. (1975). Discrimination of synthesized vowels /a/ and /i/ with varying parameters in the dog. In G. Fant & M. A. Tatham (Eds.), *Auditory analysis and the perception of speech.* London: Academic Press.

Best, C. T., Morrongiello, B., & Robson, R. (1981). Perceptual equivalence of acoustic cues in speech and nonspeech perception. *Perception and Psychophysics, 29,* 191–211.

Blumstein, S. E. (1986). On acoustic invariance in speech. In J. S. Perkell & D. H. Klatt (Eds.), *Invariance and variability in speech processes.* Hillsdale, NJ: Lawrence Earlbaum Associates.

Bond, Z. S., & Garnes, S. (1980). Misperceptions of fluent speech. In R. A. Cole (Ed.), *Perception and production of fluent speech* (pp. 115–132). Hillsdale, NJ: Lawrence Erlbaum Associates.

Bond, Z. S., & Robey, R. R. (1983). The phonetic structure of errors in the perception of fluent speech. In N. J. Lass (Ed.), *Speech and language: Advances in basic research and practice, Vol. 9.* New York: Academic Press.

Brown, R. W., & Hildum, D. C. (1956). Expectancy and the perception of syllables. *Language, 32,* 411–419.

Brudick, C. K., & Miller, J. D. (1975). Speech perception by the chinchilla: Discrimination of sustained /a/ and /i/. *Journal of the Acoustical Society of America, 58,* 415–427.

Carrell, T. D. (1984). Contributions of fundamental frequency, formant spacing, and glottal waveform to talker identification. *Research on speech perception, tech report no. 5.* Speech Research Laboratory, Indiana University, Bloomington, IN.

Carrell, T. D., Smith, L. B., & Pisoni, D. B. (1981). Some perceptual dependencies in speeded classification of vowel color and pitch. *Perception and Psychophysics, 29,* 1–10.

Chomsky, N., & Miller, G. A. (1963). Introduction to the formal analysis of natural languages. In R. D. Luce, R. Bush, & E. Galanter (Eds.), *Handbook of mathematical psychology, Vol. 2* (pp. 269–321). New York: Wiley.

Cole, R. A., Coltheart, M., & Allard, F. (1974). Memory of a speaker's voice: Reaction time to same- or different-voiced letters. *Quarterly Journal of Experimental Psychology, 26,* 1–7.

Cole, R. A., & Jakimik, J. (1978). Understanding speech: How words are heard. In G. Underwood (Ed.), *Strategies of information processing.* London: Academic Press.

Cole, R. A., & Jakimik, J. (1980). A model of speech perception. In R. A. Cole (Ed.), *Perception and production of fluent speech* (pp. 133–163). Hillsdale, NJ: Lawrence Erlbaum Associates.

Connine, C. M. (1986). *Modularity and auditory word recognition. Unpublished doctoral dissertation,* University of Massachusetts, Amherst.

Connine, C. M., & Clifton, C. (1987). Interactive use of lexical information in speech perception. *Journal of Experimental Psychology: Human Perception and Performance, 13,* 291–299.

Cotton, S., & Grosjean, F. (1984). The gating paradigm: A comparison of successive and individual presentation formats. *Perception and Psychophysics, 35,* 41–48.

Craik, F. I. M., & Kirsner, K. (1974). The effect of speaker's voice on word recognition. *Quarterly Journal of Experimental Psychology, 26,* 274–284.

Cutting, J. E. (1974). Two left-hemisphere mechanisms in speech perception. *Perception and Psychophysics, 16,* 601–612.

Cutting, J. E. (1978). There may be nothing peculiar to perceiving in a speech mode. In J. Requin (Ed.), *Attention and performance VII.* Hillsdale, NJ: Lawrence Erlbaum Associates.

Eimas, P. D., & Miller, J. L. (1980). Contextual effects in infant speech perception. *Science, 209,* 1140–1141.

Eimas, P. D., Siqueland, E. R., Jusczyk, P. W., & Vigorito, J. (1971). Speech perception in infants. *Science, 171,* 303–306.

Elman, J., & McClelland, J. (1986). Exploiting lawful variability in the speech wave. In J. S. Perkell & D. H. Klatt (Eds.), *Invariance and variability in speech processes* (pp. 360–380). Hillsdale, NJ: Lawrence Erlbaum Associates.

Fodor, J. (1983). *The modularity of mind.* Cambridge, MA: MIT Press.

Fox, R. A. (1984). Effect of lexical status on phonetic categorization. *Journal of Experimental Psychology: Human Perception and Performance, 10,* 526–540.

Fry, D. B., Abramson, A. S., Eimas, P. D., & Liberman, A. M. (1962). The identification and discrimination of synthetic vowels. *Language and Speech, 5,* 171–189.

Ganong, W. F. (1980). Phonetic categorization in auditory word perception. *Journal of Experimental Psychology: Human Perception and Performance, 6,* 110–125.

Garner, W. R. (1974). *The processing of information and structure.* Hillsdale, NJ: Lawrence Erlbaum Associates.

Garnes, S., & Bond, Z. S. (1976). The relationship between semantic expectation and acoustic information. *Phonologica, 3,* 285–293.

Grosjean, F. (1980). Spoken word recognition processes and the gating paradigm. *Perception and Psychophysics, 28,* 267–283.

Grosjean, F., & Lane, H. (1981). Temporal variables in the perception and production of spoken and sign languages. In P. D. Eimas & J. L. Miller (Eds.), *Perspectives on the study of speech* (pp. 207–238). Hillsdale, NJ: Lawrence Erlbaum Associates.

Grunke, M. E., & Pisoni, D. B. (1982). Some experiments on perceptual learning of mirror-image acoustic patterns. *Perception and Psychophysics, 31,* 210–218.

Hillenbrand, J. (1984). Perception of sine-wave analogs of voice onset time stimuli. *Journal of the Acoustical Society of America, 75,* 231–240.

Jusczyk, P. W., Pisoni, D. B., Reed, M. A., Fernald, A., & Myers, M. (1983). Infants' discrimination of the duration of rapid spectrum changes in nonspeech signals. *Science, 222,* 175–177.

Jusczyk, P. W., Pisoni, D. B., Walley, A., & Murray, J. (1980). Discrimination of relative onset time of two-component tones by infants. *Journal of the Acoustical Society of America, 67,* 262–270.

Kewley-Port, D., & Luce, P. A. (1984). Time-varying features of initial stop consonants in auditory running spectra: A first report. *Perception and Psychophysics, 35,* 353–360.

Kuhl, P. K. (1979a). Speech perception in early infancy: Perceptual constancy for spectrally dissimilar vowel categories. *Journal of the Acoustical Society of America, 66,* 1668–1679.

Kuhl, P. K. (1979b). Models and mechanisms in speech perception. *Brain, Behavior, and Evolution, 16,* 375–408.

Kuhl, P. K. (1981). Discrimination of speech by nonhuman animals: Basic auditory sensitivities conductive to the perception of speech-sound categories. *Journal of the Acoustical Society of America, 70,* 340–349.

Kuhl, P. K. (1983). Perception of auditory equivalence classes for speech in early infancy. *Infant Behavior and Development, 6,* 263–285.

Kuhl, P. K. (1986a). Theoretical contributions of tests on animals to the special-mechanisms debate in speech. *Experimental Biology, 45,* 233–265.

Kuhl, P. K. (1986b). Reflections on infants' perception and representation of speech. In J. S. Perkell & D. H. Klatt (Eds.), *Invariance and variability in speech processes* (pp. 19–30). Hillsdale, NJ: Lawrence Erlbaum Associates.

Kuhl, P. K., & Miller, J. D. (1975). Speech perception by the chinchilla: Voiced-voiceless distinction in alveolar-plosive consonants. *Science, 190,* 69–72.

Kuhl, P. K., & Miller, J. D. (1978). Speech perception by the chinchilla: Identification functions for synthetic VOT stimuli. *Journal of the Acoustical Society of America, 63,* 905–917.

Kuhl, P. K., & Padden, D. M. (1982). Enhanced discriminability at the phonetic boundaries for the voicing feature in macaques. *Perception and Psychophysics, 32,* 542–550.

Kuhl, P. K., & Padden, D. M. (1983). Enhanced discriminability at the phonetic boundaries for the place feature in macaques. *Journal of the Acoustical Society of America, 73,* 1003–1010.

Lasky, R. E., Syrdal-Lasky, A., & Klein, R. E. (1975). VOT discrimination by four to six-and-a-half month old infants from Spanish environments. *Journal of Experimental Child Psychology, 20,* 213–225.

Liberman, A. M. (1970a). Some characteristics of perception in the speech mode. In D. A. Hamburg (Ed.), *Perception and its disorders, proceedings of A.R.N.M.D.,* Baltimore: Williams and Wilkins.

Liberman, A. M. (1970b). The grammars of speech and language. *Cognitive Psychology, 1,* 301–323.

Liberman, A. M. (1982). On finding that speech is special. *American Psychologist, 37,* 148–167.

Liberman, A. M., Cooper, F. S., Shankweiler, D. P., & Studdert-Kennedy, M. (1967). Perception of the speech code. *Psychological Review, 74,* 431–461.

Liberman, A. M., Delattre, P. C., & Cooper, F. S. (1952). The role of selected stimulus variables in the perception of the unvoiced stop consonants. *American Journal of Psychology, 52,* 127–137.

Liberman, A. M., Delattre, P. C., Cooper, F. S., & Gerstman, L. H. (1954). The role of consonant-vowel transitions in the perception of the stop and nasal consonants. *Psychological Monographs, 68,* 1–13.

Liberman, A. M., Harris, K. S., Hoffman, H. A., & Griffith, B. C. (1957). The discrimination of relative-onset time of the components of certain speech and nonspeech patterns. *Journal of Experimental Psychology, 54,* 358–368.

Liberman, A. M., Harris, K. S., Kinney, J. A., & Lane, H. (1961). The discrimination of relative-onset time of the components of certain speech and nonspeech patterns. *Journal of Experimental Psychology, 61,* 379–388.

Liberman, A. M., Isenberg, D., & Rakerd, B. (1981). Duplex perception of cues for stop consonants: Evidence for a phonetic mode. *Perception and Psychophysics, 30,* 133–143.

Liberman, A. M., & Mattingly, I. G. (1985). The motor theory of speech perception revised. *Cognition, 21,* 1–36.

Lieberman, P. (1963). Some effects of semantic and grammatical context on the production and perception of speech. *Language and Speech, 6,* 172–179.

Lieberman, P. (1984). *The biology and evolution of language.* Cambridge, MA: Harvard University Press.

Lisker, L., & Abramson, A. S. (1970). The voicing dimension: Some experiments in comparative phonetics. In *Proceedings of the sixth international congress of phonetic sciences* (pp. 563–567). Prague: Academic Press.

Lisker, L., Liberman, A. M., Erickson, D. M., Dechovitz, D., & Mandler, R. (1977). On pushing the voice-onset-time (VOT) boundary about. *Language and Speech, 20,* 209–216.

Luce, P. A., & Pisoni, D. B. (1987). Speech perception: New directions in research, theory, and applications. In H. Winitz (Ed.), *Human communication and its disorders, a review.* Norwood, NJ: Ablex.

MacDonald, J., & McGurk, H. (1978). Visual influences on speech perception processes. *Perception and Psychophysics, 24,* 253–257.

Marslen-Wilson, W. D., & Tyler, L. K. (1980). The temporal structure of spoken language understanding. *Cognition, 8,* 1–71.

Marslen-Wilson, W. D., & Welsh, A. (1978). Processing interactions and lexical access during word-recognition in continuous speech. *Cognitive Psychology, 10,* 29–63.

Massaro, D. W., & Cohen, M. M. (1983). Phonological context in speech perception. *Perception and Psychophysics, 34,* 338–348.

Mattingly, I. G. (1972). Speech cues and sign stimuli. *American Scientist, 60,* 327–337.

Mattingly, I. G., & Liberman, A. M. (1986). Specialized perceiving systems for speech and other biologically significant sounds. In G. M. Edelman, W. E. Gall, & W. M. Cowan (Eds.), *Functions of the auditory system.* New York: Wiley.

Mattingly, I. G., Liberman, A. M., Syrdal, A. K., & Halwes, T. (1971). Discrimination in speech and nonspeech modes. *Cognitive Psychology, 2,* 131–157.

Mattingly, I. G., Studdert-Kennedy, M., & Magen, H. (1983). Phonological short-term memory preserves phonetic detail. *Journal of the Acoustical Society of America, 73,* Suppl. 1, S4.

McGurk, H., & MacDonald, J. (1976). Hearing lips and seeing voices. *Nature, 264,* 746–748.

Miller, G. A., Heise, G. A., & Lichten, W. (1951). The intelligibility of speech as a function of the context of the test materials. *Journal of Experimental Psychology, 41,* 329–335.

Miller, G. A., & Isard, S. (1963). Some perceptual consequences of linguistic rules. *Journal of Verbal Learning and Verbal Behavior, 2,* 217–228.

Miller, J. D., Wier, L., Pastore, R. E., Kelly, W., & Dooling, R. (1976). Discrimination and labeling of noise-buzz sequences with varying noise-lead times: An example of categorical perception. *Journal of the Acoustical Society of America, 60,* 410–417.

Miller, J. L. (1981). Effects of speaking rate on segmental distinctions. In P. D. Eimas & J. L. Miller (Eds.), *Perspectives on the study of speech* (pp. 39–74). Hillsdale, NJ: Lawrence Erlbaum Associates.

Miller, J. L., Green, K., & Schermer, T. (1984). On the distinction between prosodic and semantic factors in word identification. *Perception and Psychophysics, 36,* 329–337.

Miller, J. L., & Liberman, A. M. (1979). Some effects of later-occurring information on the perception of stop consonant and semi-vowel. *Perception and Psychophysics, 25,* 457–465.

Miyawaki, K., Strange, W., Verbrugge, R., Liberman, A. M., Jenkins, J. J., & Fujimura, O. (1975). An effect of linguistic experience: The discrimination of [r] and [l] by native speakers of Japanese and English. *Perception and Psychophysics, 18,* 331–340.

Morse, P. A., & Snowdon, C. T. (1975). An investigation of categorical speech discrimination by rhesus monkeys. *Perception and Psychophysics, 18,* 9–16.

Mullennix, J. W., Pisoni, D. B. & Martin, C. S., (in press). Some effects of talker variability on spoken word recognition. *Journal of the Acoustical Society of America.*

Nearey, T. M. (1978). *Phonetic feature systems for vowels.* Doctoral dissertation, University of Alberta. Reprinted by Indiana University Linguistics Club, Bloomington, IN.

Nusbaum, H. C. (1984). Possible mechanisms of duplex perception: "chirp" identification versus dichotic fusion. *Perception and Psychophysics, 35,* 94–101.

Nusbaum, H. C., Schwab, E. C., & Sawusch, J. R. (1983). The role of "chirp" identification in duplex perception. *Perception and Psychophysics, 33,* 323–332.

O'Shaughnessy, D. (1986, October). Speaker recognition. *IEEE ASSP Magazine,* 4–17.

Oshika, B. T., Zuc, V. W., Weeks, R. V., Neu, H., & Auerbach, J. (1975). The role of phonological rules in speech understanding research. *IEEE transactions on acoustics, speech, and signal processing, ASSP-23, 104–112.*

Parker, E. M., Diehl, R. L., & Kleunder, K. R. (1986). Trading relations in speech and nonspeech. *Perception and Psychophysics, 39,* 129–142.

Pastore, R. E. (1981). Possible psychoacoustic factors in speech perception. In P. D. Eimas & J. L. Miller (Eds.), *Perspectives on the study of speech* (pp. 165–206). Hillsdale, NJ: Lawrence Erlbaum Associates.

Pastore, R. E., Ahroon, W. A., Buffuto, K. J., Friedman, C., Puleo, J. S., & Fink, E. A. (1977). Common-factor model of categorical perception. *Journal of Experimental Psychology: Human Perception and Performance, 3,* 686–696.

Pastore, R. E., Harris, L. B., & Kaplan, J. K. (1982). Temporal order identification: Some parameter dependencies. *Journal of the Acoustical Society of America, 71,* 430–436.

Pastore, R. E., Morris, C., & Layer, J. K. (1985). Duration effects on labeling of tonal analogs to F1-cutback. *Journal of the Acoustical Society of America, 78,* Suppl.1, S69.

Pisoni, D. B. (1977). Identification and discrimination of the relative onset time of two component tones: Implications for voicing perception in stops. *Journal of the Acoustical Society of America, 61,* 1352–1361.

Pisoni, D. B. (1979). On the perception of speech sounds as biologically significant signals. *Brain, Behavior, and Evolution, 16,* 330–350.

Pisoni, D. B., Aslin, R. N., Perey, A. J., & Hennessy, B. L. (1982). Some effects of laboratory training on identification and discrimination of voicing contrasts in stop consonants. *Journal of Experimental Psychology: Human Perception and Performance, 8,* 297–314.

Pisoni, D. B., Carrell, T. D., & Gans, S. J. (1983). Perception of the duration of rapid spectrum changes in speech and nonspeech signals. *Perception and Psychophysics, 34,* 314–322.

Pisoni, D. B., & Sawusch, J. R. (1975). Some stages of processing in speech perception. In A. Cohen & S. Nooteboom (Eds.), *Structure and process in speech perception.* Heidelberg: Springer-Verlag.

Pollack, I., & Pickett, J. M. (1963). The intelligibility of excerpts from conversation. *Language and Speech, 6,* 165–171.

Pomerantz, J. R., Sager, L. C., & Stoever, R. J. (1977). Perception of wholes and of their component parts: Some configurational superiority effects. *Journal of Experimental Psychology: Human Perception and Performance, 3,* 422–435.

Ralston, J. V. (1986). *Auditory and phonetic perception of stop consonant place of articulation information.* Unpublished doctoral dissertation, State University of New York at Buffalo.

Ralston, J. V., & Sawusch, J. R. (1984). *Perception of sinewave analogs of stop consonant place information.* Paper presented at the 108th meeting of the Acoustical Society of America, Minneapolis.

Ralston, J. V., & Sawusch, J. R. (1986). *Auditory and phonetic codes in stop-consonant perception.* Paper presented at the 27th annual meeting of the Psychonomic Society, New Orleans.

Reddy, R. (1980). Machine models of speech perception. In R. A. Cole (Ed.), *Perception and production of fluent speech* (pp. 215–242). Hillsdale, NJ: Lawrence Erlbaum Associates.

Reddy, R., & Newell, A. (1974). Knowledge and its representation in a speech understanding system. In L. W. Gregg (Ed.), *Knowledge and cognition.* Hillsdale, NJ: Lawrence Erlbaum Associates.

Remez, R. E., Rubin, P. E., Pisoni, D. B., & Carrell, T. D. (1981). Speech perception without traditional cues. *Science, 212,* 947–950.

Repp, B. H. (1982). Phonetic trading relations and context effects: New experimental evidence for a speech mode of perception. *Psychological Bulletin, 92,* 81–110.

Repp, B. H. (1983). Trading relations among acoustic cues in speech perception: Speech-specific but not special. *Haskins laboratories status report on speech research SR-76* (pp. 129–132). New Haven, CT: Haskins Laboratories.

Repp, B. H. (1984). Against a role of ''chirp'' identification in duplex perception. *Perception and Psychophysics, 35,* 89–93.

Repp, B. H., Milburn, C., & Ashkenas, J. (1983). Duplex perception: Confirmation of fusion. *Perception and Psychophysics, 33,* 333–337.

Salasoo, A., & Pisoni, D. B. (1985). Sources of knowledge in spoken word identification. *Journal of Memory and Language, 24,* 210–231.

Samuel, A. G. (1981a). Phonemic restoration: Insights from a new methology. *Journal of Experimental Psychology: General, 110,* 474–494.

Samuel, A. G. (1981b). The role of bottom-up confirmation in the phonemic restoration illusion. *Journal of Experimental Psychology: Human Perception and Performance, 7,* 1124–1131.

Samuel, A. G. (1986). The role of the lexicon in speech perception. In E. C. Schwab & H. C. Nusbaum (Eds.), *Pattern recognition by humans and machines, Vol. 1: Speech perception* (pp. 89–112). Orlando, FL: Academic Press.

Sawusch, J. R. (1986). Auditory and phonetic coding of speech. In E. C. Schwab & H. C. Nusbaum (Eds.), *Pattern recognition by humans and machines, Vol. 1: Speech perception* (pp. 51–88). Orlando, FL: Academic Press.

Sawusch, J. R., & Nochajski, T. H. (1982). *Stimulus integrality in the auditory coding of speech.* Paper presented at the 23rd annual meeting of the Psychonomic Society, Minneapolis.

Schouten, M. E. H. (1980). The case against a speech mode of perception. *Acta Psychologica, 44,* 71–98.

Schwab, E. C. (1982). Auditory and phonetic processing for tone analogs of speech. *Dissertation Abstracts International, 42,* 3853B.

Sinnott, J. M., Beecher, M. D., Moody, D. B., & Stebbins, W. C. (1976). Speech-sound discrimination by monkeys and humans. *Journal of the Acoustical Society of America, 60,* 687–695.

Stevens, K. N., & Blumstein, S. E. (1978). Invariant cues for place of articulation in stop consonants. *Journal of the Acoustical Society of America, 64,* 1358–1368.

Stevens, K. N., & Blumstein, S. E. (1981). The search for invarianct acoustic correlates of phonetic features. In P. D. Eimas & J. Miller (Eds.), *Perspectives on the study of speech* (pp. 1–38). Hillsdale, NJ: Lawrence Erlbaum Associates.

Strange, W., Verbrugge, R. R., Shankweiler, D. P., & Edman, T. R. (1976). Consonant environment specifies vowel identity. *Journal of the Acoustical Society of America, 60,* 213–224.

Streeter, L. A. (1976). Language perception of 2-month-old infants shows effects of both innate mechanisms and experience. *Nature, 259,* 39–41.

Studdert-Kennedy, M., Liberman, A. M., Harris, K. S., & Cooper, F. S. (1970). Motor theory of preparation: A reply to Lane's critical review. *Psychological Review, 77,* 234–249.

Studdert-Kennedy, M., & Shankweiler, D. P. (1970). Hemispheric specialization for speech perception. *Journal of the Acoustical Society of America, 48,* 570–594.

Summerfield, Q. (1975). Acoustic and phonetic components of the influence of voice changes and identification times for CVC syllables. *Report of speech research in progress, No. 2* (pp. 73–98). The Queen's University of Belfast, Belfast, Ireland.

Summerfield, Q. (1981). Articulatory rate and perceptual constancy in phonetic perception. *Journal of Experimental Psychology: Human Perception and Performance, 7,* 1074–1095.

Summerfield, Q., & Haggard, M. P. (1973). Vocal tract normalisation as demonstrated by reaction times. *Report on research in progress in speech perception, 2* (pp. 1–12). The Queen's University of Belfast, Belfast, Ireland.

Tomiak, G. R., Mullennix, J. W., & Sawusch, J. R. (1987). Integral processing of phonemes: Evidence for a phonetic mode of perception. *Journal of the Acoustical Society of America, 81,* 755–764.

Tyler, L. (1984). The structure of the initial cohort: Evidence from gating. *Perception and Psychophysics, 36,* 417–427.

Trehub, S. (1976). The discrimination of foreign speech contrasts by infants and adults. *Child Development, 47,* 466–472.

Verbrugge, R. R., Strange, W., Shankweiler, D. P., & Edman, T. R. (1976). What information enables a listener to map a talker's vowel space? *Journal of the Acoustical Society of America, 60,* 198–212.

Warren, R. M. (1970). Perceptual restoration of missing speech sounds. *Science, 167,* 392–393.

Waters, R. A., & Wilson, W. A. Jr. (1976). Speech perception by rhesus monkeys: The voicing distinction in synthesized labial and velar stop consonants. *Perception and Psychophysics, 19,* 285–289.

Werker, J. F., Gilbert, J. H. V., Humphrey, K., & Tees, R. C. (1981). Developmental aspects of cross-language speech perception. *Child Development, 52,* 349–355.

Werker, J. F., & Tees, R. C. (1983). Developmental changes across childhood in the perception of nonnative speech sounds. *Canadian Journal of Psychology, 37,* 278–286.

Werker, J. F., & Tees, R. C. (1984). Cross-language speech perception: Evidence for perceptual reorganization during the first year of life. *Infant Behavior and Development, 7,* 49–63.

Williams, D. R. (1986). *Role of dynamic information in the perception of coarticulated vowels.* Unpublished doctoral dissertation, University of Connecticut.

Williams, L. (1977). The perception of stop consonant by Spanish-English bilinguals. *Perception and Psychophysics, 21,* 289–297.

Editorial Comments on Carterette and Kendall

The topics represented in this book define the framework overarching the comparative psychology of complex acoustic perception. The picture would not be complete without a discussion of one of the highest forms of complex acoustic perception, namely, the perception of music. Music joins language as a process that reaches its highest development with the human species. In that sense both music and language stand at the end of the comparative continuum of complex acoustic perception. However, there are indications (see chapters by Hulse and Moody and Stebbins in this volume) that at least some primitive aspects of music perception may be represented in nonhuman animals as well—such as the capacity to process absolute as compared with relative, frequency-modulated pitch. Perhaps we can learn much about human music perception from the contrast which a comparative perspective affords. By the same token, perhaps we can learn much about complex acoustic perception in nonhuman animals if we draw upon data and theory borrowed from human music perception.

In this chapter Carterette and Kendall survey the field of music perception with a broad brush. Their treatment renders the topic accessible to those who are not familiar with the principles lying behind the production and perception of music. The discussion ranges from the physics of the musical stimulus to a discussion of scales and to considerations involving memory for music, its learning, and its neurological representation. The discussion of the development of music perception in babies and children, a research topic truly in its infancy, is especially valuable. That is so given that distinctions between the capacities of adults and children is in the best tradition of comparative psychology (see chapter 13 by Kuhl for a salient example).

The chapter offers a rich resource for anyone who is interested in music perception not only for its own sake, but also for the ideas and possibilities it offers for comparative studies of acoustic perception.

5 Human Music Perception

Edward C. Carterette
Roger A. Kendall
University of California, Los Angeles

INTRODUCTION

Our purpose here is to give a brief survey of the perceptual and cognitive processes involved in sensing, perceiving, remembering, learning, and performing music. Many different aspects of music are touched upon, including acoustics, psychophysics, cognitive development, neurology, and performance.

I. ELEMENTS OF MUSICAL PERCEPTION

On the Origins of Music

My (ECC) earliest musical memories go to the backwoods and sandy plains of North Carolina. The field hands sang, intoned, and hummed as they cropped tobacco leaves or strung them on sticks for drying in the barn. We children made pan pipes of swamp bamboo and single-reed whistles by inserting a piece of hard green leaf into a cleft stick and bull roarers by whirling a lath on a thong. Workers were called for meals by the blowing of a large conch shell or cowhorn, or by the clanging of a metal rod or of a bell. At night a man walking back from town or a distant farm through the swampy woods kept away fear by "hollering" a lonely monody or shouting. I could tell uncles, cousins, and strangers apart by style or vocal timbre. Wild and domestic animals called; birdsong was everywhere. Most disturbing to me was the eerie vibrato of the guinea fowl for it was said, when they cried at night, that someone had died. Occasional music was hymns, marches, and ballads played on a mechnical victrola; and my grandfather had an Edison machine that played cylinders. An uncle played a raucous five-string banjo, eliciting a shuffling dance, or "stomp." A rare event was a visiting fiddler. In church we sang to the laments of a pump organ. The following notion of Einstein (1954) fits well with my early musical experiences.

> To the man who in prehistoric times first perceived musical sound as it originated in the beating of a hollow object or by the swing and whir of a staff, it was something incomprehensible and therefore mysterious and magical. The mere sound of percussion instruments excited him to the pitch of intoxication. From them he discovered the power of rhythm, which inflamed and ordered the ritual dance and also co-ordinated the movements of labor and, as if by magic, lightened toil. (pp. 3–4)

Practically nothing is known about the origin of language or speech or music. Signs of the artistic impulse are to be seen in paintings on the walls of caves. Said to be some 40,000 years old, one scene (Trois-Frères, Ariege, France) shows a man in animal mask and skin behind a follow of deer. The person appears to be bowing a single-stringed instrument and perhaps dancing, as are the deer, or even singing.

Music must be far older than what is known from history. Paintings, figures, and hieroglyphics of the 4th millenium BCE (Before Common Era) show that the Egyptians were musical. We know about Greek ritual and epic songs from about the 9th century BCE. Chinese music goes back at least as far as the 18th century, BCE. Bell founding was well established by about 1000 BCE in China, and acoustic theory informed esthetics, philosophy, government, and measurement by 600 BCE. For example, length and weight were implicitly defined by frequency, which was itself defined by the number of millet seeds held in a joint of bamboo (Needham, 1962).

The history of music is a vast topic which cannot be reviewed here. Two sources give entree to the field: *The New Grove Dictionary of Music and Musicians* (1980) and *The New Harvard Dictionary of Music,* edited by Don Randel (1986). For sources of musical acoustics and psychoacoustics I recommend three excellent books: J. R. Pierce (1983), *The Science of Musical Sound;* B. C. J.

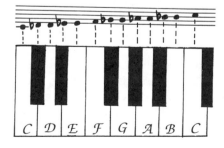

FIG. 5.1. The white keys CDEFGAB of the piano give the seven notes of the C major diatonic scale. (Notes are natural unless preceded by an accidental, here a flat.)

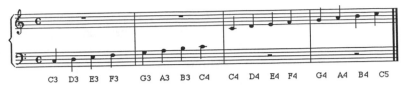

FIG. 5.2.   The treble (G) clef is shown on the top stave and the bass (F) clef on the bottom stave.

Moore (1982), *The Psychology of Hearing;* and J. G. Roederer, *Introduction to the Physics and Psychophysics of Music* (1974). Deutsch (1982), *The Psychology of Music* is the standard review of research on music perception.

In touring the domain of music it is essential to have a map of its features and a program for action. A piano should be at hand either physically or mentally. A simple electronic keyboard (such as Casio CZ-1000) will be very useful. One octave of the keyboard is shown in Fig. 5.1. Two staves of music (Fig. 5.2) show the layout of the treble (G) clef and the bass (F) clef.

The Psychological Dimensions of Sounds

Descartes, following Galileo's footsteps, explicitly separated mind and body (*res cogitans et res extensu*). However, the most powerful impact on the emerging experimental psychology of the mid-19th century was to be from the force of his concept of the world-machine, coupled with his invention of symbolically representing natural phenomena in analytical geometry. Among the first systematic studies in experimental psychology were those made by the German psychophysicists whose goal was to "establish the as yet non-existent measure of psychic magnitudes" (Fechner, 1860, p. xii). Thus, the essential framework of study arose as the search for "lawful" relations between variables, which were measured in the physical and perceptual frames of reference. In music the relations were of: (1) frequency to pitch; (2) amplitude to loudness; (3) spectrum to timbre; and (4) time to duration.

H. von Helmholtz (1877) extended research to physiological as well as acoustical and psychoacoustical factors. In the United States, Seashore (1938) approached music psychology specifically in terms of the above four pairs of variables. Hence his test of musical talent was based on "elemental capacities" for detecting changes in the perceptual variable as it depended on changes in the physical variable.

But problems arose with this spare model of isomorphic mappings. Difference limens (thresholds), measurements of the average smallest change in a physical variable that yielded a change in sensation, proved not to be reliable in several cases. Also, there were many interactions among pairs of variables. For example, frequency influenced not only pitch but loudness as well (Fletcher & Munson, 1933). Following, we explore each of the variable pairs in turn.

In music the most important qualities of sound are four: pitch, duration, loudness, and timbre. Duration and loudness are unidimensional, timbre is complex and multidimensional. Pitch is often said to be unidimensional, but many now view pitch as complex and multidimensional.

Loudness.   Intensity of a tone is the physical correlate that underlies the perception of loudness. It is complicated to assess loudness if sound energy is present in more than one critical band (see below), which is a very common situation. Loudness variations play an important role in music, but are less important than pitch variations.

Loudness is denoted in music by piano (p) and forte (f), which mean soft and loud in Italian. When teamed up with mezzo (m, middle), a more or less smooth scale is generated, from ppppp through mp to fffff. Dynamics were not regularly marked in music until about the 17th century. (I once saw a California sports car whose license read "ppp < fff" meaning "very soft to very loud.")

Duration.   Duration, or subjective time, is dealt with in the section entitled "Patterns in Time."

Timbre.   Timbre is the subjective code of the sound source or of its meaning. We speak of the timbre of a vowel, of musical instruments, the sound of a door slamming, etc. According to the American Standards Association (Acoustical Terminology, S1.1, 1960) "Timbre is that attribute of auditory sensation of which a listener can judge that two steady-state tones having the same pitch and loudness are dissimilar." Especially important is the relative amplitude of the harmonics. Recent research has shown that temporal characteristics of tones may have a profound influence on timbre as well. Both onset and steady state effects are important factors. Onset effects include rise time, presence of noise or inharmonic partials during onset, unequal rise of partials, characteristic shape of rise curve, etc. Steadier-state effects are important factors in recognizing a tone and thus in timbre: vibrato, amplitude modulation, gradual swelling, pitch instability, and so on.

There is no single scale of timbre. Rather, timbre is a multidimensional attribute of the perception of musical and vocal sounds. If middle C is sounded for 500 ms at a level of 70 dB Sound Pressure Level, first on a saxophone (a single-reed woodwind), then on an oboe (a double-reed woodwind), the two tones sound different and are said to have a different timbre. A plot of the spectrum (amplitude vs. frequency) of saxophone is not the same as that of oboe Fig. 5.3). This is because of differences in materials, reeds, cavities, and sound radiation properties, at least.

A soprano voice has a different timbre from a tenor voice and the timbre of a soprano's /how?/ is different from her /who?/. Interestingly, vocal and musical

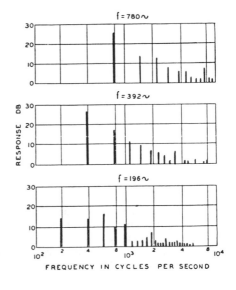

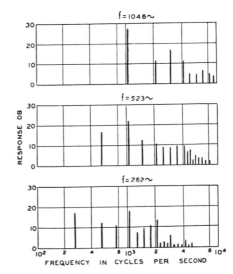

FIG. 5.3. (a) The acoustic spectrums of three tones of an alto saxophone. (b) The acoustic spectrums of three tones of an oboe.

sounds both can be described by "formants." A formant is a local maximum in a spectral plot. The similarity of voice formants (Fig. 5.4) and instrument formants (Fig. 5.3) is easy to see.

Dimensioning Timbre. Methods of multidimensional scaling (Shepard, 1987) help in discovering deep or hidden or subtle aspects of instruments and voices. Plomp (1976) asked listeners to judge the similarities among steady-state

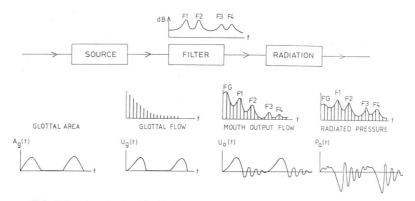

FIG. 5.4. A voiced sound (/a/ as in father) may be conceived of as the acoustic radiation of a filtered sound source (top row). The pulsed air flow from the vocal folds (glottis) has a triangular time wave form (bottom row). The line spectrum of glottal flow is filtered by the continuous spectrum of mouth output flow through the vocal tract to give rise to the (continuous) radiated pressure spectrum (middle row). The peaks F1, F2, F3 and F4 are the first four speech formants of /a/. FG is the frequency of the vocal fold vibration. (Drawing adapted by permission from G. Fant & T. V. Ananthapadmanabha, Quarterly Progress and Status Report 2-3, 1982, Speech Transmission Laboratory, Royal Institute of Technology, Stockholm, Sweden). Also see Fig. 5.6.

sounds of brasses, strings, and woodwinds. He found that the timbres were closely related to the spectral distribution of sound energy, particularly the positions of formants. Slawson (1968) had already shown this for steady-state vowel timbre.

Miller and Carterette (1975) synthesized tones of different frequencies with various envelopes and attack-decay functions, such as strong attack, sustained tone (brass-like) or strong attack, fast decay (piano-like) or trapezoidal onset-offset. A three-dimensional solution was obtained from similarity judgments: In order of strength these were fundamental frequency (pitch), piano-like versus nonpiano-like, and strong attack versus trapezoidal onset and offset. In another part of the study, frequency was kept constant to remove the dominance of pitch. Three variables of tones were the number of harmonics, the overall attack envelope, and the pattern of relative onset time of harmonics. In the scaling solution, the first two dimensions mapped out harmonic number, and the third dimension ordered attack envelope by piano, brass, and smooth.

By digitizing both transient and steady–state portions of actual instrument tones, a scaling solution of three dimensions was obtained from similarity judgments (Grey, 1977; Grey & Gordon, 1978; and Gordon & Grey, 1978). One

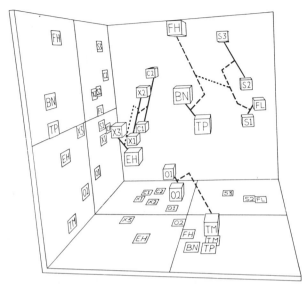

FIG. 5.5. These points in three-dimenions arose from a multidimensional scaling solution of numerical ratings of the similarity of pairs of instrumental sounds. (E.g., FH = French horn; BN = bassoon; TP = trumpet; O1 and O2 = oboe; X1, X2, X3 = saxophones; EH = English horn; FL = flute; TM = trombone; S1, S2, S3 = strings.)From a clustering method, groups of instruments were related and are connected by lines. Two-dimensional projections of the cubes show as squares on the walls (up-down and forward-back on left wall; forward-back and left-right on the bottom wall). From Pierce (1983); after J. M. Grey (1977).

dimension mapped steady-state spectral energy (Fig. 5.5). A second dimension showed that spectral onset patterns separated single-reeds from other instruments. A third dimension mapped noisiness of attack and separated high-frequency attack noise (flute and oboe) from low-frequency attack noise.

The comparative study of real and synthetic instruments by scaling methods shows what is and is not important in the perceptual judgment of timbre. One finding is that in musical context subtle variations in spectral features are not heard. Another finding (Grey & Gordon, 1978) is that, e.g., spectral envelope can be varied independently of other features; thus a bassoon can keep its vocal color yet be imbued with a plosive brass attack. A general conclusion from such scaling studies is that the main forces which determine timbre are spectral content and attack. However, Kendall (1986) found that attack transients, when embedded in musical context, were not critical for timbral categorization.

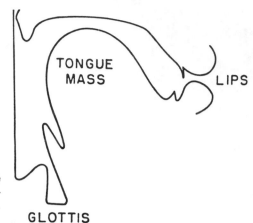

FIG. 5.6. Section through the vocal tract during the production of a vowel. Also see Fig. 5.4.

Perception of Singing

According to Sundberg (1982) most research on singing is based mainly on the acoustic correlates of certain types of voices or phonations, and has perceptual relevance. The three basic components of the vocal organ are (1) the respiratory system whose excess air pressure drives (2) the vocal folds which chop the air stream from the lungs into a sequence of quasi-periodic air pulses; (3) the vocal tract which gives each sound its characteristic spectral shape and thus its timbral identity.

The Voice Spectrum.   The chopped air stream (or voiced source) is a complex tone composed of a number of harmonic partials (Fig. 5.4). The frequency of the fundamental is the same as the air-pulse rate, and determines the perceived pitch. The amplitude of the partials fall off at about a 12-dB/octave rate. The spectrum of a given voiced sound (i.e., its fundamental and partials) is changed by the resonances of the vocal tract. The position of the jaw, tongue, lips, and the size of the mouth opening causes the voiced sound to be filtered so that there are amplitude peaks at four main frequencies. These formant peaks are somewhat independent of the partials or harmonics (Fig. 5.6).

The Soprano.   A soprano singer must sing at fundamental frequencies as high as 1000 or 1400 Hz; the first four formant peaks in this case may lie at 1000, 1500, 2500, and 4000 Hz. Indeed, when singing with an orchestra which typically plays at an intensity of 90–100 dB SPL, the soprano learns to be heard by putting energy into the 1000 and 2000–3000 Hz range so as to be 5 to 15 dB above the orchestra in those frequency ranges. Also, a rise in pitch of the fundamental must be accompanied by a rise in formant frequencies if vowel quality is to be preserved.

The Male Singer's Voice.   The pitch of bass, baritone, and tenor is about 330, 392, and 523 Hz, respectively. The male singer's voice can be heard above an orchestra because the singer has learned to place several formants high enough so that there is a peak, called the "singer's formant" between 2500 and 3000 Hz. This strategy is also consonant with research on masking, which shows that low frequencies mask higher frequencies rather than the other way round. Also, lower frequencies are radiated spherically from the mouth whereas high frequencies radiate along the axis of the mouth cavity and so lose less power in the listener's direction. Thus we see that, for reasons of articulation and masking, singers are driven to use the high frequency band between 2500 and 4000 Hz for effective vocal communication.

Finally, it appears that when a vocalist sings so as to achieve different qualities (timbres) the heard differences may depend on changes in the singers' formants. Furthermore, when vocal effort is increased, the amplitudes of the higher overtones increase at a faster rate than the amplitude of the fundamental. In short, the amplitude of the "singer's formant" (2500–4000 Hz) increases faster than SPL when vocal effort is raised.

Vibrato.   It has been suggested that *vibrato* or deviations from theoretically perfect pitch and steady amplitude is used as an expressive means in singing as in instrumental playing, for example, of the saxophone. Vibrato allows the singer a greater freedom of choice of fundamental frequency, as it eliminates beats with the sound of the accompaniment.

Phrasing.   Emotion is conveyed by singers by *phrasing,* one of the most essential aspects of singing and music in general. Joy, sorrow, fear, anger, and neutral emotions are conveyed by singers by such acoustical means as loudness, syllable duration, slow or rapid tone onsets, and unvoiced intersyllabic times. It is not unreasonable, suggests Sundberg (1982) that the acoustic characteristics of emotion in singing are the same as those in emotional speech.

Singing, Speech, and the Vocal Tract.   Sundberg (1982) considers two types of facts about singing: (1) Singers learn to adopt certain acoustic characteristics of vowel sounds which deviate in typical ways from normal speech (pitch-dependent choice of formant frequencies, "singer's formant," and vibrato) such that "singing differs from speech in a highly significant manner" (emphasized in original); (2) The acoustic correlates of various voice classifications (e.g., tenor, baritone, bass, vocal efforts, and register), which are based on perception probably arise from the form differences of vocal tracts rather than from the acoustic properties of voice sounds. "We seem to interpret the sounds in terms of how the voice organ was used in producing the sounds."

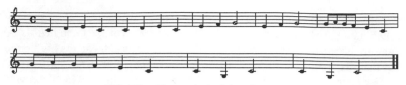

FIG. 5.7.   The melody Frère Jacques.

Pitch, Scales, and Intervals

Pitch.   Pitch is related to the frequency of a pure tone and to the fundamental frequency of a complex tone. In its musical sense, pitch has a range of about 20 to 5000 Hz (the range of the fundamental frequencies of strings and organ pipes). Some five to seven harmonics of a complex tone can be heard out individually by paying close attention. There is a dominance region for pitch perception, roughly from 500 to 2000 or 3000 Hz. Partials (harmonics) falling in the dominance region are most influential with regard to pitch.

The ability to detect small changes in the frequency of sounds not only is important for musical listeners and performers, but it is a significant factor in the perception of speech. The relative difference limen (the smallest detectable change in hertz (df) divided by the frequency in Hz (f), i.e., df/f) increases linearly with age, and so with sensorineural impairment, between 25- and 55-years-of-age, and more rapidly after age 55. This worsening of the df/f is greatest at frequencies below and above 1000 Hz.

Pitch is the perceived sound quality associated with a physical frequency. For example, a string which vibrates at 256 Hz is heard by a musician as the piano tone whose name is C. The left key labeled 1 in Fig. 5.1 sounds C, and so does the right key which sounds an octave higher. Pressing C-E in succession sounds a musical interval, which in this case is a rising interval because the pitch of E is higher. So, pressing E-C would give a falling interval. Intervals which sound at the same time are called chords. Pressing C-E-G all at once sounds the C-major triad, which is made up of a major third (C-E) and a minor third (E-G). The interval (C-G) sounds more *consonant* than does a major or minor third, and the zero interval (unison) or the interval of an eighth (octave) sound the most consonant.

Sing the tune of Fig. 5.7 ("Frère Jacques") or play it on the keyboard. Notice that it is marked in 4/4 time, that is, there are four quarter-note values per bar. The sum of the time values add up to four in each bar. Each bar, or measure, is marked off by a vertical line. An open note with stem is a half-note. A solid note with stem is a quarter note, and an eighth-note stem bears a flag (here the flags are connected to make a notational grouping). In all, only three different time values occur, but possibilities range from a whole note (4 quarter-note values) to sixteenth-notes or even smaller (a hemidemisemiquaver is a sixty-fourth note, so how much is a quaver?).

What we call the beginning is often the end
And to make an end is to make a beginning.
The end is where we start from.

These lines of T. S. Eliot (*The Four Quartets: Little Gidding*) are apt. Frère
Jacque begins on C (1) which is called the tonic and ends on C (1), the tonic. If
we let +, −, and 0 refer to the direction of pitch change the contour of the song
is {+ + −0+ + − + + + − . . . − +}. This tonal motion of the notes of varying
time values guided by a metrical beat is the essence of melody and rhythm. The
printed score is a program for generating music. Timbre could be added by
specifying an instrument (soprano), and by adding another simultaneous timbre
line (e.g., tenor), simple octave harmony would arise.

Critical Bandwidth, Beats, Roughness and Combination Tones.   The perceptual attributes of simultaneous tones includes beats and roughness. The critical bandwidth around a certain frequency roughly measures the range within
which this frequency interacts with others. The width of a critical band is about
one-third of an octave above 500 Hz and about 100 Hz below 500 Hz (see Fig.
5.8).

If two primary tones have equal frequency, they fuse as one. If they are
slightly different in frequency, fluctuations in loudness (beats) are heard. When
two frequencies are separated by 20 Hz or more a rattling sensation or roughness
is heard. Beats and roughness happen if the two primary tones are not resolved

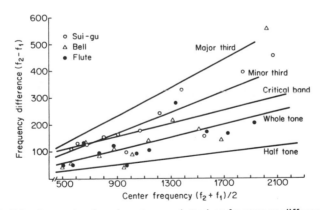

FIG. 5.8.   Intervals of various tones plotted as frequency differences
(f2−f1), in hertz, as a function of the center frequency [(f2+f1)/2] between tones (abscissa). The critical bandwidth of the ear as well as that
of some important musical intervals are shown as straight lines. The
points labelled "sui-gu" and "Zhou" are data from Chinese bronze
bells and the filled circles are data from a bamboo flute. As an example, the bell interval whose center frequency is about 1500 lies on the
whole-tone line of the equal-temperament scale.

by the ear; if the frequency difference is greater than the critical band, the tones are perceived separately and no interference is heard.

Combination tones arise from distortion in the ear and are not present in the acoustic signal though they are perceived as if they were. The ear cannot distinguish between *real* and combination tones. The most important combination tones are the first-, second-, and third-order difference tones. Since combination tones are a distortion product, individuals will differ greatly in hearing them.

Musical Scales.   The discrete scale steps of pitch are a kind of category system. All other attributes are smoothly variable, and there is no fixed level, or *zero,* in the cases of loudness, time, timbre, or consonance. In virtually all cultures, there is some canonical pitch like C and the next step up or down is a discrete, fixed interval. The size of the interval varies among cultures but the basic step is everywhere the octave. The discrete steps of pitch have an analog in speech, where each vowel, in English say, keeps to its own region as in /a e i o u/ or the consonants /p t k b d g . . . . /. Though continuous variations are possible it is a nearly universal property of languages that the sounds cluster in fixed categories. Von Helmholtz (1877) held that the musical scale was for the listener a standard against which she could judge interval size and melodic motion.

The scale of discrete pitch steps is also a cognitive device for coding the pitches and intervals of a melody into memory and, later, for retrieving. By means of the musical scale the listener hears, stores, analyzes, recodes, retrieves, and produces music as constrained by memory and attention. A small number of categories with relatively fixed relations makes the scale an efficient device for sending and receiving musical ideas. Furthermore, a categorical scale endows a musical line with an identify among other lines and a robustness in adverse noise.

The Western Scale and Equal Temperament.   There are some obvious properties that a scale ought to have if it is to be useful and endure. Rational scales, like the Pythagorean, satisfied mathematics but not listener or players. Our scale should satisfy at least four conditions:

1. It should be easy to tell successive, different pitches apart;
2. If a tone has a frequency f1, then a tone having frequency $f2 = 2 \times f1$ or $f1/2$ should seem very similar;
3. The number of different pitches in the scale interval should be about 7;
4. All intervals of a scale should be constructible from a series of minimal intervals of equal size.

The Western scale and its tuning is called Equal Temperament. Its smallest pitch interval, the semitone, is a frequency difference of about 6%. Since humans can discriminate 1%, condition (1) is satisfied. In Western music the sequence of Cs are 16.35, 32.70, 65.4, 130.8, 261.6, 523.3, 1046.5, 2093, 4186 Hz (Backus, 1969). Each pitch of the sequence C0, C1, . . . , C8, is called "C" and each has the relation $fn + 1/fn = 2$, hence condition (2) is satisfied. The so-called diatonic scale has seven pitches, C, D, E, F, G, A, and B, which meets condition (3). And condition (4) is satisfied because each octave interval, e.g., 2093–4186 Hz is divided into the 12 semitones of the chromatic scale.

A tuning system is a slight modification of a "just" or acoustically pure interval. Tuning systems have evolved over the millenia in order to satisfy the perceptual needs of the listener, to keep the number of pitches small, and to make it possible to modulate easily among modes or keys. In equal temperament all intervals are built from semitones. Our Western equal temperament system dates from the early 17th century and is based on a formal discovery in China of the late 16th century (Needham, 1962).

Frequency ratios of two to one are roughly equal psychologically. If each octave is made up of 12 pitch intervals of equal size a logarithmic scale is implied (see Dowling & Harwood, 1986, chapter 4), in which the minimal step is the 12th root of 2, $2^{1/12}$, equal to about 1.059463, which we will call a toot. Now the G is 7 semitones above C, or $toot^7$ higher. So if C = 261.63 Hz, then $f(G) = C \times toot^7 = 261.63 \times toot^7 = 261.63 \times (1.059463)^7 = 392.00$ Hz, which is the frequency of G. Note that this is an additive scale in logarithms. Thus, $\ln G = \ln C + 7(\ln toot) = 5.5669 + 7(.4043) = 5.9713$. The antilog of 5.9713 = 391.00, as advertised. In short to move from a given pitch any number k of semitones above or below simply multiply or divide the pitch by $toot^k$, respectively.

The preference for the logarithmic system with an octave base appears to have its roots in biology, since octaves and logarithmic intervals are virtually a cultural universal (Dowling & Harwood, 1986). Octave judgments of successive tones are made precisely everywhere, as is the transposition of logarithmic scale intervals. Even the slight stretching of the octave with higher frequencies (with ratio of 2.009:1 in middle range) is universal to musicians and nonmusicians and is attested by the fact that pianos are tuned with stretched octaves.

On Scaling the Dimensions of Pitch.   Two pitches near each other in frequency which sound similar (property 1, above) are similar in pitch height. Two pitches an octave apart which sound similar (property 2, above) have the same chroma. This idea is embodied in a spiral model of the pitch scale (Fig. 5.9). Similar chromas lie on the spiral above each other (vertical line) whereas pitch heights lie near each other on the spiral. This model accounts for the paradox that C1 is more similar to C2 (an octave interval) than C1 is similar to G1 (a fifth interval).

Though equal temperament is not used by most of the world's cultures as the base of their tonal scale systems, their scales are based on the octave, and this leads to a logarithmic frequency scale. Generally, their interval sizes cannot be mapped onto our semitone. But, as with equal temperament, other scales have a

FIG. 5.9. The diatonic scale shown as points on an ascending spiral. C', C'', C'''. . . lie close to each other and are perceived as similar, and so too for the others. C' and G' are closer in frequency than are C' and C'' but C' and C'' sound more similar than C' and G'.

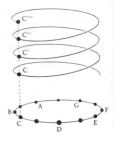

variety of interval sizes which allows for melodic variation and interest. For example, the pentatonic scale of Chinese and Tibetan music (similar to the five black notes of the piano) generates 8 semitone-like intervals. Western equal-tempered scale has more variety since the major scale of 7 pitches generates 11 intervals. The smallest number of pitches which gives all of the possible intervals (completeness) was shown to be seven by Balzano (1980).

The spiral model of Fig. 5.9 has some support from similarity judgments, as well as from experiments which measured the degree to which an extraoctave pitch was a good completion of a major-scale sequence minus one note (Krumhansl & Shepard, 1979). But there are more than two dimensions of pitch relations, for example, key distance, and the equal-appearing intervals of the major scale which are actually of different size. Shepard (1982) has captured multifarious dimensions of musical pitch in his double helix model. Non-Western scale systems on different pitch sets cannot be directly explained by the double helix, but Dowling and Harwood (1986) suggest that the single helix model depicts well the way in which pitch is organized for all cultures.

Consonance and Musical Intervals.   Musical consonance in Western polyphonic and harmonic music is clearly based on perceptual consonance of complex (harmonic) tones. Intervals with simple frequency ratios are consonant; those with nonsimple frequency ratios are dissonant. Dissonance occurs if the frequency separation of two tones is less than a critical bandwidth, the most dissonant interval being about a quarter of a bandwidth.

In respect of intervals, scales, and tuning, the evidence strongly favors that musical-interval categories are learned rather than being the direct result of properties of the auditory system. An important line of evidence for this conclusion is the relative inability of musically untrained subjects to perform musical interval identification or discrimination experiments.

II.   PERCEPTION OF MUSICAL PATTERNS

Selective Attention and Schemas

How do we recognize what one person is saying when others are speaking at the same time? This is the "cocktail party problem" (Cherry, 1953). In music this problem arises in listening, playing, and composing. How does the ear sort out violin, cello, and piano in a trio? Of course different *voices* have different timbres; perhaps the ear has timbre filters. Expectancy plays a role, too. We know where a melodic line begins, suspect where it is going, like mild surprises, but know when the line is over (more or less where it began). We follow a motif (a handful of notes) under its variations or aliases, and notice larger forms to which it gives rise: The detail of the pattern is movement. The immediate present, the past, and the future all seem to be involved. We shall take up the moment of nowness, short-term memory, long-term memory, schemas, and attention.

The late Sir Frederick Bartlett (1932) used the term "schema" to refer to the active organization of past reactions or experinces. He thought of schemas as active organized settings which could be at lower levels (visual, auditory) or higher levels (art, science, music). Attention is guided by schemas. A musical schema can be as particular as knowing the rhythmic structure of a waltz or as general as knowing the fused scalar and melodic properties of the ragas of North Indian music, or of Western polyphonic music.

An example from Dowling and Harwood (1986) may clarify the how selective attention is guided by schemas. Figure 5.10a shows "Frère Jacques" (filled notes) interleaved with "Twinkle, Twinkle" (open notes), in different pitch ranges. Figure 5.10b shows the two melodies in the same pitch range. If each note of Fig. 5.10b is played successively at about 7 notes per sec, each melody can be heard clearly, but if you listen to one, you cannot listen to the other. Even in Fig. 5.10b where the pitch range of the two melodies is the same, you can attend to one or the other of the two melodies if they differ in timbre, or loudness, or spatial location, or if one line is played faster than the other line. All these devices have been used by composers from the ancients to the moderns: Brass choirs are placed in opposite balconies (Gabrielli); chorales are made up of several voices but also grouped spatially; a recitative moves swiftly against the slower harmonic accompaniment of the continuo (bass line); in a piano trio, the piano, violin, or cello is each important, and so contrast in pitch-range and timbre.

Now if two new interleaved melodies are played to you the "tune" seems meaningless. Dowling (1973) played interleaved tunes to two groups of listeners.

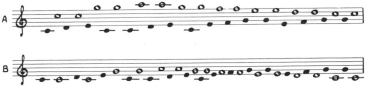

FIG. 5.10. The notes of "Frères Jacques" (filled notes) interleaved with the notes of "Twinkle, Twinkle" (open notes) (a) in different pitch ranges, and (b) in the same pitch range.

One group was armed with true, the other with false, labels for the tunes. The true-labels group almost always identified the tunes, but the false-labels group almost never reported hearing the labeled tune nor correctly recognized the actual tune. These results fit with the idea that if a schema or schemas are active they serve as expectancies for focusing attention.

What is a melody schema like? Because a familiar melody can be recognized when played fast or slowly or in any octave or key, the schemas must map something more abstract than specific pitches and time intervals. Dowling and Harwood (1986) suggest some mappings onto schemas:

1. contour plus tonal scale locus;
2. sequence of logarithmic pitch intervals;
3. sequence of do-re-mi labels in a movable-do system.

From the evidence, Harwood and Dowling argue that schemas of familiar tunes are mapped as sets of relative pitch chromas which are rhythmically organized. These schemas can be accessed by labels and global melodic features such as contour.

Attitudes and Strategies of the Listener: Set.   A listener can know or process music only in a surface way or very deeply in achieving a cognitive grasp of a piece. Each local pattern is heard as an instance if the listener makes no effort at integration or if the piece is new. The opera can't be heard for the arias. At the other extreme, the listener tries to weave the themes together into a global pattern and store the whole in semantic memory.

A listener can sink into the music and be swept along by the sound and feeling, making no effort to note the details or formal structure. This subjective attitude contrasts with the objective, detached strategy, such as a critic or student might take in an effort to know the composer's intent or to see the conductor's interpretation. Most listeners take the subjective view.

Schemas Guide Expectancies.   The global invariants of a work clearly affect what is expected. My knowledge of music, composers, styles, and works are mental schemas that set me up to expect a range of pieces, and these schemas set the stage with invariants against which I match and contrast the actual against the expected event. Beethoven's 33 variations on a simple waltz of Diabelli are a case in point. My knowledge of the waltz and of Beethoven's works and style are mental schemas. I expect variations on rhythm, key, tempo, and the like; also general, nonspecific variations. I hear what I expect, variations, but often with unexpected, brilliant solutions. Even after many hearings of the variations I am still surprised by the serious, somber mood from variation 28 to the end.

Expectancy is an assumption of signal detection theory: A preview of the tone to be detected improves accuracy; known word sets are learned to asymptote more quickly than are unknown sets (Green & Swets, 1966). Musical contexts set up expectancies which depend on such factors as musical training or culture. For example, when presented with a musical scale and a note from another octave, novices rate congruity of scale and note on pitch height proximity, but musicians rate on triadic concordance (Krumhansl & Shepard, 1979). Dowling and Harwood (1986) suggest that attention is under control of rhythmic invariants, as well as pitch invariants; indeed, many schemas tend to operate at once. Using real music, Carlsen (1981) showed that dictation errors made by expert listeners were inversely related to expectancy of success.

Therefore, it is possible to speak of two types of musical knowledge: explicit and implicit. Explicit knowledge is that which is verbalizable and usually involves the manipulation of symbols according to notatable rules. An example of an explicit musical rule is that for the construction of a scale or chord, as delineated above. Implicit knowledge is, in contrast, not generally open to introspection. The unconscious schemata of Dowling and Harwood (1986), which guide the expectancies of the individual, are examples.

Much musical behavior is the manifestation of implicit, rather than explicit, knowledge, and such implicit knowledge is often obtained through modeling. Musical performance, for example, cannot be learned exclusively from a book. The acquiring of the rules for appropriate stylistic interpretation and expression must be handled by one-on-one instruction by example.

The explicit/implicit knowledge dichotomy fits well with the subsymbolic orientation of cognitive science, in which explicit awareness is the single interpretation of the state of the neural network. Kendall (1987) argues that such a model accounts for the interpretation of musical illusions (Deutsch, 1975) in terms of gestalt processes, and that the gestalt "laws" are simply examples of implicit rules.

Memory for Melody

Memory for Pitch.   Krumhansl (1979) played to a listener a brief standard tone (a G, say), then a sequence of seven pitches and, finally, either the standard tone (target) or one a semitone away. If the pitch sequence was from the same key as the target, the target was remembered well (95% correct) but if the pitch sequence was not in any key, performance fell to 80% correct. If the target was outside the tonal scale of interfering pitches (e.g., a G#), the results were reversed, that is, tonal interference was more disruptive than atonal interference. Dowling and Harwood (1986) review this and other studies on memory for pitch. Briefly, it can be said that memory for a pitch is affected by the context in which it is heard. If the context is a tonal scale, pitches which fit the context are remembered well, whereas, pitches which do not fit the context are detected well.

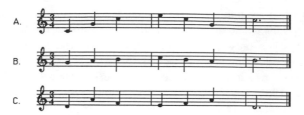

FIG. 5.11.   The note sequences (a) and (b) have the same contour, but the note sequence (c) has a different contour from either (a) or (b).

Memory for Contour.   Two melodies have the same contour if the sequence of up and down intervals are the same even if the interval sizes differ. In Fig. 5.11, A and B have the same contour but C has a different contour from either A or B.

Contour dominates in the immediate recognition of melodies whose scale is not well established or is atonal. Dowling and Fujitani's (1971) listeners heard pairs of 5-note atonal melodies. The comparison melody was an exact transposition, or a same-contour imitation, or a different-contour comparison (Fig. 5.12). Listeners easily told transpositions and imitations from the melodies with altered contour. But listeners could not tell transpositions and imitations from each other. Listeners apparently used similarity of contour in making their judgments, but could not detect changes in interval size. Dowling (1978), using tonal melodies found similar results except that tonal transpositions and atonal imitations could be told apart, especially by experienced musicians. Thus, in the case of a constant tonal scale frame, contour also dominates in the immediate recognition of novel melodies.

Psychological Reality of Key Distance.   One key is related to another mainly by the number of pitches in common. This can be as many as six and as few as one. In this sense the keys of C and G are very close, whereas the keys of F and B are maximally distant (Fig. 5.13). Experiments of Bartlett and Dowling (1980) show that key distance affects the recognition of melodies. A standard melody was heard followed by a comparison melody which was the standard, or by either

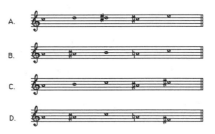

FIG.   5.12.   Atonal   melodies used in Dowling and Fujitani's (1971) study. See text.

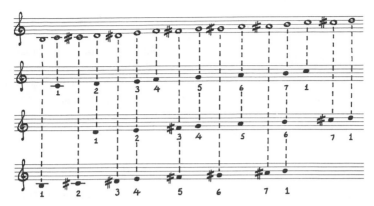

FIG. 5.13.   Keys which are closely related share more pitches than distantly related keys. Thus the keys of C major and D major are close to each other, sharing all but two pitches. C major and B major are distant, having only two pitches in common.

a transposition or a tonal imitation in either a near key or in a far key. It was found that as the key distance of transformations went from same to near to far, the pairs were less confusable and easier to reject. This key-distance effect was put down mainly to better rejection of imitations in a far key rather than to better recognition of transpositions in a far key. If the keys of a pair are close both contour and chroma are shared, so it is hard to reject an imitation. If the keys of a pair are distant, chroma is not shared, hence the imitation is not confusing. Bartlett and Dowling suggest that listeners can solve the task in part by using schematic scale information.

Memory for Intervals and Chromas.   Contour dominates in the listener's immediate memory for novel melodies. But if you try to pick out a well-known melody on the keyboard you will instantly sense a distorted interval. In one of their experiments Bartlett and Dowling (1980) tested immediate recognition of melodic phrases drawn from familiar and unfamiliar folk songs. The listeners scored very much better with familiar than with unfamiliar phrases in telling same-contour imitations and transpositions apart.

Chroma or interval information, which is more detailed and constrained than contour, dominates in long-term memory. Why not contour here also? (Keep in mind that 30 sec is about the upper limit of short-term memory.) Dowling and Bartlett's (1981) listeners heard sequences from Beethoven string quartets made up of themes, repetitions (imitations), and excerpts not related to themes. After a pause of 5 min listeners heard a series which included exact themes, their imitations, and excerpts not heard before. A theme and its imitation had the same contour but different intervals and chromas. The task of the listener was to tell both themes and imitations from other excerpts. Though listeners could tell themes from other excerpts in three-fourths of the cases (chance was one-half), surprisingly they could not tell same-contour imitations of the themes from other excerpts, scoring at chance level. This was surprising because imitation and theme had the same contour, were close neighbors in the score, and had very similar tempo, loudness, and timbre. Apparently long-term memory was used in recognizing chromas or interval-size patterning of a novel melody but could not be used in recognizing contour. The results of Dowling and Fujitani (1971) suggest that if contour is to be useful in retrieval from long-term memory, a melody must be both familiar and very well learned.

Summary of Features Important in Memory for Melody.   Key roles in remembering and perceiving melody are played by pitch intervals or chroma (patterns of intervals), contour, and tonal scale. Two major points are emphasized by Dowling and Harwood (1986). First, the importance of a given feature depends on the demands of the task. So, in short-term memory alternative choices are few and contour is a useful feature. But in long-term memory where many melodies share a given contour, interval-size is an important feature in retrieval choice. Second, any theory of music cognition must allow for individual differences in development for it is clear that the use of tonal scales and other complex schemas depends on training. Further data on this second point can be found in the section on Performance.

The Organization of Melody: Local, Global and Hierarchical

"La donna è mobile" (Verdi's "Rigoletta") is a familiar sequence of 24 notes (Fig. 5.14), which can be heard as a perceptual schema having local and global features, to use the notion of LaBerge (1981). Local features are such as interval or stress, e.g., the first two intervals are zero. Global features, those which extend across more than two notes, are such as contour and rhythm. Thus, the first set of 6 notes (A) has the same contour and rhythmic pattern as the second set of 6 notes (A'). This same relation holds for the third and fourth sets of 6 notes (B) and (B'). A simple hierarchy also exists, extending over pairs, in that a pattern is succeeded at once by its imitation, thus (AA'BB'); note, however that the rhythmic pattern is the same for each set of notes.

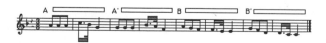

FIG. 5.14.   La donna è mobile (Verdi's "Rigoletta") can be heard as a perceptual schema having local and global features, AA*BB*. See text.

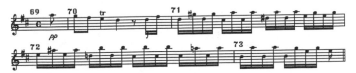

FIG. 5.15. The perceived melody breaks into two lines yet the notes are played singly, one after the other (from a Concerto Grosso of G. F. Handel).

Local and Short-Range Features

Propinquity. In the first movement of Beethoven's Fifth Symphony, a famous pattern of four notes is repeated twice, in the form (rrrp) or (rrrq) where p is a major third down and q is a minor third down in pitch from r. Though there are some larger intervals between patterns in this particular piece, a rule of the world's music is that pitch steps are small. Over all cultures, it appears that pitch-interval sizes of five semitones or less account for about 90% of all observed interval sizes (Dowling & Harwood, 1986, Fig. 6.2).

If this rule of proximity is broken, the musical pattern may be hard to follow, as in music of the 12-tone school where jumps of six semitones are not rare. If jumps are too large and closely spaced in time, the music seems to fly apart, or *fission.* When two pitches are trilled rapidly in an interval of three semitones or more, a perceptual splitting occurs. Composers have used fission for effect, so that an organ of two manuals could be made to sound like one of three. Figure 5.15 shows an excerpt from a Concerto Grosso of Handel in which the perceived melody breaks into two melodic lines, even though the notes are played singly one after the other. The threshold size of interval at which fission occurs depends on such factors as rate and timbre. Thus, fast sequences of 8 to 10 notes/sec fission at three semitones. For slower sequences attention can be directed so as to achieve one or two melodic lines. When two lines are heard one appears as figure, the other as ground.

"Rhythmic fission" (van Noorden, 1975) can also occur. On a keyboard play each of the following quarter-note sequences:

(1) E~~F~~E~~F~~ . . . . .   [~ = ⅛ rest; ~~ = ¼ rest; B',b'
(2) E~FE~FE~ . . . . .   = a fifth + an octave above E,e;
(3) E~B'E~B'E~ . . . .   e,b,f = eighth notes; E, B, F =
(4) E~~B'E~~B'E~~ . . . .   quarter notes; (4) is twice as fast as
(5) E~~FE~~FE~~ . . .   (3) and (5) is twice as fast as (2).]

(1) is heard as two alternating regular pitches. (2) is heard as a halting rhythmic pattern, as is (3). But in (4) the halting rhythm disappears perceptually as the

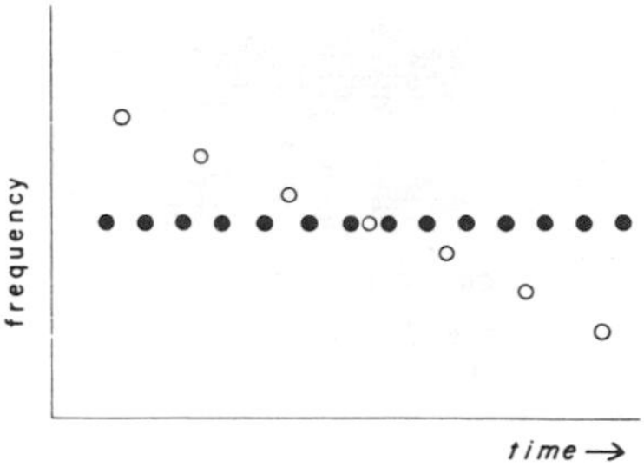

FIG. 5.16. The repeating notes (filled circles) capture the notes of the descending scale (open circles).

temporal integration fails, only to return in (5) as the pitch difference returns to that of (1). There is a tradeoff between tempo and pitch interval. Rhythm can be integrated over large pitch intervals if tempo is slow, but not if tempo is fast. And at fast tempos perception of the halting rhythm recovers if pitch interval is reduced.

As might be intuited, if distance or contrast can somehow be lessened, pitch and rhythmic fission will be reduced or disappear. For example, Bregman and Dannenbring (1973) showed that fission is reduced or disappears by gliding in frequency between notes (glissando).

Gestalt Properties.   The most general perceptual law of Gestalt psychology was the law of pregnance [Praegnanz], which says that every gestalt becomes as good as possible. This notion of "good continuation" is to say the least, a fluid, subjective concept which seems to work best over sets of elements. Thus, if I play the first five notes of a rising scale, CDEFG . . . , a good continuation is . . . ABC. As an organizing principle, good continuity is fragile in coping with the forces of proximity. For example, if the odd notes in a regular temporal sequence alternate with notes from a scale sequence (Fig. 5.16), the scale seems to be captured by the repeating notes (van Noorden, 1975). Dowling and Harwood (1986) point out that good continuation of pitch also can be deranged easily by similarity of timbre, as in the case of melodies arranged by pattern of timbres. Generally, rapid changes in timbre are hard to follow, but rapid changes in pitch pattern can be followed at prestissimo rates.

From the notions and facts so far reviewed, it is fair to conclude that the local features which figure in musical patterning are direct and automatic functions of the perceptual mechanisms. Global features on the other hand are functions of memory, knowledge and training.

Invariants: Organization of Global Features

What makes a waltz a waltz? "The Blue Danube" and "The Emperor Waltz" epitomize the waltz, now a polished form which arose from a folk dance. The hallmark of the waltz is an invariant, a recurring triple beat. Another invariant is the opening notes of Beethoven's Fifth Symphony pppr (see above) that form a recurring contour pattern in which the interval pr is variously 1, 3, 4, 5, and 7 semitones. The pitch contour pppr is imitated by the time contour (sssl) where s = short and l = long. The time interval sl varies as well, but the relative time contour is an invariant. A liason of time and pitch, this pattern returns again and again over the eight minutes of the first movement.

The structure of a piece of music is perceived by the listener through its invariants. An ever-changing surface flow of pitch-time patterns is generated out of the underlying structural constancies. Some invariants are local, like the prosaic waltz tune of Diabelli on which Beethoven composed 33 variations. But waltz, like other compelling rhythmic forms such as samba or meringue or tango, is a global invariant across many pieces. Common invariants within a piece are meter, key, or instrumentation. An example of the last is Prokofiev's "Peter and the Wolf" in which each of the characters of a children's story recurs as a specific tune and instrument—Peter as a string quartet. Invariants over sets of pieces, such as relative consonance and dissonance, may identify a composer or style.

A listener must grasp a complex of invariant structures if she is to understand a piece of music. Even a very local note pattern depends on the invariants of the given piece. "The meaning of the note [pattern] lies in the sets of invariants it invokes" (Dowling & Harwood, 1986, p. 162). At another level, the composer may order sets of constancies so as to induce tension, to create ambiguity or to set a mood.

Knowing and Remembering Musical Form.   The vast domain of memory can be divided into procedural and propositional memories (Tulving, 1983). Procedural knowledge is of operations, of knowing how to do a thing. An expert skill like playing the saxophone is procedural knowledge (which is discussed in the section on performance). Propositional memory has two aspects, episodic and semantic memories. The recording and retrieval of memories of personal events and doing is episodic memory. Knowledge of the world which is independent of one's identity or past is semantic knowledge.

Almost everyone can hear in her mind the familiar air "Greensleeves" and many can hear the main motif of the "The Trout" ("Die Forelle") in Schubert's Quintet in A Major. These salient, memorable themes are episodic. On the other hand, the overall, semantic meaning of a larger work involves working themes into a larger structure of repeated patterns, with names like chaconne, rondo, or sonata form. Within sonata form—(Introduction-Exposition-Development-Recapitualation-Coda)—the parts have subpatterns. Thus, Exposition may contain a primary theme with a transition into a secondary theme, then a closing theme. The exposition is "a highly flexible interaction of tonality, thematic material, and large-scale rhythmic motion" (The Harvard Dictionary of Music, 1986).

Memory for a piece of music is a sequential pattern of (memorable) episodes of varying lengths. The meaning, or semantic memory of the piece is more than the sum of the episodic encounters. Semantic memory of a piece of music concerns "a grasp of the broad pattern invariants of pieces and styles" (Dowling & Harwood, 1986, p. 165).

Hierarchical Organization: Music, Language, and Meaning

How shall we tie together local and global aspects of music? As mentioned earlier, "La donna e mobile" reveals a simple hierarchy which relates two local patterns A and B and the imitations A' and B' in the form AA'BB'. This simple structure could be a unit within a family of various hierarchies. The idea of parsing local-local, local-global, and global-global relationships is explicit in Rameau (1722) and Schenker (1906/1954). Chomsky (1956) used hierarchical tree structures in his influential theory of transformational grammars. The surface structure of observed sentences were generated from underlying deep structures using rewrite rules (equivalent to tree structures). It was natural for musicians to try such methods for generating melodies from primitive motifs; Sloboda (1985) discusses these attempts.

The psychological reality of hierarchies can be seen in both melody and rhythm. Dowling and Harwood (1986) show how the melodic structure of "Three Blind Mice" can be represented in a tree: That melody begins ". . . with a repeated phrase, followed by a translation of the whole pattern to another level of the scale with a slight rhythmic elaboration." Restle (1970) asked observers to learn (by anticipating) sequences of light which were patterned in time. He found that errors tended to follow breaks between constituents in the structure, that simple continuations were wrongly anticipated, and that when preview was allowed, performance was better to the degree that the preview sequences were temporally "in phrase" with the phrase structure. Using a melodic dictation task, Deutsch (1980) found that copying errors tended to be low when boundaries of temporal and phrase structure groups coincided. Copying errors tended to be high when temporal phrasing conflicted with phrase structure.

The Language of Music.   The influence of global and local structure on perception and performance raises the question of whether Music is a Language. Sloboda (1985) lists some similarities between music and language. Both: are universal and specific to humans; can generate an infinity of novel strings; can be learned by children by example alone; are primarily audio-vocal; are notated by many but by no means all cultures and notational literacy usually must be taught; are understood earlier than produced. Sloboda (1985) remarks that "Although literacy is hard to acquire, its acquisition can profoundly alter cognitive functioning" (p. 19). Forms of natural language and natural music differ among cultures, yet some universal features exist.

Natural language is used for telling or asking about states of the world, about the objects in it and the relationships among the objects and states, in short, for social interaction. Music has no obvious domain and purpose. Analogies between language and music should not be pressed too far but are useful devices for sharpening musical theory and practice.

Most agree that language has three components: phonology, syntax, and semantics. Most tend to agree that music also can be analyzed naturally into the same three components. Sloboda (1985) shows that it is fruitful to consider music in relation to language. Musical phonology is based on the notions of scale and meter and, like language, is governed by category perception, that is, discrimination between categories is more keen than discrimination within categories.

The rules of melody, harmony and rhythm provide temporally local constraints, but as musical syntax these cannot account for larger structures, such as repetition. This is a grave defect since repetition, both exact and inexact, pervades music in the form of motifs, pitch transposition, inversion, contraction, expansion, and other transforms. Sundberg and Lindblom (1976) wrote a generative grammatical program which makes Swedish nursery rhymes. Longuet-Higgins (1976) described a computer program which transcribed the rhythmic and tonal features of sophisticated classical melodies. A major effort at giving a generative theory of tonal music (Lehrdahl & Jackendoff, 1983) turns out to be a formal system for analysis of musical sequences, a model of the listener, rather than a generative model of the composer. There is an abyss between the parsing of a sentence or melody and the composing of a symphony. "A generative grammatical approach could hardly succeed . . . unless it were founded on musical insights as deep as, and more explicit than, those of Bach himself" says Longuet-Higgins (1976).

The evidence is clear that, in language, semantics is king. We remember the the gist of a proposition, not its form. Does music have meaning beyond its form? Clearly it does, for a listener carries away from a concert feelings and memories outside the music, even when she is unable to retrieve a single specific musical pattern. Some music frankly mimics nature or is symbolic or programmatic, yet seems to mean more than these referents. Do musical patterns denote emotional states? Definitely, yes, says Cooke (1959), whose ideas are reviewed with sympathetic care by Sloboda (1985). Cooke argues that diatonic scale intervals evoke emotional states. For example, major sequences of triads evoke pleasure; movement toward the tonic is restful. Certain recurring interval motifs evoke emotional qualities (like "restless sorrow"), and so on, as attested by over 300 years of Western music. These ideas imply that the mapping of musical forms onto emotions can be discovered, and that unnatural pairings of musical forms and emotions should be hard to learn.

Patterns in Time

But there is one source of evidence that is always available, even when there are no words, when the notes are of indefinite pitch, and when the performance is devoid of accent, phrasing, or rubato: even in such impoverished conditions the listener may still arrive at a rhythmic in-

terpretation of the passage based solely on the relative durations of the notes.

—H. C. Longuet-Higgins & C. S. Lee (1984)

Rhythm is too much neglected as an organizing force in music perception yet its role may be more basic than that of pitch. A hundred years ago William James (1890) noted that a tune could be told from its rhythmic pattern. Rhythm turned out to be a dimension more salient than pitch in a task where listeners rated similarities of melodies (Carterette, Monahan, Holman, Bell, and Fiske, 1982).

The Window of Time Present.   Play on a keyboard the theme and its repetition (8 notes in all) of the first movement of Beethoven's Fifth Symphony. This handful of notes seems to heard in the here and now. The evidence, reviewed by Fraisse (1978, 1982), is that the psychological present endures at least a few sec but its upper limit is about 5 sec, with the most extreme estimate being 10 sec. Such estimates arise from studies in which listeners reproduce or recognize the durations of sequences, and from the lengths of phrases of songs and poetry. Dowling (1984) arrived at similar estimates from his analysis of phrase length in the songs of children and adults.

As might be expected on physiological and mechanical grounds psychological pace has a natural rate of events of about 1.5 per sec, which corresponds to a metronome rate of 80–100 beats/sec, and fits well with musician's intuition of a moderate tempo. Of course the duration of time-present and the tempo of natural pace will depend on the task, which in turn invokes different psychological mechanisms (Dowling & Harwood, 1986).

Time's Topology.   Play four octaves up, then four octaves down on the white keys of a piano in 20 seconds, a moderate pace of about 350 ms per keypress. Or play CDCDCD . . . . CD at the same rate for 20 sec. Subjectively the four octave scale sounds more interesting and shorter than the repeating sequence of CDs. Dowling and Harwood (1986) give a good discussion of the rubber-ruler aspects of musical time. If the pace of a piece is tied directly to the clock it moves in ontological time. A composer or performer can alter the pace of a piece so that its apparent (virtual) time is slower or faster than clock time. Most of Telemann's music appears to move regularly, obeying ontological time. In music where key, intensity, melody, rhythm, complexity, and change of pace are made to contrast strongly, virtual time controls, as in North Indian music (Jairazbhoy, 1971) and in many of Beethoven's pieces.

Rhythmic Interpretation of Music.   Meter is the most basic organizing level and tells when to accent beats. A beat is a pulse that marks off equal durations, the tempo is rate of pulsing. Duration is the perceptual unit of time which may vary from clock time. A pattern of related durations and accents refers to rhythm. Just as pitch motifs repeat and set up expectancies so do rhythms. Any of meter, rhythm, or tempo can be varied separately from the others.

For a sequence of beats spaced at 600 ms, a listener can detect a change of about 15 ms in spacing, or about 2.5%, whereas the just-noticeable difference for pitch is less than 1%. Musicians have good accuracy in producing steady patterns of beats or of complex rhythms (Monahan, 1984). Both Povel (1981) and Monahan (1984) believe that in music metrical beat patterns are used as cognitive invariants for producing or perceiving precise rhythmic patterns. "Metric structure thus functions as the temporal analog of the pitch scale . . ." (Dowling & Harwood, 1986).

Perception of Rhythmic Patterns.   In the note durations of Western music, close to 90% of their temporal ratios are as 2:1 and, furthermore, the times of the longer notes range between 300 and 900 ms. Asked by Povel (1981) to tap out repetitions of a repeated rhythmic pattern whose intervals varied over ratios of 4:1 to 5:4, his listeners gave copies, which tended strongly to be assimilated by a ratio of 2:1. The task was quite difficult as prototype ratios approached 5:4, and wrong copies tended to be split between ratios of 2:1 and 1:1. With beat structures like 4:4:1, which are not typical of Western music, listeners assimilated the second and third notes to the ratio 2:1. However, when a context was given, both novices and musicians copied accurately and without assimilation.

Povel argues that the listener encodes a rhythmic pattern in a dual schema, a hierarchy of beat schema with rhythmic subschemas. Monahan (1984) showed that in judging similarity of melodies which varied in both temporal and rhythmic contour, listeners could use relative rhythmic information. She suggests that rhythmic subschemas are encoded as rhythmic contour having relative, not absolute, temporal relations and, furthermore, that metric structure is the temporal analog of pitch scale schema whereby relative melodic information is used.

A given melody played with different duration patterns usually does not sound like the same melody. Neither does the same dance rhythm played with different melodies sound like the same rhythm. The opening of Schubert's Symphony No. 8 ("Unfinished") and the opening of a popular television series, "Dragnet" sound very different, yet the pitches are the same! In an experiment on pitch and duration as determinants of musical space (Monahan & Carterette, 1985) asked musicians to rate the similarity of pairs of brief melodies on a 9-point scale. Four melodies and their inversions were played in each of four rhythmic patterns (anapestic, dactylic, iambic, and trochaic) for a total of 1024 pattern pairs. Multidimensional scaling and cluster analysis both showed that at least five dimensions were need for a good accounting of the perceptual space of these melodies. Surprisingly, the major dimensions found were rhythmic (Fig. 5.17): (I) two-element patterns (Iamb and Trochee) from three-element patterns (Anapest and Dactyl); (II) initial-accent patterns (Trochee and Dactyl) from final-

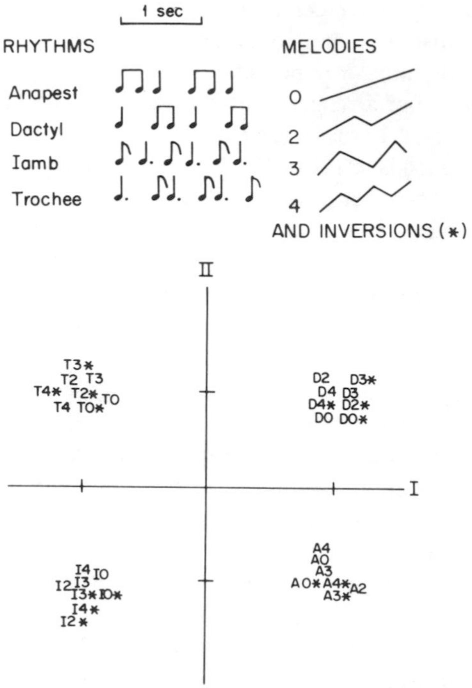

FIG. 5.17. A plot of Dimensions I and II of the best-fitting INDSCAL solution. Dimension I is duple versus triple rhythm, and Dimension II is accent first versus accent last. A given point (e.g., D3) specifies a rhythm and melody. A = anapest, D = dactyl, I = iamb, and T = trochee. The numerals refer to the number of changes in pitch motion. Thus the point D3 is a dactyl rhythm with three changes in the direction of pitch motion. Starred points are inversions. Thus D3* is the inversion of dactylic melody D3.

accent patterns (Iamb and Anapest). In the next ranking dimensions of melodic features surfaced. III sorted out patterns with rising global pitch contours from those with falling pitch contours. And IV ordered pitch contours from uninflected melodies ("0") to highly inflected ("4"). In this study rhythm was more important in determining the responses of the listeners than was pitch patterning.

Music Performance

> We have been, let us say, to hear the latest Pole
> Transmit the Preludes, through his hair and finger-tips.
> —T. S. Eliot (1917), Portrait of a Lady

"To read an orchestra score is like reading at the same time fifteen lines of type, some of which are in different languages" (Peyser, 1987). The great American performer, composer, and conductor Leonard Bernstein had a stunning facility for sight-reading, simultaneous transposition, an an uncanny musical memory, and other unteachable techniques. What skills lie under such expert performing?

The first step in performing is sight-reading a musical score. Next, many rehearsals of the score lead to better performance. The final stage of the expert is polished performance. Some experts can totally memorize a score. Sight-reading a musical score differs from sight-reading a written text. For one thing, score reading is not taught so widely or with the same rigor as book reading. And it is usually enough to know the gist or meaning of a text, but the reading of music is tied to complex responses that must be reasonably true to the score.

Sight-Reading a Musical Score.   An expert reads a book by a series of brief fixations of about 250 msec in rapid sweeping saccades of about 50 msec. Not all sweeps are left-right, but vertical and horizontal leaps and retracings are common. There is evidence that rather immediate cognitive control of reading guides fixations to salient features and away from (often) redundant words like *the*. Cognitive requirements of the reader and linguistic aspects of the text interact in reading.

Reading a musical score is similar to reading a book. Consider piano reading. A piano reader can't read both staves at once (Fig. 5.18). One strategy would be to read down, sweep right and up, and so on. Another would be to sweep across the top stave, down and left to the beginning of the second stave, then across, and so on. Experiments (Weaver, 1943) show that the nature of the music governs the sequence of eye fixations. Fixations in chordal music follow the first, or sawtooth pattern, whereas fixations in contrapuntal music (two or more melodic lines) follows the second, or Greek frieze pattern.

A fixation is useful in sight-reading because it gives to the reader a preview of the structural elements of a text which are then organized in fluent, skilled performance. If a touch-typist is given a preview of no more than the next eight characters, his performance is equal to that with an unlimited preview, or about 600 characters a minute (Shaffer, 1976). There may be two qualitatively differ-

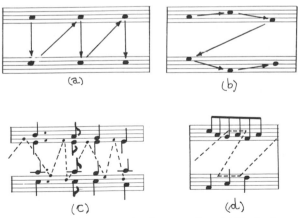

FIG. 5.18.   Fixation sequences in piano reading. (a) Vertical sequence. (b) Horizontal sequence. (c) An example of an actual fixation sequence in chordal piano music. (d) An example of an actual fixation sequence in contrapuntal piano music. Both (c) and (d) are taken from Weaver (1943), and adapted from Sloboda (1985).

ent regions in visual search, a decision region, and a preview region of about six and eight letters, respectively (Rayner & Fisher, 1987).

No one appears to have manipulated musical preview, for technical reasons. However, Sloboda (1974, 1977) found that instrumentalists reading one-line melodies could produce up to seven correct notes after the score was removed. Thus about seven consecutive notes are sufficient to organize a fluent performance. This span length appeared to shrink or stretch when phrase boundary occurred just before or just after an average span. Apparently the musical unit, call it "musit," is something less than a phrase, which is typically longer than 7 notes. Also, the size of a musit depends on the musical context. Musits become shorter if normal harmonic progression is lacking or if rhythmic divisions between phrases are cluttered by passing notes. And poor readers have musits only half the size of good readers. In short, musit size depends on phrasal rhythms and harmony, and on expertise.

Sloboda (1985) suggests that musits are not very much like words; there is no received lexicon of musical patterns, though recurrent scales, pitch movements, and rhythms come to be recognized. Even so the musician must have some general strategy for organizing groups of notes. A good candidate strategy is a metrical unit, or frame. "The same frame can be applied to any metrically regular piece of music, bar by bar" (p. 73). This notion explains variable musit length: ". . . take the bar as the performance unit, unless it contains more than seven notes, in which case take the half-bar" (p. 73). Sloboda's metrical frame is consistent with the view that the prime difficulty in sight-reading is rhythm more often than notes (Newman, 1974).

Misprints occur in scores but are more likely to be played by the novice than by the expert. The latter fails to see the misprint because he plays the musically *correct.* Sloboda (1976) altered certain notes by one pitch step in contexts where such errors were inappropriate. Sight-readers showed the proofreader's error by playing some notes as they should be played, even though noticing some notational errors. As readers do with words, the players restored alterations in the middle more often than at the beginning or end of phrases. From this, Sloboda argues that attention is guided by phrase boundaries. Furthermore, on a second playing the proportion of proofreader's errors increased, which suggests that as a player discerns the structure of a piece she is more likely to infer the expected notes.

In other experiments Sloboda (1976, 1978) showed short runs of notes for brief times and asked both nonmusicians and musicians to record the notes on a music stave. At exposures of less than 100 ms neither group got more than one note right. But when forced to guess, musicians recorded better approximations to contour than did nonmusicians. Accuracy increased as exposure duration increased. Musicians were able to record six correct notes from a single flash, whereas the nonmusician recorded only three correct notes. Musicians are able to code and store notes as music whereas nonmusicians must code and store the notes as visual patterns.

Halpern and Bower (1982) found that musicians performed better with *good* than with bad melodies, whereas nonmusicians did no better with one type than with the other. Sloboda (1985) suggests that structure "is not the whole story" because in the experiments of Chase and Simon (1973), masters reproduced *bad* chess positions as poorly as novices. Actually, both experts and novices were superior to masters in reproducing random chess positions. I suggest that the inferior performance by masters arises from inference to a position, a case of the proofreader's error.

Conveying Expressiveness. Without expressiveness a master sight-reader would be of no more interest than a computer program. A master pianist varies expressiveness within even a new piece and these variations are similar on successive playings of the piece. What are her *rules?* A pattern which is repeated with rising or falling pitch may mark an ensuing climax or relaxing to which the pianist responds by an increase or decrease in keypress force. She must notice and remember such markers over a large scale. Variations within a bar are only loosely tied to the large-scale structure. Sloboda (1983) asked masters to play two versions of a short melody embedded in other melodies. The two were identical except for notated stress, but the two performances were significantly different, as shown by analysis of timing and intensity. A (not notated) "half-bar" effect guided expressiveness which showed up in the playing as accent, slurring, and tenuto (sustaining) of notes. Sloboda suggests that these devices are cued rapidly and almost automatically because they are used on the first reading. And different performers use different mixes of devices and in this way each shows her style.

Nakamura (1987) showed that performers communicate their intentions fairly well. If a crescendo was intended and intensity was gradually increased, most listeners recognized the crescendo. Perception of crescendo was enhanced by rising pitch whereas perception of decresendo was enhanced by falling pitch. Crescendo was easier to play and to recognize than decrescendo. Though dynamics marks (p and f) mean relative, not fixed, intensity levels, a performer's intent to observe the marks was conveyed fairly well to the listeners. Nakamura suggests that her findings imply a context which is common to playing and listening.

A violinist (Mariko Senju) played a concerto with the aim of conveying to an audience 10 different nuances set by expression words: weak, powerful, bright, sad, sophisticated, beautiful, dreamy, fashionable, simple, and deep (Senju & Ohgushi, 1987). Listeners rated each nuance by on each expression. A multidimensional scaling analysis of the data revealed that on the whole the player's intention and the listener's impression were in general agreement.

How does the expert assign expressive variation? First, a mental map of the music is made from features to be marked. A four-beat bar is subdivided. A pattern repeats at higher pitches (so play more loudly) or at lower pitches (an echo, so play more softly). Second, the player develops a lexicon of expressive variations. Some are based on auditory grouping mechanisms which belong to every listener, such as interval consonance, loudness, or accent. Others are set by the culture, for example, a resolution (final cadence) is signaled by a slowing, possibly with crescendo. Third, motor programming is set up. This is a sequence of commands which tells the muscles how to embody in the sound the expressive devices of the lexicon. Two features are of concern here. One is that elementary sequential acts overlap variably in time—a finger must be ready to play the $n+1$ note in an arpeggio but has no time for a cue from the nth note. Another is that the goal of playing a given note at a set loudness may be achieved by many different movements, and these depend on the hand position before and the hand position to follow. Thus we are forced, says Sloboda (1985) to realize "performance is the result of an interaction between a mental *plan* which specifies features of the intended output and a flexible programming system" (p. 89).

This conception implies that a mental plan is separate from the motor program which is to execute it, and helps to explain a number of aspects of playing and listening. A performer can know how a passage should sound but be unable to play it correctly—the plan is fine but the program is not. A pupil swears that he played a passage but the teacher swears he did not. This is because the teacher monitored the output (program) whereas the pupil monitored his mental plan. And, if one wants to attain a high degree of musical skill it is necessary both to listen and analyze a great deal of music and to practice one's instrument in a systematic way over a very long time.

Rehearsal: It Takes More Than Practice to Make Perfect.   "Play it again, Sam!"   "Once more now—from the top!" Sloboda (1985) points out that not much is known about how much or what kind of rehearsal is done by masters, yet practice is what they do most of. Expert teachers and masters agree on at least three points. First, productive rehearsal requires the dissection of problem passages. Second, a master's knowledge of a piece allows entry at any point, whereas a lesser player can enter at only certain points. The master's assured knowledge of a musical rests on having multiple mappings of it so that the piece can be written out from memory or mentally sight-read through. Third, there is a learning-to-learn effect. The rehearsal of one piece now lessens the need for rehearsal on other pieces later.

The rehearsal of musicians has not been well studied. Sloboda (1985) cites in some detail a study by Gruson (1981). She found that the greatest portions of total practice time were taken up by (a) uninterruped playing, 25%; (b) repetition of a single note, 17%; (c) repetition of a bar, 17%; and (d) errors, 14%. Repetitions of sequences larger than a bar accounted for less than 3% of the time, and playing with hands separately only 1% of the time. There were 40 piano students in Gruson's study covering 10 levels from beginner to proficient amateur; each level adds about 1 year of instruction. Gruson correlated skill levels against incidence in the categories of piano rehearsal. Correlated significantly and positively with skill were (a) repetition of sections larger than a bar; (b) playing hands separately; (c) self-guiding verbalizations; and (d) time spent actually practicing a piece. And correlated significantly and negatively with skill were (a) errors; (b) repeating single notes; and (c) pauses of longer than two seconds. Gruson concludes that the achieving of expert performance takes thousands of hours of practice spread over a wide variety of pieces.

The Musical Performance of Experts.   Composers almost always start out as performers, and expert performers are almost always skilled sight-readers. A flawless, fluent, expressive rendition of a piece of music obviously demands the integration of separate skills. Timing, meter, rhythm, and correct fingering are subskills of playing any instrument. Some instruments have special demands, e.g., the oboist must maintain tone quality over a large dynamic range, tongue easily and quickly, control breath, keep a relaxed embochure, and control vibrato ("the soul of the sound") (Goosens & Roxburgh, 1977). As Sloboda (1985) points out, an expert sustains these skills in the service of the whole piece. Each subskill requires attention but the attentional resources are limited. Has "Somehow, the expert . . . managed to escape these limits"? Only in the sense that each skill has become more automatic, requiring less attention.

How does the expert make automatic each of the subskills? First some of the skills she learns are general and arise from increasing musical knowledge. Highly useful and often indispensable is memorization, a skill which is based on an ability to encode by structures and groupings. A present pattern can be related to an earlier or familiar pattern. Bernstein was asked to play the piano part in a blind orchestral score. He saw a tune in the woodwinds that he had learned to recognize in grammar school by a bit of doggerel and so knew at once that it was The Academic Festival Overture of Brahms (Peyser, 1987). A new pattern may be no more than a transposition of an old or a simple change in fingering. In brief, "effective musical memory familiar depends on the ability to represent music in terms of groupings of notes which can be related to familiar stylistic patterns and structures, and also to other sequences within the same piece" (Sloboda, 1985, p. 95).

When the subskills have all become nearly automatic, attention can be devoted to expression, interpretation, and nuance. Finally, the fingers seem to walk unaided through the landscape of the music. New, strange, or difficult music becomes easier to play because the performer has implicit heuristic fingering rules. Because what has been memorized is a plan, the fingering may differ in two performances. Many pieces may be in memory and yet a new piece can be mastered quickly because only the new information is learned and put into a plan to be guided by general musical knowledge. Variability may (and does) arise in performance partly because plans are incomplete and partly because the expert chooses to emphasize a particular parameter (legato, sustenato, speed, or intensity), especially when a pattern is ambiguous.

Finally, the expert performer has a grasp of the whole musical structure, and knows its architecture which she reveals in the consistency of playing and the control over speed and dynamics. In short: The expert performer on any instrument knows the larger picture in terms of patterns and hierarchical groupings. She has flexible and automatic control over local events. She can monitor her playing and change it by means of an error-correcting feedback control system.

You can now understand better what makes Ms Luisa de Larrocha play like an angel.

Development of the Perception of Musical Patterns

Infants' Perception of Musical Patterns. Asking an infant questions about music takes time and patience and the right probe. Studies of very young infants can use surprise as shown by heart rate. If a melody repeats, the heart rate settles down to a steady rate (no surprise). If that melody continues, no further decrease in heart rate is seen but if a new melody is heard, the heart rate increases again (surprise!). Though tedious, the surprise or startle method works. Another method that can be used with infants aged 6 months or older is to train the infant to turn her head toward a comparison sound (melody) if it is different from a repeating sound. It is inferred from change in heart rate or head turn that the comparison melody differs in some way from the repeating melody.

Adults recognize a familiar melody mainly on the basis of intervals, or the relations between notes, and an unfamiliar melody from melodic contour. How does an infant deal with melodies? Trehub (1987) reviews her own and other work in answering this question. The musical material consisted of transformed six-tone melodies: (a) transposition, wherein both interval and contour were preserved; (b) alteration which preserved contour; and (c) alteration which violated contour. At retention intervals less than a second infants detected all transformations. This suggests that infants perceive exact pitch cues, which suffice for all of these detections. But for retention intervals between about 3 and 15 sec, the infants detected only alterations which violated contour. Thus at short retention intervals, infants behave as adults and children do with familiar melodies, that is, as if they encoded interval relations between notes. And at longer retention intervals, infants behave as do adults with unfamiliar melodies, that is, as if they encoded contour.

In other experiments (Trehub, 1987), it was found that infants categorize tone sequences by using global, relational properties, the most salient being contour. Indeed, it turns out that infants are able to detect directional pitch changes of a semitone, which is the smallest interval of relevance in Western music. This evidence that an infant has an abstract image of the contour of a musical pattern is echoed by findings on the role of pitch contours in speech perception and production.

Adults and even 6-year-olds detect semitone changes in brief melodies but as melodies diverge from diatonic structure so do errors increase. Do infants, ignorant of our diatonic tradition, perform in this way? The answer is a bit complicated. Infants can detect deviations from diatonic structure, but less well than young children. Trehub, Bull, and Thorpe (1984) suggest that infants do have innate skills which facilitate the mental mapping of our Western, tonal music. The major triad with its simple ratios of 4:5:6 may be especially salient because it induces neurally a bass fundamental or periodicity pitch (Moore, 1982; Rameau, 1722). It is surely the case that the human auditory system, and perceptual and cognitive needs led to the invention of tonal music and its forms.

Rhythm, Meter and Streaming: Motion in Time.   Given a temporal row of sounds, an adult feels compelled to subgroup the elements of the row by frequency or duration or intensity or timbre, and will do so whether the elements are tones, clicks, thumps, or groans. Subgroups appear to be temporally cohesive. If an infinite train of equally spaced clicks changes in timbre after every kth click, the durations between clicks within a timbre will appear shorter than the durations between clicks of different timbre. It is likely that temporal grouping exists in infancy for the crucial role that it plays in organizing sensory and cognitive structures, particularly speech and memory.

Work of Trehub, Bull, and Thorpe (1984) showed that infants grouped melodies into rhythmic patterns even though notes and internote durations were equal. The infants were able to use similarities of frequency or of timbre. For example, infants detected the disparity in six-note sequences like TTTSSS where T is a sawtooth and S a sinusoid waveform, both at 440 Hz. Since T has many harmonics and S has none, harmonic structure (timbre) is the basis of the infant's detection in this case.

Eimas and Miller (1980) showed that overall syllable duration affects an infant's perception of the duration of formant transitions of speech. If alterations in the timing of multitone sequences are made, children, like adults, find the alterations to be hard to detect when overall group structure is kept (Trehub, 1984). Also, infants can tell simple rhythms apart over a range of tempi (e.g., uus vs. suu, where s = stressed, u = unstressed); and simple temporal patterns apart (– – vs. — -) over a range of tempi (Thorpe, Trehub, & Cohen, 1986). Thus, infants have a general ability to encode relations in temporal patterns no matter what the durations, which parallels their ability to encode the pitch contours of melodies.

A sequence of alternating high and low tones splits into two lines for infants (stress segregation) (Demany, 1982). Infants cannot track ordered elements across streams at rates that allow the ordering of elements within streams. In these two aspects they behave like adults (Demany, 1982), which implies that pitch proximity is what holds melodies together just as it does for adults.

In short, infants are able to perceive elementary melody and rhythm much as adults perceive them. Infants are blessed with skills by means of which they can represent the tonal and temporal scales of Western music, and probably of all the world's music.

Musical Learning and Development.   Taking account of extensive observations of Moog (1979b) as well as his own, Sloboda (1985) detects four main strands in a child's musical development between ages 1 and 5: (1) Imitation increases in the order, words, melodic fragments, whole songs; (2) Free note-play is bent by musical culture; diatonic intervals appear, then phrases from well-known songs and then precise imitation; (3) Skill grows in being able to organize songs by tonal and metrical rules; (4) Implicit knowledge of harmony and meter is not easily used in perception or judgment tasks in that, e.g., beating time to music is not reliable and gross dissonance may not be noticed.

Musical development from 5- to 10-years-of-age shows up mainly as an increasing ability of the child to be able to deal explicitly with implicit skills and knowledge. Thus, a 5-year-old can change speed or pitch in singing, but does not make good perceptual judgments about what she does easily. Sloboda (1985) reports trends as assessed by perceptual tests. Gross dissonances (in hymn harmony) were noticed at 5, and more subtle dissonances (as in single chords) at 7. Only at about age 11 did the child near an adult's ability to detect violations of normal sequential structure, such as in musically ordered sequences of chords. Sloboda (1985) noted that girls did better than boys on most tests and at most ages. Because music lessons made no difference on test scores, Sloboda feels strongly that the tested skills are "true products of enculturation" (p. 213).

At 6-years-of-age, the child compares one musical piece with another in direct sensory terms but at age 14 the child compares two pieces using many dimensions and at many levels (Gardner, 1973). The 6-year-old's base similarity judgments on pitch, intensity, or speed. Eight-year-olds could explain judgments in (nonmusical) terms like "happy" or "like a funeral." At 14 a young person can tell pieces apart by complex aspects of style, instrument, period, composer, or idiom, using terms like "baroque," "jazzy," or even "sonata form" and "duple meter."

Neuropsychological Aspects of Music

"The optimistic view of classical neurology that musical functions are clearly localized has not been verified" (Marin, 1982, p. 469).

A common finding in neurological disorders is that of dissociation of functions. For example, a severe blow to the head may render a person aphasic: She cannot speak at all but has no trouble in writing or reading books and can sight play a Chopin etude. A brilliant mathematician struck in mid life by Alzheimer's disease may not know the day or date and cannot tell time from an analog clock. Yet she can read her digital watch. If asked whether cosine x is a transcendental function, she says "yes," smiling brightly. Deep and automatic skills resist decay.

Amusia.   Aphasia is an impairment in receiving or manipulating or expressing the symbolic content of language owing to brain damage (Walsh, 1978). Amusia is an acquired clinical disorder which involves musical cognition or performance. Almost any possible mix of sensory, perceptual, cognitive, and motor disorders has been reported as can be seen in Marin's (1982) review of neurological aspects of music perception and performance. There can be amusia with aphasia, amusia without aphasia, and aphasia without amusia. It is hard to tell how much amusia and aphasia are dissociated owing to problems of method, case selection, assessment, and defining criteria. Theories of brain laterality confuse the issue as well.

If aphasia and amusia are strongly linked clinically, strong inferences can be drawn about the locus in the brain of musical functions since language and speech are very strongly lateralized, mainly in the left cerebral hemisphere. Amusia and aphasia often do go together as is to be expected of cognitive, information processing skills. However, care must be taken not to confuse sensory-perceptual effects with symbolic language effects. A close look at clinical cases suggests that amusia and aphasia can be dissociated. In one well-known case (Wertheim & Botez, 1961) a violinist who suffered a sensori-motor right hemiparesis and a receptive aphasia had impaired musical skills. He was able to deal well with perception of pitch, chord, timbre, rhythm, and melody. Whereas musical symbols and isolated notes could be read, he did not understand these, could not read sequential music, played badly, and was poor at recognizing composers, pieces or styles. There have been amusiacs who could neither read nor recognize music but who could sing well-known melodies and lyrics or play pieces spontaneously. In short, musical functions may be intact at the perceptual level but deranged at the level of identifying and naming.

There are many cases of speechless aphasiacs who could sing with words. As Marin (1982) emphasizes, an inability to initiate new cognitive tasks yet in contrast being able to run off automatic skills is the hallmark of neurological disorder. For example, an aphasiac who could play melodies on his violin but not on the less familiar piano is cited as a parallel to the finding in language that a complex skill is spared but a simpler one is lost. The paradox disappears if expert performance depends on highly automatized motor schemas that run off without loading selective attention (see the section on Performance).

In comparing amusia and aphasia it becomes clear at once that great care must be taken in concluding that the two are similar or depend on the same neural substrates. Musical alexia is different from verbal alexia at least because they differ in symbol systems and semantic referents, and probably they also differ in visuospatial functions. Errors in the sequential ordering of music may be interpreted in two or more ways. Do they arise from the same source as do syntactic word order errors of aphasia, or from the difficulty of selective attention owing to a spatial visual derangement?

Aphasia without Amusia and Conversely. Cases exist of musicians with aphasia but whose musical abilities did not appear to be affected (Marin, 1982). One aphasiac was a composer and professor of music who had severe sensory aphasia from a stroke. He continued to compose new works which were judged by musical peers to be of excellent quality. From this and a number of other cases it must be inferred that musical functions do not depend on neural structures which, when damaged, bring about aphasia. And, conversely, clinical cases exist of amusia with no aphasia. Mainly musical memory, discrimination or perception were affected, and lesions tended to be in the right temporal brain regions. However, a careful study of 26 patients (Dorgeuille, 1966, cited in Marin, 1982), of whom about two-thirds were amusiacs, led to no definitive relation between lesion site and the behavioral defect. Lesions were on both sides, mainly in anterior temporal lobes.

Auditory Perceptual Defects.   Sensory, or receptive, aphasia is produced by lesions in the auditory association cortex of the left side. Acoustic agnosia, associated with lesions of the right hemisphere or of both hemispheres (especially temporal cortex; Marin, 1982) is an inability to distinguish nonverbal sounds. A person who is afflicted with acoustic agnosia hears external sounds as confused or loud or noisy and may hear illusory sounds or voices. Generally, acoustic agnosiacs discriminate time or rhythm poorly, cannot tell or reproduce rhythmic patterns, and are "usually hopelessly defective" in recognizing timbre and complex sounds (Marin, 1982). This syndrome has not been studied well enough to point up its musical aspects. Marin (1982) reviews the bewildering evidence and suggests that as the number of levels of analysis increase, there is a shift toward specialized laterality of the perceptual apparatus.

So, simple sound analysis is bilateral, but phonetic analysis of speech features is lateralized, which accounts for a patient's hearing sounds but not words. Words, syntax, and meaning require more processing at more levels, and schemas which are organized in hierarchies appear. As musical functions move toward schemas such as themes, motifs, complex harmonies, rhythmic patterns, and structured forms, so should varieties of amusia resemble the disorders of cognitive processing. But keep firmly in mind that most music is heard for pleasure in the moment. Most musical responses are more emotional and perceptual than cognitive, involve short-term memory, require little in the way of processing, and make light demands on the allocation of attention.

Brain Structures and Musical Functions.   Marin (1982) gives an informative, readable review of the relation between localizations of brain lesions and disorders of musical performance and perception. Generally, sensory and perceptual disorders involve temporal lobe lesions in either hemisphere. Sensory amusia without aphasia tends to go with lesions on the right side. When aphasia and amusia are mixed and amusia ranges from perceptual to symbolic, lesions tend to be on the left side. Expressive amusia is a complex disorder and shows no strong association with locus of lesion. Lesions are typically on the left side when musical disorders are of schemas involving temporal order or language or vocalization.

Beware the belief that deranged perception of music goes with lesions on the right but deranged expression of music goes with lesions on the left side of the brain. As the operations of perceiving or expressing specialize, function tends to laterality as does the loci of the neural substrates. It can be said broadly that wholistic functions of music and language tend to a preferred side (usually the left) whereas operational functions of music and language tend to a preferred side (usually the right) (Bever, 1980). Though brain function and laterality have much biological fixedness, lateralization is fluid in infancy and childhood, can be altered by lesions, and varies among individuals (Lenneberg, 1967; Marin, 1976).

The traditional clinical types of disorders of musical functions are too broad, says Marin (1982), who suggests a way out of assigning a category name to symptoms of different levels of complexity. Using principles of neuropsychology, and the psychology of language and music, he orders musical defects in 6 levels: (1) acoustical-psychophysical; (2) precategorical perception; (3) categorical perception; (4) perception of musical schemas; (5) symbolic musical processes; and (6) the learning of musical perceptual or executive functions. As an example, level (1) includes disorders in the perceiving of intensity, pitch, onset or offset of sound, etc. Problems such as note naming, and identifying or naming intervals, chords, and rhythms belong to level (5). Highest level (6) disorders include those like recognizing style, composers or musical form, and dealing with transforms of melodic or rhythmic themes and hierarchies.

REFERENCES

American Standards Association (1960). *Acoustical terminology*, S1.1.

Backus, J. (1969). *The acoustical foundations of music*. New York: W. W. Norton.

Balzano, G. J. (1980). The group-theoretic description of 12-fold and microtonal pitch systems. *Computer Music Journal, 4*, 66–84.

Bartlett, F. C. (1932). *Remembering*. Cambridge, England: Cambridge University Press.

Bartlett, J. C., & Dowling, W. J. (1980). The recognition of transposed melodies. *Journal of Experimental Psychology: Human Perception & Performance, 6*, 501–515.

Bever, T. (1980). Broca and Lashley were right: Cerebral dominance is an accident of growth. In D. Caplan (Ed.), *Biological studies of mental processes*. Cambridge, MA: MIT Press.

Bregman, A. S., & Dannenbring, G. L. (1973). The effect of continuity on auditory stream segregation. *Perception & Psychophysics, 13*, 308–312.

Carlsen, J. C. (1981). Some factors which influence melodic expectancy. *Psychomusicology, 1*, 12–29.

Carterette, E. C., Monahan, C. B., Holman, E., Bell, T., & Fiske, R. A. (1982). Rhythmic and melodic structures in perceptual space. *Journal of the Acoustical Society of America, 72*, S11.

Chase, W. G., & Simon, H. A. (1973). The mind's eye in chess. In W. G. Chase (Ed.), *Visual information processing*. New York: Academic Press.

Cherry, E. C. (1953). Some experiments on the recognition of speech with one and with two ears. *Journal of the Acoustical Society of America, 25*, 975–979.

Chomsky, N. (1956). *Syntactic structures*. The Hague: Mouton.

Cooke, D. (1959). *The language of music*. London: Oxford University Press.

Demany, L. (1982). Auditory stream segregation in infancy. *Infant Behavior & Development, 5,* 261–276.

Descartes, R. (1955). *Philosophical works.* (E. S. Haldane & G. R. T. Ross Translators). (2 Vols.). New York: Dover.

Deutsch, D. (1975). Musical illusions. *Scientific American, 233,* 92–104.

Deutsch, D. (Ed.). (1980). *The psychology of music.* New York: Academic Press.

Dowling, W. J. (1973). The perception of interleaved melodies. *Cognitive Psychology, 5,* 322–337.

Dowling, W. J. (1978). Scale and contour: Two components of a theory of memory for melodies. *Psychological Review, 85,* 341–354.

Dowling, W. J. (1984). Development of musical schemata in children's spontaneous singing. In W. R. Crozier & A. J. Chapman (Eds.), *Cognitive processes in the perception of art* (pp. 145–163). Amsterdam: North Holland.

Dowling, W. J., & Bartlett, J. C. (1981). The importance of interval information in long-term memory for melodies. *Psychomusicology, 1,* 30–49.

Dowling, W. J., & Fujitani, D. S. (1971). Contour, interval, and pitch recognition in memory for melodies. *Journal of the Acoustical Society of America, 49,* 524–531.

Dowling, W. J., & Harwood, D. L. (1986). *Music cognition.* New York: Academic Press.

Eimas, P. D., & Miller, J. L. (1980). Contextual effects in infant speech perception. *Science, 209,* 1140–1141.

Einstein, A. (1954). *A short history of music* (4th American Ed.). New York: Vintage Books.

Fechner, G. H. (1860). *Elemente der Psychophysik* (Vol. 1, 2d Ed.). Leipzig: Breitkopf und Haertel.

Fletcher, H., & Munson, W. A. (1933). Loudness, its definition, measurement, and calculation. *Journal of the Acoustical Society of America, 5,* 82–108.

Fraisse, P. (1978). Time and rhythm perception. In E. C. Carterette & M. P. Friedman (Eds.), *Handbook of perception* (Vol. 8, pp. 203–254). New York: Academic Press.

Fraisse, P (1982). Rhythm and tempo. In D. Deutsch (Ed.), *The psychology of music* (pp. 149–180). New York: Academic Press.

Gardner, H. (1973). Children's sensitivity to musical styles. *Merrill-Palmer Quarterly of Behavioral Development, 19,* 67–77.

Goosens, L., & Roxburgh, E. (1980). *Oboe* (2d Ed.). London: Macdonald.

Gordon, J. W., & Grey, J. M. (1978). Perception of spectral modifications on orchestral instrument tones. *Computer Music Journal, 2,* 24–31.

Green, D. M., & Swets, J. A. (1966). *Signal detection theory and psychophysics.* New York: Wiley.

Grey, J. M. (1977). Multidimensional perceptual scaling of musical timbres. *Journal of the Acoustical Society of America, 61,* 1270–1277.

Grey, J. M., & Gordon, J. W. (1978). Perceptual effects of spectral modifications on musical timbres. *Journal of the Acoustical Society of America, 63,* 1493–1500.

Halpern, A. R., & Bower, G. H. (1982). Musical expertise and melodic structure in memory for musical notation. *American Journal of Psychology, 95,* 31–50.

Handel, S., & Lawson, G. R. (1983). The contextual nature of rhythmic interpretation. *Perception & Psychophysics, 34,* 103–120.

Helmholtz, H. von (1877). *On the sensations of tone.* (A. J. Ellis, Trans.). New York: Dover (1954 reprint).

Jairazbhoy, N. A. (1971). *The rags of North Indian Music: Their structure and evolution.* Middletown, CT: Wesleyan University Press.

James, W. (1890). *The principles of psychology,* (Vol 1). New York: Holt.

Kendall, R. A. (1986). The role of acoustic signal partitions in listener categorization of musical phrases. *Music Perception, 4,* 185–213.

Kendall, R. A. (1987). Model building in music cognition and artificial intelligence. *Proceedings of the 1st Annual Artificial Intelligence and Advanced Computing Conference,* East Wheaton, IL: Tower Conference Management, 183–196.

Krumhansl, C. L. (1979). The psychological representation of musical pitch in a tonal context. *Cognitive Psychology, 11*, 346–374.

Krumhansl, C. L., & Shepard, R. N. (1979). Quantification of the hiearchy of tonal functions within a diatonic context. *Journal of Experimental Psychology: Human Perception & Performance, 5*, 579–594.

LaBerge (1981). Perceptual and motor schemas in the performance of musical pitch. In *Documentary report of the Ann Arbor Symposium*. Reston, VA: Music Educators National Conference, pp. 179–196.

Lehrdahl, F., & Jackendoff, R. (1983). *A generative theory of tonal music*. Cambridge, MA: MIT Press.

Lenneberg, E. H. (1967). *Biological foundations of language*. New York: Wiley.

Longuet-Higgins, H. C. (1976). The perception of melodies. *Nature, 263*, 646–653.

Longuet-Higgins, H. C., & Lee, C. S. (1984). The rhythmic interpretation of monophonic music. *Music Perception, 1*, 424–441.

Marin, O. S. M. (1976). Neurobiology of language: An overview. *Annals of the New York Academy of Sciences, 280*, 900–912.

Marin, O. S. M. (1982). Neurological aspects of music perception and performance. In D. Deutsch (Ed.), *The psychology of music*. New York: Academic Press.

Miller, J. R., & Carterette, E. C. (1975). Perceptual space for musical structures. *Journal of the Acoustical Society of America, 58*, 711–720.

Moog, H. (1976). *The musical experience of the pre-school child* (C. Clarke, Trans.). London: Schott.

Moore, B. C. J. (1982). *The psychology of hearing* (2d Ed.). New York: Academic Press.

Monahan, C. B. (1984). *Parallels between pitch and time: The determinants of musical space*. Unpublished doctoral dissertation, University of California, Los Angeles.

Monahan, C. B., & Carterette, E. C. (1985). Pitch and duration as determinants of musical space. *Music Perception, 3*, 1–32.

Monahan, C. B., Kendall, R. A., & Carterette, E. C. (1987). The effect of melodic and temporal contour on recognition memory for pitch change. *Perception & Psychophysics, 41*, 576–600.

Nakamura, T. (1987). The communication of dynamics between musicians and listeners through musical performance. *Perception & Psychophysics, 41*, 525–533.

Needham, J. (1962). *Science and civilisation in China* (Vol 4, Part 1). Cambridge, England: Cambridge University Press.

New Grove Dictionary of Music and Musicians (1980). London: Macmillan.

Newman, W. S. (1974/1984). *The pianist's problems*. New York: Da Capo Press. [Unabridged republication of the 3d expanded edition (New York: Harper & Row, 1974) supplemented with a new preface and author's corrections.]

Newman, W. S. (1984). *The pianist's problems*, (4th Ed.). New York: Da Capo Press.

Peyser, J. (1987). *Bernstein: A biography*. New York: William Morrow.

Pierce, J. R. (1983). *The science of musical sound*. New York: Scientific American Books.

Pitt, M. A., & Monahan, C. B. (1987). The perceived similarity of auditory polyrhythms. *Perception & Psychophysics, 41*, 534–546.

Plomp, R. (1976). *Aspects of tone sensation*. New York: Academic Press.

Povel, D.-J. (1981). The internal representation of simple temporal patterns. *Journal of Experimental Psychology: Human Perception & Performance, 7*, 3–18.

Rameau, J.-P. (1772). *Treatise on harmony*. New York: Dover (reprint, 1971).

Randel, D. (1986). *The new Harvard dictionary of music*. Cambridge, MA: Harvard University Press.

Rayner, K., & Fisher, D. L. (1987). Letter processing during eye fixations in visual search. *Perception & Psychophysics, 42*, 87–100.

Restle, F. (1970). Theories of serial pattern learning: Structural trees. *Psychological Review, 77,* 481–495.

Roederer, J. G. (1974). *Introduction to the physics and psychophysics of music.* New York: Springer-Verlag.

Schencker, H. (1906/1954). *Harmony* (O. Jones, Editor; E. M. Borgese, Translator). Chicago: University of Chicago Press. [Reprinted, Cambridge, MA: MIT Press.]

Seashore, C. E. (1938). *Psychology of music.* New York: McGraw-Hill.

Senju, M., & Ohgushi, K. (1987). How are the player's ideas conveyed to the audience? *Music Perception, 4,* 311–323.

Shaffer, L. H. (1976). Intention and performance. *Psychological Review, 83,* 375–393.

Shepard, R. N. (1980). Multidimensional scaling, tree-fitting, and clustering. *Science, 210,* 390–398.

Shepard, R. N. (1987). Toward a universal law of generalization for psychological science. *Science, 237,* 1317–1323.

Slawson, A. W. (1968). Vowel quality and musical timbre as functions of spectrum envelope and fundamental frequency. *Journal of the Acoustical Society of America, 43,* 87–101.

Sloboda, J. A. (1974). The eye-hand span. An approach to the study of sight reading. *Psychology of Music, 2,* 4–10.

Sloboda, J. A. (1976). The effect of item position on the likelihood of identification by inference in prose reading and music reading. *Canadian Journal of Psychology, 30,* 228–236.

Sloboda, J. A. (1977). Phrase units as determinants of visual processing in music reading. *British Journal of Psychology, 68,* 117–124.

Sloboda, J. A. (1978). Perception of contour in music reading. *Perception, 6,* 323–331.

Sloboda, J. A. (1983). The communication of musical metre in piano performance. *Quarterly Journal of Experimental Psychology, 35,* 377–396.

Sloboda, J. A. (1985). *The musical mind: The cognitive psychology of music.* Oxford: The Clarendon Press.

Sundberg, J. (1982). Perception of singing. In D. Deutsch (Ed.), *The psychology of music* (pp. 59–98). New York: Academic Press.

Sundberg, J., & Lindblom, B. (1976). Generative theories in language and music descriptions. *Cognition, 4,* 99–122.

Thorpe, L. A., Trehub, S. E., & Cohen, A. J. (1986). *Infant's categorization of rhythmic form.* Paper presented at meeting of the Canadian Psychological Association, Toronto.

Trehub, S. E. (1987). Infants' perception of musical patterns. *Perception & Psychophysics, 41,* 635–641.

Trehub, S. E., Bull, D., & Thorpe, L. A. (1984). Infants' perception of melodies: The role of melodic contour. *Child Development, 55,* 821–830.

Tulving, E. (1983). *Elements of episodic memory.* Oxford: The Clarendon Press.

Van Noorden, L. P. A. S. (1975). *Temporal coherence in the perception of tone sequences.* Unpublished doctoral dissertation. Technische Hogeschool Eindhoven, The Netherlands.

Walsh, K. W. (1978). *Neuropsychology: A clinical approach.* Edinburgh: Churchill Livingstone.

Weaver, H. E. (1943). A study of visual processes in reading differently constructed musical selections. *Psychological Monographs, 55,* 1–30.

Wertheim, N., & Botez, M. I. (1961). Receptive amnesia: a clinical analysis. *Brain, 84,* 19–30.

Editor's Comments on Gerhardt

Acoustic pattern recognition is a universal behavioral problem for hearing organisms. Especially for organisms that communicate by sound, from the simplest insect to the most sophisticated of vertebrates, there is an awesome challenge in deciding quickly, efficiently, and accurately which sounds must be attended to because they are essential to survival and which can be ignored. Viewed in this way, it is obvious that acoustic pattern recognition abilities do not arise in a vacuum but rather are intimately tied to an organism's ecology and evolutionary history.

In this chapter, Gerhardt reviews behavioral and physiological studies of acoustic pattern recognition in anuran amphibians. These studies reveal a rich and complex acoustic communication system involving sex differences in perception, ecological correlates, and temperature dependence of both vocal production mechanisms and auditory perceptual mechanisms.

6 Acoustic Pattern Recognition in Anuran Amphibians

H. Carl Gerhardt
University of Missouri, Columbia

INTRODUCTION

My goal is to review acoustic pattern recognition in anuran amphibians. The majority of behavioral studies have exploited natural responses to sounds, and frogs and toads of both sexes usually responded selectively. Playback experiments using synthetic signals have demonstrated that frogs, especially females, can discriminate among acoustic patterns that differ in very subtle ways. This is hardly surprising in view of their natural history. Frogs must often recognize and localize other individuals of the same species against a background generated by many other individuals of the same and of different species. Moreover, the signals of several pairs of species are similar enough to elicit appropriate responses by individuals of both species (Gerhardt, 1982), so that even species recognition is usually not merely a function of audibility.

Although the auditory modality dominates anuran communication systems, behavioral analyses of the general hearing abilities of frogs have been limited because of the resistance of these animals to conditioning. This is perhaps surprising since fish are readily conditioned to respond to sound (e.g., Hawkins, 1981). Simmons and her colleagues (Megela-Simmons, Moss, & Daniel, 1985; Moss & Simmons, 1986) have recently adapted the reflex modification technique originally described by Yerkes (1904) in order to derive audiograms and to estimate masked thresholds of anurans. Although this technique has seldom been used to provide data directly bearing on the discrimination of two or more audible sound patterns, estimates of behavioral thresholds and masked thresholds are comparable with estimates derived from neurophysiological studies and some experiments with unconditioned subjects.

After reviewing specific approaches to hearing and pattern recognition in anurans, I shall review the literature within a parametric framework. That is, I discuss the kinds of physical properties of sounds used to differentiate among different biologically significant classes of acoustic signals, the minimum differences that are discriminated, and the dynamic range in terms of sound pressure level (SPL in decibels [dB] re 20 μ Pa) of discrimination. I shall then indicate how these data are pertinent to current knowledge about sensory mechanisms. I have discussed the evolutionary implications of this work in detail elsewhere (Gerhardt, 1982, 1986, 1987, 1988).

I. EXPERIMENTAL APPROACHES TO SOUND PATTERN RECOGNITION IN ANURANS

Natural Behavior

The courtship pattern of many species of frogs and toads is relatively simple. The male calls at night, usually from a stationary position. The female typically initiates sexual contact with him. Males use the same vocal signals to attract females and to mediate some interactions with other males, sometimes even across species (e.g., Schwartz & Wells, 1984). For this reason, Wells (1977) proposed that the term "advertisement" call be used instead of "mating" call.

In many of the species that have been studied males do not produce calls randomly with respect to the calls of their neighbors. Antiphonal calling is the usual pattern, but in some species males may attempt to synchronize calls, presumably to make it more difficult for predators to locate them (Tuttle & Ryan, 1982). Male anurans of many species also have "aggressive" calls in their repertoires. Aggressive calls are elicited when a neighbor produces advertisement calls that exceed some threshold intensity, related to the distance by which males usually space themselves in a chorus (Wells & Schwartz, 1984).

Whereas the male is both vocal and indiscriminate in that he attempts to mate with most other frogs of comparable size that touch or move near him, the female is usually silent and selective. Moreover, phonotactic behavior can be elicited from gravid females merely by playing back appropriate sounds; visual, olfactory, and tactile cues are thus unnecessary for localization and identification of the male even though they could augment the acoustic information. Mismating has been observed in nature, and females of the green treefrog (*H. cinerea*), which were attracted to a speaker playing back conspecific calls, sometimes attempted to induce amplexus (mating) with a tethered male of another species (Gerhardt, 1982). A female generally does not or cannot dislodge a male that has clasped her. Testimony to this fact is the widespread occurrence of so-called "satellite" males in some species. The male does not call, but situates himself near a calling male and attempts to intercept the female as she moves toward the caller (Perrill,

Gerhardt, & Daniel, 1978; Roble, 1985). This would be a very ineffective strategy if the female could easily dislodge any male that clasped her.

Playback Experiments with Male Frogs

Capranica (1965), in a pioneering study, exploited the vocal responses of a laboratory colony of male bullfrogs to the playbacks of synthetic sounds in order to identify relevant acoustic properties of communication signals. The detection of nonrandom vocal responses to the playbacks of conspecific calls or synthetic calls can be used to estimate "thresholds" of various sorts, even in nature. However, these thresholds are not necessarily equivalent to hearing thresholds because there is no reason to suppose that a male gains anything from calling antiphonally with another male located at some distance from him. That is, the male could hear another male at a distance, but because the competitor's calls would be of such low intensity, they would not interfere acoustically with the male's own calls. Thus, we might expect thresholds derived from natural, unconditioned responses to be higher than thresholds derived from psychophysical and neural data (e.g., Megela-Simmons et al., 1985).

As mentioned earlier, increases in the SPL of a neighbor's call (or an experimenter's playback) may also elicit a switch from advertisement calls to aggressive calls, indicating a higher probability of further aggressive behavior. Estimates of thresholds for the change of call type are available for several species of frogs (e.g., Robertson, 1984).

Playback Experiments with Female Frogs

Behavioral thresholds for phonotactic responses by females have seldom been estimated (Gerhardt, 1976). The main drawback is that phonotaxis depends very much on the reproductive state of the female. Individuals that are not gravid or that have just laid their eggs are unresponsive to playbacks of conspecific advertisement calls, even at fairly high SPLs. The development of hormonal recipes for eliciting phonotactic behavior in nonreproductive females should encourage more studies of phonotactic behavior in single-stimulus presentations (Schmidt, 1985).

Most studies of female frogs have employed the two-stimulus playback design, the so-called "discrimination test" of Littlejohn and Michaud (1959). A gravid female is placed between two loudspeakers, each of which plays back a different sound. The female indicates her preference by moving toward, and usually touching one of the speakers. Unfortunately, the results of many of these tests cannot be compared directly because of differences in the acoustics of the playback environment or because multiple tests of individual females were not documented. Usually, an individual female is tested just once in a given two-stimulus test; the responses of a sample of females constitute the data for testing the null hypothesis of no preference. When females have been tested multiple times, their pattern of choices has usually been similar to the pattern of a sample of females. That is, if, in their initial test, some females responded to one of two alternatives and other females, to the other alternative, then individual females, tested multiple times, did not consistently choose one or the other of the alternatives. As an individual female may be tested in a number of two-stimulus experiments having at least one stimulus in common, there is still the chance that her previous exposure could bias her one way or another. For example, finding a loudspeaker rather than a male could bias a female against responding to the same sound pattern later. A detailed analysis of this question is presented for the green treefrog, *H. cinerea* (Gerhardt, 1981a). There was no indication that subsequent choices of females were influenced by their choices in previous tests, even when these occurred within minutes.

Electrodermal Responses

Strother (1962) first used changes in skin potentials in response to acoustic stimulation, also called galvanic skin responses, to estimate auditory thresholds in frogs. Brzoska (1981, 1984) used this technique not only to estimate auditory thresholds, but to assess the responsiveness of European ranid frogs to species-specific vocalizations. The main drawback of the technique is the large variability in the magnitude and latency of responses from one animal to another and seasonally. Moreover, thresholds estimated from this procedure were considerably higher than those obtained neurophysiologically or by the reflex modification technique (see next section). In *R. temporaria* there were considerable differences in the shapes of threshold curves derived from neurophysiological studies and electrodermal responses even when the same acoustic stimuli were used (Brzoska, Walkowiak, & Schneider, 1977).

Reflex Modification

The presentation of one stimulus just before another stimulus may modify the magnitude or latency of an animal's response to a second stimulus. The response to the second stimulus is a reflexive one, usually a startle response, and the prestimulus modifying stimulus may be of an entirely different modality (Hoffman & Ison, 1980). Megela-Simmons et al. (1985) administered mild electric shocks to frogs placed in small containers partially filled with water and recorded flexion of the hind legs. The amount of flexion, quantified by measuring the voltage output of a movement detector, is reduced (inhibited) by the presentation of an acoustic stimulus prior to the shock. The optimum lead-time, or time of sound presentation before the shock that resulted in maximum inhibition, is apparently species or size-specific. For example, in bullfrogs, *R. catesbeiana*, it was 400 ms; in green treefrogs, it was 200 ms.

As pointed out by Megela-Simmons et al. (1985) the reflex modification technique does not depend on prior learning and requires no instrumental response. The fact that a response inhibition is seen on the first trial distinguishes reflex modification from classical conditioning, at least in other animals. Nevertheless, reflex modification yields sensitivity functions that resemble those derived from classical and operant conditioning paradigms. There are two important advantages of this procedure in comparison with studies of natural behavioral responses to sound. First, behavioral data about hearing can be obtained using sound patterns and frequencies that normally do not elicit natural behavior. Second, the responses do not depend importantly on the sex and reproductive condition of the animal, and experiments can always be conducted under controlled laboratory conditions.

II. HEARING CAPABILITIES

Audiograms

Megela-Simmons et al. (1985) provide audiograms based on the reflex modification technique for two species of frogs. The bullfrog is most sensitive (estimated thresholds of less than 20 dB) between about 300 Hz and 1800 Hz. The thresholds rise to about 60 dB at 100 Hz and to about 70 dB at 3000 Hz. The audiogram of the green treefrog reveals two, disjunct peaks of maximum sensitivity, one around 900 Hz (estimated threshold of about 25 dB) and the other, at about 3000 Hz (estimated threshold of 35–45 dB). Estimated thresholds rise to about 50 dB at about 200 Hz and to about 60 dB at 4000 Hz. In comparison with the several species of fish (e.g., Coombs & Popper, 1979; Fay, 1969; Myrberg & Spires, 1980) the two frogs have lower absolute thresholds and broader ranges of hearing, but they are distinctly limited in these respects in comparison with birds and mammals.

Masked Thresholds and Critical Bands

One way of assessing the frequency selectivity of an animal is to estimate critical bands, either directly by band-narrowing experiments, or indirectly, by estimating masked thresholds (e.g., Scharf, 1970). Moss and Simmons (1986) used the reflex modification procedure to estimate masked thresholds for the green treefrog at frequencies between 0.3 to 5.4 kHz; the spectrum level of a broadband masker was either 25 or 35 dB RMS/Hz. Thresholds increased with masker spectrum level so that critical ratios remained about the same.

The maximum frequency selectivity (minimum critical ratio) is comparable to that estimated in other vertebrates, but the pattern of change in critical ratios with frequency is unusual in that it roughly resembles the pure tone audiogram. That is, frequency selectivity is maximal at the frequencies to which the animals are most sensitive: 900 and 3000 Hz. These two frequencies correspond to the two regions of the audio spectrum that are emphasized in the advertisement and aggressive calls of *H. cinerea.* As Moss and Simmons (1986) point out, other unusual patterns of critical ratio change with stimulus frequency also appear to be specializations for the detection and processing of species-specific vocalizations (e.g., in parakeets, Dooling & Saunders, 1975, and in bats, Long, 1977).

Comparisons of the Results of Reflex Modification Studies and Other Behavioral Studies

Estimated thresholds for phonotactic responses for the green treefrog to tone bursts are limited to relatively few stimulus frequencies and tonal combinations, representing the typical spectral peaks in the advertisement calls of the male. About one-third (of more than 100 animals) of the females responded to tone bursts of 900 Hz or 900 + 3000 Hz at 48 dB (Gerhardt, 1981a). Only six females, which had responded rapidly at 48 dB, were tested at 42 dB, but four of them showed phonotactic responses. Females responded to the combination of 2700 + 3000 Hz at about 70 dB (Gerhardt, 1976). In the latter experiments females were placed at 1 meter from a speaker, and a positive response was tabulated if they oriented toward the speaker and moved to within 30 cm. A much lower phonotactic threshold at 3000 Hz, estimated at about 54 dB, was obtained by placing a female midway between two speakers and offering her the choice of a tone burst of 900 Hz and one of 900 + 3000 Hz. The SPL of the 900 Hz-component of the combination tone was equalized to that of the 900 Hz-stimulus. Females did not show a preference for the combination tone at 48 dB, but they did so at 54 dB (Gerhardt, 1981a).

These results indicate that the green treefrog's phonotactic thresholds are higher than their hearing thresholds, as estimated by the reflex inhibition procedure. This is hardly surprising as even the definitions of threshold are different and arbitrary. Both kinds of estimates show, however, that the animals are more sensitive (responsive) to frequencies corresponding to the low-frequency spectral peak in the natural communication signals than they are to frequencies typical of the high-frequency peak. A comparison of thresholds in *H. cinerea* estimated from the reflex inhibition technique, the electrodermal response, phonotactic behavior and neurophysiological studies is presented in Fig. 6.1.

Gerhardt and Klump (1988) have recently estimated phonotactic thresholds in the barking treefrog, *H. gratiosa,* to chorus sounds, which have a prominent spectral peak at 400–500 Hz. This peak corresponds to the low-frequency spectral peak in the male's advertisement call, and it propagates effectively (43 − 47 dB in the 500 Hz octave band) to distances of at least 160 meters from the chorus, especially at night along the ground. Females reliably moved toward the sound source at playback levels of about 40 dB. By contrast, females of *H.*

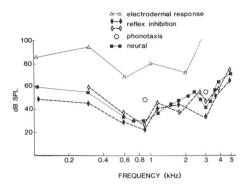

FIG. 6.1. Comparisons of audiograms of the green treefrog (*Hyla cinerea*) based on behavioral and electrodermal responses (Weiss & Strother, 1965), the reflex modification procedure (Megela-Simmons et al., 1985), and evoked potentials in the midbrain (neural thresholds; Lombard & Straughan, 1974). Also indicated are estimated thresholds for phonotaxis at two frequencies prominent in the advertisement call. A few females, tested at 900 Hz and 42 dB SPL, also showed positive phonotactic responses (Gerhardt, 1981a, unpublished data).

cinerea were not reliably attracted to conspecific chorus sounds played back at 70 to 75 dB, even though there was a prominent 900 Hz-spectral peak in the stimulus. This comparison serves to emphasize that hearing capabilities do not necessarily predict if particular sounds will elicit specific behaviors. Green treefrogs obviously can hear chorus sounds at much lower levels than 70 dB, and estimated thresholds of auditory neurons in *H. gratiosa* suggest that this species is no more sensitive to 400–500 Hz-sounds than is *H. cinerea* to 900 Hz-sounds (Capranica & Moffat, personal communication).

In contrast to the differences between estimated thresholds for reflex inhibition and phonotaxis, the two techniques yielded remarkably similar estimates of critical ratios (Fig. 6.2). Again, the phonotactic study was restricted to frequencies that were prominent in the advertisement call. The critical ratios estimates (group averages) obtained by Moss and Simmons (1986) were about 20–22 dB at 900 Hz, and 22–26 dB at 3000 Hz; spectrum levels of the masker were 25 and 35 dB. Ehret and Gerhardt (1980) estimated critical ratios of 22 dB at 900 Hz and 21.5 dB at 3000 Hz. The estimate at 900 Hz was based on the average masked spectrum level necessary to abolish phonotactic behavior in response to a tone burst at 65 dB SPL. In eight of ten animals, a spectrum level of 25 or 35 dB was sufficient; a level of 45 dB was necessary for two animals. The estimate at 3000 Hz was made by offering females a choice between a signal of 900 + 3000 Hz at 65 dB SPL, played back from one speaker, and the same signal plus high-frequency noise (masking the 3000 Hz-component only), from another speaker. Females reliably chose the unmasked signal when the masker spectrum level was 46 dB but not when it was 41 dB. The masked threshold was taken to be the

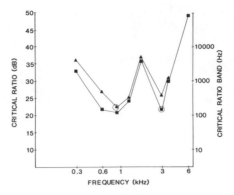

FIG. 6.2.   Masked auditory thresholds in the green treefrog as a function of stimulus frequency. The curves are taken from Moss and Simmons (1986) and are based on reflex modification with masker spectrum levels of 25 dB/Hz (squares) and 35 dB/Hz (triangles). The circles at 900 Hz and 3000 Hz show the values of estimated critical ratios based on phonotaxis (Ehret & Gerhardt, 1980). Masker spectrum levels were mostly 35 dB/Hz or less.

average, or 43.5 dB. Additional masked thresholds at 900 Hz, determined at signal levels of 65 and 75 dB, yielded estimates of critical ratios of 25 and 30 dB. The difference of 3 dB between signal levels of 65 and 75 dB probably reflects measurement errors, primarily due to variability in female responsiveness. The CR-band estimate of 30 dB was probably attributable both to measurement error and to the high noise spectrum levels, which were mostly 45 dB or greater, that were necessary to mask the 900 Hz-signal at 75 dB SPL. Scharf and Meiselman (1977) found that in humans CR-bands above 1000 Hz widened when masker levels exceeded 40 dB, which has been the usual maximum level in animal studies. Hence, the reflex inhibition technique and the phonotactic one were also consistent in finding that critical ratios did not change very much, if at all, at different masker spectrum levels below 40 dB.

Narins (1982a) estimated critical ratios of 31–40 dB at 1000 Hz for evoked calling by males of the Co-Qui (*Eleutherodactylus coqui*), a leptodactylid frog from Puerto Rico. However, the high ambient noise levels in the natural environment, where the experiments took place, precludes direct comparisons with the work on the green treefrog.

III.   ACOUSTIC BASES OF RECOGNITION

Here, I discuss the acoustic properties of natural communication signals that mediate differential responses in frogs. Because most of the studies have been restricted to unconditioned responses, the data do not bear on the issue of whether or not the failure to respond differentially indicates limitations of the auditory system. I restrict my treatment to studies that have used synthetic acoustic stimuli, in which various properties have been varied in a systematic fashion. I have reviewed experimental studies of the effects of the gross rate of calling elsewhere (Gerhardt, 1988).

Sound Pressure Level

Females of *H. cinerea* chose the louder of two synthetic calls that differed by 3 dB at moderate SPLs (63 versus 60 dB and 73 versus 70 dB); at a higher level, a 6 dB-difference (86 versus 80 dB) was necessary (Gerhardt, 1987). Zelick and Narins (1983) provide comparable (4 to 6 dB) estimates for intensity discrimination by males of *E. coqui* in Puerto Rico.

Spectral Differences

The spectral patterns of anuran vocalizations range from simple pure tone bursts to complex, frequency-modulated, harmonic spectra. Other frogs produce noise-like sounds. Differences in some of these spectral patterns are the primary ways in which the calls of closely related species can be recognized.

Dominant Frequency.   Two-stimulus experiments with females indicate that a 10% difference in frequency may elicit selective phonotaxis in the spring peeper (*H. crucifer*) (Doherty & Gerhardt, 1984). In most other species, selective responses were obtained only when frequency differences were about 15% or more (*H. cinerea, H. gratiosa, Physalaemus pustulosus*) (Gerhardt, 1981b, 1987, 1988; Ryan, 1983a). In the green treefrog, the frequency differences (150 Hz) that were discriminated at about 1000 Hz were consistent with the critical band estimates discussed above (Gerhardt, 1988a).

Frequency preferences were abolished by relatively small changes (6 to 12 dB) in the relative SPLs of the alternatives in *H. crucifer* and *H. cinerea*. Indeed, in *H. cinerea,* some frequency preferences even depended on the absolute SPL to which the two alternatives were equalized (Gerhardt, 1987). Thus, these amphibians are not demonstrating an ability for frequency (intensity-independent) discrimination in the context of mate choice, despite the fact that the anatomy and physiology of one of the inner ear organs indicate that frogs may possess the requisite mechanisms (see below). Moreover, estimates of frequency discrimination at a constant SPL indicate poorer selectivity than has been estimated psychophysically in fish, which discriminate differences of about 5 to 9% (Hawkins, 1981).

Frequency Modulation.   Many anurans produce vocalizations with frequency-modulated components. Ryan (1983b) showed that females of *Physalaemus* preferred natural, frequency-modulated "whines" to tone bursts of the same duration and constant frequency. He also found that females preferred the whine played forwards to the same call played backwards, thus reversing the direction of the frequency sweep. Unfortunately, the amplitude-time envelope of the whine is distinctly different from beginning to end, so that this experiment did not exclude the possibility that differences in amplitude-time envelopes in addition to or instead of frequency-modulation were involved in the selective phonotaxis. The amplitude-time envelopes of the tonal stimuli also did not match that of the whine.

In the gray treefrog, *H. versicolor,* males produce pulses in which frequency rises from beginning to end. Females did not, however, prefer synthetic calls with frequency-modulated pulses to synthetic calls in which pulse frequency remained constant (Gerhardt, 1978a). Similarly, Doherty and Gerhardt (1984) found that females of the spring peeper did not prefer a frequency-modulated synthetic call (a tone burst) to one of constant frequency. However, the percentage change in frequency in the advertisement call of this species is quite modest (about 12 to 15%) compared with *Physalaemus* and other tropical species.

Spectral Patterns.   In many anurans the advertisement call contains two or more spectral peaks. In *H. cinerea* females preferred a synthetic call with two components of 900 and 3000 Hz of equal relative amplitude (the standard stimulus) to alternatives in which the relative amplitudes of these two components differed by 6 or 12 dB (Gerhardt, 1981a; Fig. 6.3). When the 900 Hz-component was 12 dB down relative to the 3000 Hz-component, females preferred the standard sound at absolute SPLs from 48 dB to 85 dB. When the 3000 Hz-component was attenuated by 12 dB relative to the 900 Hz-peak, females preferred the standard stimulus only at playback levels above about 70 dB SPL. Qualitatively similar results were obtained for the barking treefrog, *H. gratiosa* (Gerhardt, 1981b). Schwartz (1987) found that spectral patterns were also relevant in the neotropical species, *H. microcephala.*

Temporal Differences

The advertisement calls of closely related species that breed in the same place and time are more likely to differ in their temporal structure than in their spectral patterns. Here, I consider differences in duration, envelope shape, pulse-repetition rate (pulse rate) and waveform periodicity. The distinction between the last two of these acoustic properties is arbitrary. When vocalizations are made up of distinct sound pulses separated by silent intervals and produced at slow rates, the pulsed nature of the sound is obvious, even to human ears. More rapidly produced pulses may be resolved only by an oscilloscopic analysis, and the spectra of such sounds reflect the fine-temporal patterns in that side-bands at difference-frequencies corresponding to the pusle-repetition rate appear around the carrier

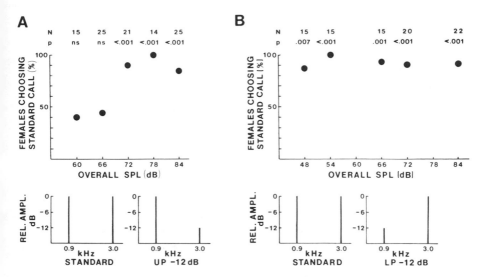

FIG. 6.3. Selective phonotaxis in the green treefrog as a function of the relative amplitudes of the two prominent spectral peaks in the advertisement call. (A) Females did not prefer a synthetic stimulus with peaks of equal relative amplitude (standard call) to an alternative in which the high-frequency peak was attenuated by 12 dB unless the two playback SPLs of the two sounds were about 70 dB or higher. (B) Females preferred the standard call to an alternative in which the low-frequency peak was attenuated by 12 dB at all playback levels from 48 to 84 dB SPL. Modified from Gerhardt (1981a).

frequency or frequencies. Finally, the complex harmonic spectra of some vocalizations is reflected in the periodicity of the repeating waveform. As changes in temporal structure inevitably give rise to changes in the spectrum, even studies using synthetic sounds seldom indicate directly whether the animals are using temporal, spectral or some combination of cues in recognition tasks.

Duration.   In three species of treefrogs, females were not particularly selective with respect to stimuli that differed in duration (Doherty & Gerhardt, 1984; Gerhardt, 1988; Schneider, 1982). Sounds that had the duration of a typical conspecific call were preferred to alternatives that were 25 to 50% shorter in *H. crucifer, H. cinerea,* and *H. meridionalis.* In the first two of these species, preferences were abolished by small increases in the relative SPLs of the alternatives. Since the stimuli of "normal" duration were less than 200 msec, these results probably reflect the widespread phenomenon of temporal summation (e.g., Yost & Nielsen, 1985). Females of *H. crucifer* and *H. cinerea* preferred sounds of normal duration to alternatives that were about two and a half to three times longer; females of *H. meridionalis* did not show a preference for a synthetic call of normal duration to an alternative that was twice as long. By contrast, females of *H. regilla* and *H. versicolor* preferred synthetic calls that were longer than a typical conspecific call (Gerhardt & Doherty, 1988; Klump & Gerhardt, 1987; Straughan, 1975). Females of *H. versicolor* preferred alternatives that were as little as 50% or as much as four times longer than the average advertisement call. Females of this species were biased toward long calls even when their rate of presentation was reduced relative to that of short calls so that differences in acoustic energy were minimal (Klump & Gerhardt, 1987).

The vocal responses of male frogs to synthetic stimuli differing in duration were somewhat selective. Males of *E. coqui* responded maximally when the duration of a "co" stimulus was 100 msec, the typical duration of the species (Narins & Capranica, 1978). Shortening or lengthening the stimulus duration reduced the percentage of vocal responses. Males of *H. ebraccata,* a neotropical hylid, synchronized their vocal responses most precisely to a synthetic stimulus when its duration equaled or exceeded that of the natural advertisement call (Schwartz & Wells, 1984). Walkowiak and Brzoska (1982) observed very little effect of stimulus duration on call production in *R. temporaria.*

Shape of the Amplitude-Time Envelope.   The advertisement calls of *H. cinerea* and *H. gratiosa* have a distinctly pulsatile beginning. A synthetic call with a pulsatile beginning was more attractive than a stimulus without such a beginning in *H. gratiosa,* but not in *H. cinerea.* Moreover, playing the natural call backwards so that the pulsatile part ended rather than began the call did not reduce the attractiveness of the sound relative to the call played forwards in *H. cinerea;* females of *H. gratiosa* never chose the conspecific call played backwards (Gerhardt, 1981b).

Males of *H. cinerea* produce aggressive calls by amplitude-modulating (pulsing) the advertisement call, thus producing four to six cycles at about 50 pulses/sec. Females prefer natural advertisement calls to aggressive calls of the same male (Oldham & Gerhardt, 1975). When offered choices between a synthetic advertisement call and alternatives that were amplitude-modulated at 50 pulses/sec, females preferred the unmodulated sound only when the depth of modulation was about 40% or greater (Gerhardt, 1978c). Females also preferred unmodulated noise bursts to strongly modulated (95%) ones, thus reinforcing the idea that they use the temporal difference (envelope) rather than spectral differences (Gerhardt, 1978c). The long-term spectrum of noise is unchanged by AM.

Another study of *H. cinerea* showed that females could discriminate between synthetic signals on the basis of a one-cycle difference in amplitude-modulation (Gerhardt, 1978b; Fig. 6.4); they preferred the alternative with fewer cycles of amplitude-modulation. These results suggest that they process sounds that are acoustically intermediate between advertisement and aggressive calls in a continuous rather than in a categorical fashion. Preliminary studies of males of *H. cinerea* indicate that they are also selective in the same task. Perrill and I

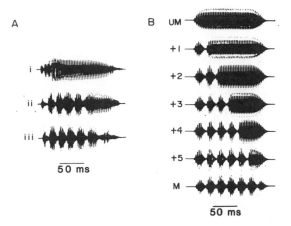

FIG. 6.4. Oscillograms of natural vocalizations of *Hyla cinerea* and a synthetic call continuum. (A) Natural vocalizations: (i) an advertisement call; (ii) a call of the same male that is intermediate in acoustic structure between (i) and an aggressive call; (iii) aggressive call of the same male; (B) Synthetic call continuum based on natural vocalizations. Females preferred natural and synthetic advertisement (UM) calls to aggressive calls (M), and in pairwise playbacks of the synthetic calls, they preferred the alternative with the fewest cycles of amplitude-modulation, even if there was only a one-cycle difference. They did not prefer the unmodulated call to the call with one cycle of amplitude-modulation. Modified from Gerhardt (1978b).

(unpublished data) placed satellite males between two speakers and found that they preferentially moved toward the source of synthetic sounds with one cycle of amplitude-modulation when the alternative stimulus had three cycles. Since satellite males situate themselves near calling ones and attempt to intercept females, a male adopting this strategy would be expected to sit near males that produce calls that are most attractive to females.

Pulse Rate.   If their calls are pulsed, closely-related species that breed at the same time and place usually produce calls that differ in pulse rate by a factor of two or more (Littlejohn, 1969). Experiments using synthetic calls have confirmed that female frogs readily discriminate between sounds differing in pulse rate by a factor of two (Doherty & Gerhardt, 1983; Loftus-Hills & Littlejohn, 1971; Straughan, 1975) or even less (Gerhardt, 1982; Schneider, 1982; Schwartz, 1987).

Detailed studies of pulse rate preferences in the cryptic species of gray treefrogs, *H. chrysoscelis* and *H. versicolor,* revealed that pulse rate preferences are temperature-dependent, in a fashion that roughly parallels temperature-dependent changes in pulse rate in the male's call (Gerhardt, 1978a, 1982). However, the strength of the preferences are asymmetrical and species-specific. A female of *H. versicolor* most strongly rejects alternative stimuli that have higher pulse rates than those produced by a conspecific male at the temperature at which she is tested, especially at relatively cool temperatures (16 to 20°C). A female of *H. chrysoscelis* is most selective in rejecting stimuli with lower pulse rates, even when she is tested at relatively warm temperatures (24–28°C). These are just the conditions in which a female could mistakenly respond to a heterospecific male in a mixed species chorus, if she did not take temperature into account. That is, at cool temperatures, males of *H. chrysoscelis* produce calls with pulse rates that are similar to those of *H. versicolor* at warm temperatures. A mismating is a total loss for the female because the two species differ in chromosome number and hence produce sterile hybrids. Females of *H. versicolor* tested at 20°C chose the conspecific pulse rate of 20 pulses/sec over an alternative stimulus with a rate of 40 pulses/sec, which is in the range of variation of *H. chrysoscelis,* even if the latter stimulus had a SPL that was 18 dB (a factor of 8) higher than the "conspecific" stimulus.

Male anurans are generally not very selective in their vocal responses to playbacks of stimuli that differ in pulse rate. In fact, males usually attempt to avoid acoustic overlap with sounds similar in duration to conspecific calls even if the stimulus lacks a pulsatile structure (e.g., Narins, 1982b; Schwartz & Wells, 1984; Sullivan & Leek, 1986). Walkowiak and Brzoska (1982) found some selectivity in *R. temporaria*. If the pulse rate of a synthetic stimulus was twice the normal rate, the frogs showed a reduced number of vocal responses. There was little change in evoked calling if the pulse rate of the stimulus was one-half of the normal pulse rate. Similarly, Brzoska and Schneider (1982) also found some differences in the response latency of *H. arborea savignyi* to synthetic sounds differing in pulse rate.

Waveform Periodicity. Females of *H. cinerea* preferred synthetic sounds with a waveform periodicity of about 300/sec to an alternative with a periodicity of 900/sec and especially to alternatives with periodicities of 100/sec or less (Gerhardt, 1978c). However, it was necessary that the periodicity be reflected in the amplitude-time waveform. That is, females preferred the combinations of 900 + 1200 + 3000 Hz and 900 + 2700 + 3000 Hz to an alternative of 900 + 3000 Hz. The periodicity of all three stimuli is 300/sec, but the three-component sounds have beats of 300/sec, whereas the 300/sec-periodicity of the two-component stimulus is evident only by examining the fine structure of the waveform. Moreover, females did not show a preference for a stimulus of 900 + 3000 Hz (300/sec periodicity) to one of 900 + 2700 Hz; (900/sec periodicity). In neither stimulus is the periodicity expressed strongly in the envelope of the sound.

Simmons (1988), using the reflex modification technique to study the same species, found that in the presence of broadband background noise, frogs better detected complex sounds consisting of harmonically related (e.g., 900 + 3000 Hz and 828 + 2760 Hz) components than an inharmonic complex (830 + 3100 Hz). The harmonic complexes had a periodic waveform with periodicities of

300/sec and 276/sec, respectively. Masked thresholds and critical ratios in responses to harmonic stimuli were 8 to 10 dB lower than in response to the
inharmonic stimulus. Simmons (1988) argues that the harmonic structure of the
natural advertisement call is thus an relevant species-specific acoustic feature,
and that the detection of this property must occur in the central nervous system,
rather than in the periphery. The basis for the latter conclusion is that frogs have
two inner ear organs, and each of the frequency components used in her experimental stimuli would be encoded in neurons innervating a different organ. The
inputs from the two organs converge in the central auditory system. Recent
experiments failed to corroborate these results. Females offered a choice between
the same harmonic and inharmonic sounds in the presence of broadband noise
failed to show a preference (Gerhardt, Schwartz and Allen, unpublished data).

Combinations of Relevant Properties

The use of artificial sounds can provide information about the importance of a
single acoustic property, although varying one property often alters another
property by necessity. A change in temporal properties almost always alters
spectral properties, and in terms of the natural signals of frogs, which often
consist of trains of pulses, the interdependence of two or more properties is even
more obvious. For example, if the pulse rate is changed, then the pulse duty
cycle (ratio of pulse duration to pulse period) and pulse train duration are also
changed.

More significantly, the animals themselves probably do not attend to just one
property of a communication signal, even if these properties vary independently.
The multidimensional nature of acoustic signals is advantageous precisely because different kinds of information can be encoded simultaneously.

As discussed above, females of the gray treefrog, *H. versicolor* discriminate
between signals which differ in pulse rate. At 20°C, females chose a synthetic
call with a pulse rate of 20 pulses/sec to one of 30 pulses/sec. If pulse number
was held constant so that the duration of the sound of 20 pulses/sec was by
necessity longer, then females continued to choose the stimulus of 20 pulses/sec
even when its SPL was 12 dB less than that of the stimulus of 30 pulses/sec. If,
however, pulses were added to the sound of 30 pulses/sec so that its duration was
the same as that of the call of 20 pulses/sec, then females preferred the stimulus
of 20 pulses/sec when its SPL was reduced by 6 dB but not by 12 dB relative to
the SPL of the call of 30 pulses/sec (Gerhardt & Doherty, 1987).

The stimuli discussed in the preceding paragraph were presented at the same
rate (call-repetition rate or call rate), and their phase relationship was fixed so
that the sounds did not overlap in time. In another series of experiments, both
pulse rate and call rate were varied. When the call rate of a stimulus of 30
pulses/sec was nearly double that of a stimulus of 20 pulses/sec, female *H.
versicolor* failed to show a preference. However, when the alternatives had pulse

rates of 20/sec and 40/sec, females reliably chose the stimulus of 20 pulses/sec, despite a nearly two-to-one difference in call rate. Recall that a pulse rate of 40/sec is within the range of *H. chrysoscelis* at 20°C. Doherty (1985a, 1985b) has also found that variation in "gross" temporal properties can affect preferences based on pulse rate in crickets.

These experiments show that, within limits, changes in call duration and call rate can modify preferences based on pulse rates. Moreover, these results are consistent with biologically significant priorities in mate choice. Call duration and call rate vary among conspecific males and indicate their energetic investment in calling, at least over the short term (e.g., Taigen & Wells, 1985). If pulse rate is within certain limits, females tend to choose calls that are most costly to produce, even if the sounds do not differ in acoustic energy (Klump & Gerhardt, 1987). By so choosing, females are at least certain of obtaining a male in good physical condition, because calling is an extremely costly activity. If, however, pulse rate exceeds a certain limit, falling in the range of the other species of gray treefrog (*H. chrysoscelis*), then differences in duration, call rate, and SPL, even if they strongly favor the stimulus with the "heterospecific" pulse rate, have little or no effect on female preferences for the signal with the "conspecific" pulse rate. Mating with a genetically compatible male is obviously a much more serious mistake than mating with a conspecific male of less than average fitness.

IV. DISCUSSION

Hearing Abilities and Acoustic Communication

The psychophysical approach provides information about what animals can hear and discriminate. Because no one has yet succeeded in conditioning frogs and toads to respond to sound, we know less about their basic hearing abilities than about their ability to discriminate among natural communication signals. The reflex modification technique generates functions that resemble psychometric functions derived from conditioning paradigms in other kinds of animals, and the audiograms based on reflex modification are generally consistent with neurophysiologically derived ones. Phonotactic thresholds were consistently higher than hearing thresholds, but estimates of critical ratios based on reflex modification and phonotactic assays were very similar.

The difference between hearing and phonotactic thresholds might have been expected for a number of reasons, especially since the motivation of the animal is so important for phonotactic responses. However, once phonotactically motivated animals were selected, then it is reasonable to suggest that they would use the full capabilities of their auditory system to perform the biologically significant task of extracting pertinent signals from background noise.

I emphasize that an animal's general hearing ability and its mechanisms of auditory processing merely define the limits of its capacity to recognize acoustic patterns. An analysis of the sounds that are important in its evolutionary history, day-to-day survival, and reproductive success will provide insights about the animal's use of its auditory system and the extent to which it may be specialized. Differences in auditory thresholds may not translate directly into differences in relative attractiveness of two sounds in a phonotactic context. Nevertheless, the two approaches are complementary, and each can provide information and hypotheses pertinent to the other.

Behavioral and Neurophysiological Approaches to Hearing and Recognition

As indicated in Fig. 6.1, audiograms derived from the reflex modification technique are comparable with those estimated from evoked responses or multiunit activity at the level of the midbrain in two anuran species. The sensitivity at low frequencies was, however, considerably less (by 10 to 30 dB) than would be expected from estimates of the thresholds of single auditory neurons (Megela-Simmons et al., 1985). There is another discrepancy at 3 kHz in the green treefrog. Capranica and Moffat (1983) found that the most sensitive neurons tuned to the region of the spectrum had thresholds of about 55 to 60 dB, whereas the behavioral audiograms of Megela-Simmons et al. (1985) and neural evoked-response estimates of Lombard and Straughan (1974) indicate thresholds of 35 to 45 dB. One possible reason for the discrepancy is that the behavioral and midbrain studies used free-field stimulation, whereas the eighth nerve studies employed a closed system (see, for example, Pinder & Palmer, 1983). Another possibility is that the anesthesia or immobilization of the animals for recording may lower neural thresholds.

A more fundamental reason for not finding as much correspondence between studies of central processing (including behavior) and the auditory periphery as in higher animals is that amphibians are unique in having two types of inner ear organs. The basilar papilla is a simpler organ than the amphibian papilla in terms of the numbers and orientation of hair cells, and this is reflected in the physiology of the auditory neurons innervating the two organs. Moreover, evidence for tonotopic organization and traveling waves within the amphibian papilla suggest that frequency discrimination (intensity-independent) is a definite possibility within the range of frequencies to which this organ is sensitive. Wilczynski and Capranica (1984) provide a comprehensive review. Obviously, the convergence of auditory information, already processed to some extent separately in the central nervous system, might be expected to result in response properties that are not readily predictable from the peripheral ones alone in comparison with animals having a single inner ear organ.

Moss and Simmons (1986) offer hypotheses to explain the differences in the shapes of critical ratio functions of frogs and higher animals. These authors not only refer to specific differences in inner ear morphology between frogs and higher animals, but also argue persuasively for the idea that frequency selectivity in anurans cannot be explained solely in terms of peripheral tuning.

Some aspects of phonotactic behavior are, however, consistent with fundamental differences in the two auditory organs in that selective responses to sounds differing in frequency or in the relative amplitude of low-and high-frequency components differ with playback SPL. More specifically, the amphibian papilla, tuned to low frequencies, has a greater absolute sensitivity than the basilar papilla, which is tuned to high frequencies. Females of *H. cinerea* did not prefer a stimulus with components of 900 and 3000 Hz of equal amplitude to alternatives in which the high-frequency component was attenuated by 6 to 12 dB unless the sounds were played back at about 70 dB or higher. They detected low-frequency attenuation of 12 dB at 48 dB SPL and higher, but failed to respond selectively when the low-frequency peak was attenuated by only 6 dB at about 70 dB SPL and higher (Gerhardt, 1981a). Similarly, females were more selective in responding to sounds around 900 Hz that differed in frequency when these were played back at low to moderate SPLs than at a high SPL; females were more selective in the high-frequency region around 3000 Hz at moderate to high SPLs (Gerhardt, 1987).

The relatively poor performance in the high-frequency region at low playback levels very probably reflects the fact that relatively few neurons innervating the basilar papilla are excited at low levels. The relatively poor performance in the low-frequency region at high SPLs possibly indicates saturation of a substantial proportion of the more sensitive neurons innervating the amphibian papilla.

Studies of selective phonotaxis provide no evidence for differences in the capacity of the two organs to resolve frequency differences, at least over the best ranges of playback SPL. In *H. cinerea* and *H. gratiosa* differences of 10–20% were discriminated in both the low- (amphibian papilla) and high (basilar papilla) frequency regions of the spectrum, corresponding to the two spectral peaks in the advertisement call. Although the anatomy and physiology of the two organs suggest that the amphibian papilla should be superior in this respect to the basilar papilla, the animals may not use their full frequency-resolving capabilities in this task. Thus, it will be especially important to use reflex modification or other psychophysical techniques to investigate this question.

In terms of selective phonotaxis in treefrogs and evoked calling in the bullfrog, two widely-separated frequency components, each exciting one of the two inner ear organs, are more effective than the same components presented in isolation (Capranica, 1965; Gerhardt, 1976). Moreover, a quantitative study, in which absolute as well as relative amplitudes of disjunct frequency components were varied, indicates that a phonotactically optimal stimulus evokes a particular ratio of neural activity in the two organs (Gerhardt, 1981a). Neural correlates of this convergence have been found in the central auditory system of several anuran species, mostly at the level of the thalamus (e.g., Fuzessery & Feng, 1983; Mudry, 1978; review by Wilczynski & Capranica, 1984). Evoked potentials and multiunit activity were significantly higher in response to the simultaneous presentation of disjunct frequency components than would be predicted by responses to the same components presented one at a time. Mudry (1978) also found a strong temperature effect on the frequency of the most effective low-frequency component in evoking a non-linear facilitated response in *H. cinerea*. Subsequently, Mudry and I confirmed the prediction that females of this species would prefer signals with much lower than normal low-frequency spectral peaks when tested at relatively cool temperatures (Gerhardt & Mudry, 1980). This was a counterintuitive prediction, because the spectral properties of a male's call do not change significantly with temperature, and thus the communication system of this species becomes mis-matched or uncoupled at low temperatures.

With respect to temporal properties important for call recognition, and considerable progress has also been made in the search for neural correlates. Already at the level of the torus semicircularis (midbrain) neurons that respond selectively to sounds with particular pulse rates have been described (Rose & Capranica, 1985; Walkowiak, 1984). In the gray treefrogs, *H. chrysoscelis* and *H. versicolor*, the distribution of most effective pulse rates is distinctly biased to the species-specific range, and the most effective pulse rate increases with temperature, in a qualitatively similar fashion to the way that pulse rate in the male's advertisement call changes with temperature (Rose, Brenowitz, & Capranica, 1985). These observations indicate that these neurons are probably involved in the recognition of natural communication signals. At the level of the auditory thalamus, Hall and Feng (1986) recently described neurons in *R. pipiens* that selectively respond to pulse duration as well as pulse rate.

REFERENCES

Brzoska, J. (1981). Der electrodermale Reflex auf akustische Reize beim Grasfrosch *Rana t. temporaria* (L). *Zoologisches Jahrbuch Physiologie, 85,* 66–82.

Brzoska, J. (1984). The electrodermal response and other behavioral responses of the grass frog to natural and synthetic calls. *Zoologishes Jahrbuch Physiologie, 88,* 179–192.

Brzoska, J., & Schneider, H. (1982). Territorial behavior and vocal response in male *Hyla arborea savignyi* (Amphibia, Anura). *Israel Journal of Zoology, 31,* 27–37.

Brzoska, J., Walkowiak, W., & Schneider, H. (1977). Acoustic communication in the grassfrog (*Rana t. temporaria*): Calls, auditory thresholds and behavioral responses. *Journal of Comparative Physiology, 118,* 173–186.

Capranica, R. R. (1965). *The evoked vocal response of the bullfrog.* Cambridge, MA: MIT Press.

Capranica, R. R., & Moffat, A. J. M. (1983). Neurobehavioral correlates of sound communication in anurans. In J. P. Ewert, R. R. Capranica, & D. J. Ingle (Eds.), *Advances in vertebrate neuroethology* (pp. 701–730). NATO ASI Series A, Vol. 56. New York: Plenum.

Coombs, S., & Popper, A. N. (1979). Hearing differences among Hawaiian squirrelfish (Family

Holocentridae) related to differences in the peripheral auditory system. *Journal of Comparative Physiology, 132,* 135–144.

Doherty, J. A. (1985a). Temperature coupling and "trade-off" phenomena in the acoustic communication system of the cricket, *Gryllus bimaculatus* De Geer (Gryllidae). *Journal of Experimental Biology, 114,* 17–35.

Doherty, J. A. (1985b). Trade-off phenomena in calling song recognition and phonotaxis in the cricket, *Gryllus bimaculatus* (Orthoptera, Gryllidae). *Journal of Comparative Physiology, 156,* 787–801.

Doherty, J. A., & Gerhardt, H. C. (1983). Hybrid tree frogs: vocalizations of males and selective phonotaxis of females. *Science, 220,* 1078–1080.

Doherty, J. A., & Gerhardt, H. C. (1984). Evolutionary and neurobiological implications of selective phonotaxis in the spring peeper (*Hyla crucifer*). *Animal Behaviour, 32,* 875–881.

Dooling, R. J., & Sanders, J. C. (1975). Hearing in the parakeet (*Melopsittacus undulatus*). *Journal of Comparative Physiol Psych, 88,* 1–20.

Ehret, G., & Gerhardt, H. C. (1980). Auditory masking and effect of noise on responses of the green treefrog (*Hyla cinerea*) to synthetic mating calls. *Journal of Comparative Physiology, 141,* 13–18.

Fay, R. R. (1969). Behavioral audiogram for the goldfish. *Journal of Auditory Research, 9,* 112–121.

Fuzessery, Z. M., & Feng, A. S. (1983). Mating call selectivity in the thalamus and midbrain of the leopard from (*Rana p. pipiens*): Single and multiunit analyses. *Journal of Comparative Physiology, 150,* 333–344.

Gerhardt, H. C. (1976). Significance of two frequency bands in long distance vocal communication in the green treefrog. *Nature (London), 261,* 692–694.

Gerhardt, H. C. (1978a). Temperature coupling in the vocal communication system of the gray treefrog (*Hyla versicolor*). *Science, 199,* 992–994.

Gerhardt, H. C. (1978b). Discrimination of intermediate sounds in a synthetic call continuum by female green tree frogs. *Science, 199,* 1089–1091.

Gerhardt, H. C. (1978c). Mating call recognition in the green treefrog (*Hyla cinerea*): the significance of some fine-temporal properties. *Journal of Experimental Biology, 74,* 59–73.

Gerhardt, H. C. (1981a). Mating call recognition in the green treefrog (*Hyla cinerea*): importance of two frequency bands as a function of sound pressure level. *Journal of Comparative Physiology, 144,* 9–16.

Gerhardt, H. C. (1981b). Mating call recognition in the barking treefrog (*Hyla gratiosa*): responses to synthetic calls and comparisons with the green treefrog (*Hyla cinerea*). *Journal of Comparative Physiology, 144,* 17–25.

Gerhardt, H. C. (1982). Sound pattern recognition in some North American treefrogs (*Anura: Hylidae*), implications for mate choice. *American Zoologist, 22,* 581–595.

Gerhardt, H. C. (1986). Recognition of spectral patterns in the green treefrog: Neurobiology and behavior. *Experimental Biology, 45,* 167–178.

Gerhardt, H. C. (1987). Evolutionary and neurobiological implications of selective phonotaxis in the green treefrog (*Hyla cinerea*). *Animal Behaviour, 35,* 1479–1489.

Gerhardt, H. C. (1988). Acoustic properties used in call recognition by frogs and toads. In B, Fritzsch, T. Hetherington, M. Ryan, W. Wilczynski, & W. Walkowiak (Eds.), *The evolution of the amphibian auditory system* (pp. 455–483). New York: Wiley.

Gerhardt, H. C., & Doherty, J. A. (1988). Acoustic communication in the gray treefrog, *Hyla versicolor:* Evolutionary and neurobiological implications. *Journal of Comparative Physiology A, 162,* 261–278.

Gerhardt, H. C., & Klump, G. M. (1988). Phonotactic responses and selectivity of barking treefrogs (*Hyla gratiosa*) to chorus sounds. *Journal of Comparative Physiology, A, 163,* 798–805.

Gerhardt, H. c., & Mudry, K. M. (1980). Temperature effects on frequency preferences and mating call frequencies in the green treefrog, *Hyla cinerea* (Anura: Hylidae). *Journal of Comparative Physiology, 137,* 1–6.

Hall, J., & Feng, A. S. (1986). Neural analysis of temporally patterned sounds in the frog's thalamus: Processing of pulse duration and pulse repetition rate. *Neuroscience Letters, 63,* 215–220.

Hawkins, A. D. (1981). The hearing abilities of fish. In W. N. Tavolga, A. N. Popper, & R. R. Fay (Eds.), *Hearing and sound communication in fishes* (pages 109–133). New York: Springer-Verlag.

Hoffman, H. S., & Ison, J. R. (1980). Reflex modification in the domain of startle: I. Some empirical findings and their implications for how the nervous system processes sensory input. *Psychological Review, 87* 175–189.

Klump, G. M., & Gerhardt, H. C. (1987). Use of non-arbitrary acoustic criteria in mate choice by female gray tree frogs. *Nature (London), 326,* 286–288.

Littlejohn, M. J. (1969). The systematic significance of isolating mechanisms. In *Systematic Biology,* Publ. 1692 (pp. 459–482). National Academy of Sciences, Washington, D.C.

Littlejohn, M. J., & Michaud, T. C. (1959). Mating call discrimination by females of Strecker's chorus frog (*Pseudacris streckeri*). *Texas Journal of Science, 11,* 86–92.

Loftus-Hills, J. J., & M. J. Littlejohn. (1971). Pulse repetition rate as the basis for mating call discrimination by two sympatric species of *Hyla. Copeia, 1971,* 154–156.

Lombard, R. E., Fay, R. R., & Werner, Y. L. (1981). Underwater hearing in the frog, *Rana catesbeiana. Journal of Experimental Biology, 91,* 57–71.

Lombard, R. E., & Straughan, I. R. (1974). Functional aspects of anuran middle ear structures. *Journal of Experimental Biology, 61,* 57–71.

Long, G. R. (1977). Masked auditory thresholds from the bat, *Rhinolophus ferrumequinum. Journal of Comparative Physiology, 116,* 247–255.

Megela-Simmons, A., Moss, C. F., & Daniel, K. M. (1985). Behavioral audiograms of the bullfrog (*Rana catesbeiana*) and the green tree frog (*Hyla cinerea*). *Journal of the Acoustical Society of America, 78,* 1236–1244.

Moss, C. F., & Simmons, A. M. (1986). Frequency selectivity of hearing in the green treefrog, *Hyla cinerea. Journal of Comparative Physiology, 159,* 257–266.

Mudry, K. M. (1978). *A comparative study of the response properties of higher auditory nuclei in anurans: Correlations with species-specific vocalizations.* Doctoral Thesis, Cornell University.

Myrberg, A. A., & Spires, J. Y. (1980). Hearing in damselfishes: an analysis of signal detection among closely related species. *Journal of Comparative Physiology, 140,* 135–144.

Narins, P. M. (1982a). Effects of masking noise on evoked calling in the Puerto Rican Coqui (Anura: Leptodactylidae). *Journal of Comparative Physiology, 147,* 439–466.

Narins, P. M. (1982b). Behavioral refractory period in neotropical treefrogs. *Journal of Comparative Physiology, 148,* 337–344.

Narins, P. M., & Capranica, R. R. (1978). Communicative significance of the two-note call of the treefrog, *Eleutherodactylus coqui. Journal of Comparative Physiology, 127,* 1–9.

Oldham, R. S., & Gerhardt, H. C. (1975). Behavioral isolation of the treefrogs *Hyla cinerea and Hyla gratiosa. Copeia, 1975,* 223–231.

Perrill, S. A., Gerhardt, H. C., & Daniel, R. (1978). Sexual parasitism in the green treefrog (*Hyla cinerea*). *Science, 200,* 1179–1180.

Pinder, A. C., & Palmer, A. R. (1983). Mechanical properties of the frog ear: vibration measurements under free- and closed-field acoustic conditions. *Proceedings of the Royal Society, London, B219,* 371–396.

Robertson, J. G. M. (1984). Acoustic spacing by breeding males of *Uperoleia rugosa* (anura:Leptodactylidae). *Zeitschrift für Tierpsychologie, 64,* 283–297.

Roble, S. M. (1985) Observations on satellites males in *Hyla chrysoscelis, Hyla picta,* and *Pseudacris triseriata. Journal of Herpetology, 19,* 432–436.

Rose, G. J., Brenowitz, E. A., & Capranica, R. R. (1985). Species specificity and temperature dependency of temporal processing by the auditory midbrain of two species of treefrogs. *Journal of Comparative Physiology, 157,* 763–769.

Rose, G. J., & Capranica, R. R. (1985). Sensitivity to amplitude modulated sounds in the anuran auditory system. *Journal of Neurophysiology, 53,* 446–465.

Ryan, M. J. (1983a). Sexual selection and communication in a neotropical frog, *Physalaemus pustulosus. Evolution, 37,* 261–272.

Ryan, M. J. (1983b). Frequency modulated calls and species recognition in a neotropical frog. *Journal of Comparative Physiology, 150,* 217–221.

Scharf, B. (1970). Critical bands, In J. V. Tobias (Ed.), *Foundations of modern auditory theory* (pp. 159–202). New York: Academic Press.

Scharf, B., & Meiselman, C. H. (1977). Critical bandwidth at high intensities, In E. F. Evans & J. P. Wilson (Eds.), *Psychophysics and physiology of hearing* (pp. 221–232). New York: Academic Press.

Schmidt, R. S. (1985). Prostaglandin-induced mating call phonotaxis in female American toads: facilitation by progesterone and arginine vasotocin. *Journal of Comparative Physiology, 156,* 823–829.

Schneider, H. (1982). Phonotaxis bei Weibchen des Kanarischen Laubfroches, *Hyla meridionalis. Zoologische Anzieger, Jena, 208,* 161–174.

Schwartz, J. J. (1987). Spectral and temporal properties in species and call recognition in a neotropical frog with a complex vocal repertoire. *Animal Behaviour, 35,* 340–347.

Schwartz, J. J., & Wells, K. D. (1984). Interspecific acoustic interactions of the neotropical treefrog *Hyla ebraccata. Behavioral Ecology and Sociobiology 14,* 211–224.

Simmons, A. M. (1988). Selectivity for harmonic structure in complex sounds by the green treefrog (*Hyla cinerea*). *Journal of Comparative Physiology A, 162,* 397–403.

Straughan, I. R. (1975). An analysis of the mechansisms of mating call discrimination in the frogs *Hyla regilla and Hyla cadaverina. Copeia, 1975,* 415–424.

Strother, W. F. (1962). Hearing in frogs. *Journal of Auditory Research, 2,* 279–286.

Sullivan, B. K., & Leek, M. R. (1986). Acoustic communication in Woodhouse's toad (*Bufo woodhousei*). I. response of calling males to variation in spectral and temporal components of advertisement calls. *Behaviour, 98,* 305–391.

Taigen, T. L., & Wells, K. D. (1985). Energetics of vocalization by an anuran amphibian (*Hyla versicolor*). *Journal of Comparative Physiology B, 155,* 163–170.

Tuttle, M. D., & Ryan, M. J. (1982). The role of synchronized calling, ambient light, and ambient noise, in anti-bat-predator behavior of a treefrog. *Behavioral Ecology and Sociobiology, 11,* 125–131.

Walkowiak, W. (1984). Neuronal correlates of the recognition of pulsed sound signals in the grass frog. *Journal of Comparative Physiology, 155,* 57–66.

Walkowiak, W., & Brzoska, J. (1982). Significance of spectral and temporal call parameters in the auditory communication of male greas frogs. *Behavioral Ecology and Sociobiology, 11,* 247–252.

Weiss, B. A., & Strother, W. F. (1965). Hearing in the green treefrog. *Journal of Auditory Research, 5,* 297–305.

Wells, K. D. (1977). The social behaviour of anuran amphibians. *Animal Behaviour, 25,* 666–693.

Wells, K. D., & Schwartz, J. J. (1984). Vocal communication in a neotropical treefrog, *Hyla ebraccata:* Aggressive calls. *Behaviour, 91,* 128–145.

Wilczynski, W., & Capranica, R. R. (1984). The auditory system of anuran amphibians. *Progress in Neurobiology, 22,* 1–38.

Yerkes, R. M. (1904). Inhibition and reinforcement of reaction in the frog, *Rana clamitans. Journal of Comparative Neurology and Psychology, 15,* 279–304.

Yost, W. A., & Nielsen, D. W. (1985). *Fundamentals of hearing: An introduction* (2nd ed.). New York: Holt, Rinehart & Winston.

Zelick, R. D., & Narins, P. N. (1983). Intensity discrimination and the precision of call timing in two species of neotropical treefrogs. *Journal of Comparative Physiology, 153,* 403–412.

Editor's Comments on Brown

The perception of the speech code has enjoyed a rich history of attention not only from psychologists but also from engineers and computer scientists. Much of the past work on speech has been perhaps overly influenced by technological considerations in striving to produce a speech reception machine. In spite of a huge commitment of energy and resources, a full understanding of how the human auditory system processes complex acoustic stimuli—particularly speech sounds—remains largely elusive.

In this chapter, Brown argues that our incomplete understanding of the perception of complex speech sounds stems from a failure to adequately address the *biology* of language. Brown examines the vocal repertoires, auditory sensitivities, and acoustic ecologies of Old World monkeys. Brown's findings are consistent with the idea that the form of complex vocal signals—and the perceptual processes that subserve these signals—are the result of acoustic compromises that can only be understood in the context of the organism's habitat and social milieu.

7

The Acoustic Ecology of East African Primates and the Perception of Vocal Signals by Grey-Cheeked Mangabeys and Blue Monkeys

Charles Hawkins Brown
University of South Alabama

INTRODUCTION

Two decades ago a seminal paper by Liberman et al. (1967) entitled "Perception of the speech code" drew attention to the fact that the perception of speech sounds by trained human listeners did not track the magnitude of physical variation between sounds. Perception of complex speech-like signals was not easily predicted by the response of the receptive system to the simple components of complex signals. From an engineering framework, speech perception was a nonlinear system (Capranica, 1972), and the emergence of these nonlinearities led to the idea that speech perception was special and distinct from other presumably generalized perceptual phenomena. According to this emerging view a specialized subsystem of the brain was devoted to language processing, and the peculiarities of speech perception were due to the peculiarities of this portion of the brain which evolved to promote vocal communication.

The discovery of nonlinearities in the perception of complex auditory stimuli was unexpected, yet the idea of a distinct subsystem of the brain devoted to language skills was consistent with an extensive clinical literature regarding trauma to the temporal lobe of the human brain. Damage to Wernicke's and Broca's areas of the left temporal lobe usually resulted in deficits of language perception and language production respectively. Hence, there was clinical support for the idea of specialization of function of portions of the auditory brain subserving language skills. These observations were supported by the early technical failures of applied researchers to develop speech reception machines. Failures in the machine processing of speech were paralleled by failures to develop suitable nonlinguistic substitutes for speech intended to be employed in reading machines for the blind (Liberman, 1982). Thus, observations from a variety of avenues of inquiry led investigators to gradually abandon their preconceptions about how language processing should be accomplished, and begin to study the *biology* of language.

It is to this new area of the biology of language that the research described in this chapter is devoted. Because human speech in some manner emerged from the vocal gestures of nonhuman primates, the focal subjects here are Old World monkeys. Yet for comparative purposes, comparable observations are included for human subjects as well. Many investigators, including most of those contributing to this volume, have identified phenomena or processes pertinent to the evolution of language. Yet very few studies have examined Darwin's "hostile forces of nature," those impediments to communication in the natural environment, which are the primary agents of natural selection, and which have acted to shape the form of communication systems. Because *both* the production and the perception of vocal gestures are the products of natural selection, the acoustic ecology from which these processes emerged and in which they must normally function is an area of considerable interest. This chapter, perhaps more than any other in this volume, is devoted to the interface between characteristics of the natural environment and features of vocal communication systems.

I. THE SELECTION OF STUDY SPECIES AND STUDY SITES

To assess the impact of ecology on communication systems it is strategic to select closely related organisms adapted to extremes of habitat. Primates are found in three classes of habitat: riverine forest, rain forest, and savanna. Riverine forests are narrow strips of forest found along water courses traversing arid regions. These forests are intermediate in type, sharing features of adjacent savanna regions and those of more densely wooded rain forests. The most divergent habitat types in respect to flora and fauna, humidity, rainfall, temperature, and wind are rain forests and savanna. Because sound production and perception have been most thoroughly studied for primates which reside in open habitats, especially vervet monkeys, and most of the macaque monkeys (Green, 1975; Rowell & Hinde, 1962; Seyfarth & Cheney, 1982; Stebbins, 1973), rain forest monkeys have recently received considerable attention for purposes of comparison (Brown, 1986a; Brown & Waser, 1984; Waser & Brown, 1984, 1986).

Kortlandt (1986) has argued that "typical" East African forested habitats should exhibit areas of deforestation or foliage damage caused by "bulldozer" herbivores, principally elephants. His argument is based on the idea that undisturbed forests are atypical and are the result of the artificial elimination or removal of elephants, hippos, and other large herbivores. Due to the phenomenal increase in rural human population levels throughout much of modern East Africa, natural habitats undisturbed by man have virtually vanished. In Kenya, forest reserves have been reduced to about 2% of their precolonial levels (Wolfheim, 1983). Other considerations influencing the selection of habitat study sites are accessibility, the availability of supplies and equipment, and the political stability of study areas. In September, 1986 Brown and Waser were unable to continue their work at their original riverine forest study site near Mchelelo along the Tana River due to incursions by poachers armed with automatic weapons. Hence, a variety of academic and practical factors contribute to the selection of study sites. Figure 7.1 displays some of the prominent features of habitats occupied by primates (Waser & Brown, 1986). The left panel shows western Kenya's Kakamega Forest Reserve (0° 17'N, 34° 47'E). The forest exhibits a continuous canopy at around 30 m, and a dense understory of semiwoody plants. Dry and wet seasons occur twice annually, but seasonality is not extreme, and the onset of the heavy rains varies markedly between years. Elephants are no longer found in the forest, yet the maintained trails cut through the forest, and intrusions by firewood cutters may approximate some of the disturbances caused by large herbivores. In this forest the resident primates rarely descend to the forest floor; 5 to 7 m is the lowest strata usually occupied by monkeys. Figure 7.1, center panel, displays a portion of the Mchelelo riverine forest adjacent to the Tana River (1° 50'S, 40° 10'E). This forest extends as a narrow strip, about 400 m wide, on either side of the Tana River. The forest understory is much denser than in the rain forest, and the canopy is not complete, with the number and size of individual trees being much lower than in the rain forest. The region around the Mchelelo site is arid, with highly seasonal rainfall. The integrity of the forest is dependent on seasonal flooding. The primates residing in this riverine habitat are confined to much lower elevations than those in the rain forest. Some of the primate species found here routinely descend to the forest floor. Figure 7.1, right panel, shows the savanna habitat located several hundred meters west of the Mchelelo forest study site. The vegetation here is primarily grass with small thickets and small trees as is characteristic of the *Acacia-Commiphora* thornbush found across most of eastern and northern Kenya (Lind & Morrison, 1974).

Blue monkeys (*Cercopithecus mitis*) and grey-cheeked mangabeys (*Cercopithecus albigena*), shown in Fig. 7.2, are both large arboreal rain forest monkeys. Blue monkeys are found in central, eastern, and southern Africa in evergreen and semideciduous forests. They are common or abundant in much of their range with population densities varying from 42 to 183.4 monkeys per km^2 (Wolfheim, 1983). Because grey-cheeked mangabeys require relatively undisturbed evergreen rain forests, they are more vulnerable to deforestation and are confined to more restricted regions of equatorial Africa from Cameroon's Atlantic coast to central Uganda. Though mangabeys are abundant in parts of their range, population densities are generally less than 20 monkeys per km^2 (Wolfheim, 1983). Both blue monkeys and grey-cheeked mangabeys are gregarious, residing in groups containing 12–30 individuals. Home range estimates of blue monkeys vary from 5.2 to 100 hectares (ha), which compare to those for

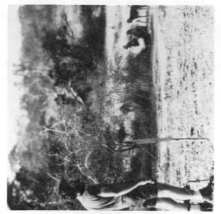

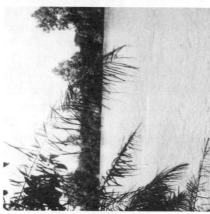

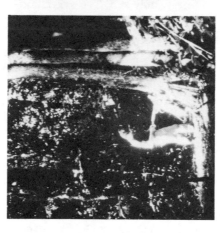

FIG. 7.1.　East African primate habitats: left panel, Kakamega rain forest, center panel, Tana River riverine forest, right panel, savanna at Mchelelo. The author is shown in the left and right panels, photographs by P. Waser. The center photograph is by the author.

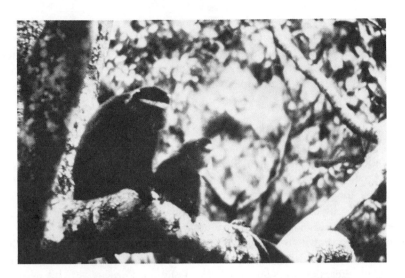

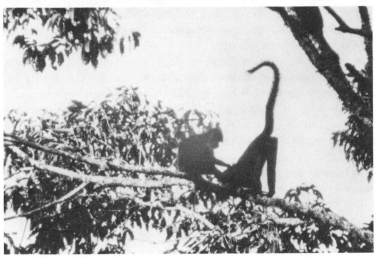

FIG. 7.2. Blue monkeys, top; grey-cheeked mangabeys, bottom. Photographs by P. Waser.

grey-cheeked mangabeys ranging from 13 to 400 ha (Wolfheim, 1983). Grey-cheeked mangabeys relative to blue monkeys exhibit low population densities, large home ranges, and are more widely dispersed both within and between groups (Waser, 1976).

Species differences in life history are paralleled by differences in their vocal repertoires. Blue monkeys are noted for their brief, punctate, stereotyped calls which satisfy the classic requirements of a "discrete" vocal repertoire (Marler,

1965, 1973, 1975). The grey-cheeked mangabey's vocalizations are principally composed of graded vocal elements like those of the baboons, and contrast distinctly with those of blue monkeys. Mangabey calls are longer in duration, and as a rule are less stereotyped, with each new rendition of a call sounding slightly different from the previous version rendered (Chalmers, 1968).

II. GRADED AND DISCRETE VOCAL CATEGORIES

The graded–discrete dimension identifies the relative degree of stereotypy of calls at production as would be determined either by the human ear or by a cluster analysis of the acoustical parameters of the signals. This dimension does not address the mode of perception of these signals. It is possible that conspecific listeners perceive signals drawn from a discrete repertoire in a categorical fashion, and those drawn from a graded one in a continuous fashion, though the converse is possible also (Green & Marler, 1979; for a discussion of categorical and graded perception see Kuhl, 1986, this volume). Furthermore, the number of call categories for either species, and the boundaries between these categories described by human listeners, may not parallel the perceptual experience of the species which utilize these signals.

It was initially argued that the more discrete signals would be superior for communication in forested environments (Marler, 1975). The density of forest vegetation necessarily restricts the possible range of visual communication signals. In addition, the number of acoustically signaling sympatric species may be highest in rain forests because of the variety of niches. As a result, a premium may be placed on the distinguishability of a species' vocal repertoire. Third, it is likely that certain classes of vocal signals are degraded in a predictable and consistent manner as a function of transmission distance. Thus the magnitude of degradation of certain stereotyped calls may function as a vocal position marker identifying the relative distance between group members out of visual contact. Though discrete, stereotyped signals may possess these advantages for species resident in forested habitats, they are also apt to have less potential for specificity and subtlety in the information communicated relative to that for graded signals possessing a fuller range of acoustic variation. Consistent with this view is the observation that primate species with discrete repertoires are more commonly found in forested habitats than in open ones (Marler, 1975; Gautier & Gautier, 1977). The blue monkeys and grey-cheeked mangabeys provide an interesting contrast because they live in sympatry in the parts of their range that overlap, yet their vocal repertoires are markedly different. It is possible that the use of vocal signals differ between species, such that the graded calls given by mangabeys are audible over only short distances, and are accompanied by corollary visual displays. Where visual contact is maintained, any ambiguity in the intent of a graded utterance may be reduced by the visual expressions that accompany vocal gestures. In this framework two questions are of interest: What is the relative audibility of various kinds of signals in habitat noise, and what is the audible distance of representative vocalizations? In a later section of this chapter both of these questions are addressed.

III. BLUE MONKEY AND MANGABEY VOCAL REPERTOIRES

Marler (1973) identified eight categories of blue monkey vocalizations: *pyow, ka, ka-train, boom, growl, grunt, chirp,* and *trill* calls. Of these categories the *growl* is the least discrete; Brown (1986a, 1989b) has studied the relative audibility of all of these categories except for the *growl* vocalization. Sound spectrograms for these calls may be seen in Fig. 7.3. The *chirp* is the shortest duration call at about 20 ms, while the longest signal at 1690 ms is the *ka-train.* Under natural conditions this signal is given almost exclusively in response to sightings of aerial predators. Furthermore, the *ka-train,* like the *ka, boom,* and *pyow* is given exclusively by adult male blue monkeys. *Grunts* are given by individuals of all age and gender classes, while *trill* and *chirp* signals are limited to juvenile and adult female vocalizers.

Chalmers (1968), Waser (1974, 1975), Waser and Waser (1977) and Brown (1989b) recognize 12 categories of mangabey calls: *whoop, gobble, bark, staccato bark, soft grunt, loud grunt, rattling grunt, normal chorused grunt, loud chorused grunt, postcopulatory grunt, scream,* and *squeal.* As already noted, these mangabey calls exhibit substantial variation and gradation between them. The audibility of four representative mangabey vocalizations has been studied by Brown (1986a, 1989b): *gobble, staccato bark, loud chorused grunt,* and *soft grunt.* Sound spectrograms of these calls are also given in Fig. 7.3. Unlike any other call described here, the *chorused grunt,* as its name implies, is produced as a group endeavor. The version Brown (1989b) studied was recorded from three adult mangabeys grunting simultaneously. Each *grunt* element is 200 ms in duration given synchronously by all members in the group. A typical *chorused grunt* bout may last 10 or more s, though the sample used here was 1 s in duration. The mean duration of the mangabey calls shown in Fig. 7.3 was 753 ms, a value more than twice that for the blue monkey signals (362 ms). The dominant frequency of the calls ranged from 160 Hz for the *gobble* or *boom* to 4 kHz for the *trill* utterance. Mangabey calls tend to be noisier or of greater bandwidth than blue monkey signals. The *staccato bark* exhibited a bandwidth greater than 5 kHz, while that for the *boom* call was only a few Hertz in width. The *whoop* and *gobble* utterances are produced exclusively by adult male mangabeys, and the *staccato bark, soft grunt,* and *chorused grunt* calls are emitted by both male and female vocalizers. *Staccato barks* are typically exchanged between individuals out of visual contact with one another, and contrast with

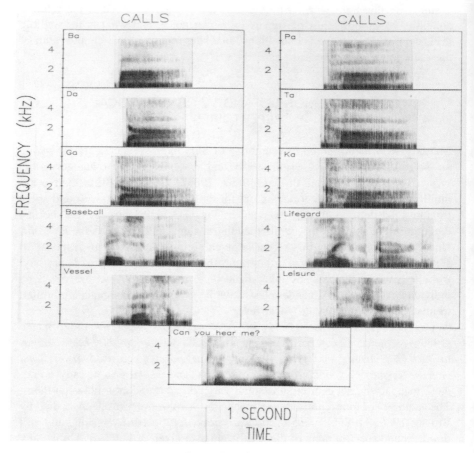

FIG. 7.3.   Sound spectrograms of grey-cheeked mangabey and blue monkey calls. Mangabey calls: *chorused grunt, soft grunt, staccato bark,* and *gobble.* Blue monkey calls: *boom, chirp, trill, ka, grunt,* and *ka-train.* Horizontal bar represents 1 s time. From Brown (1986a).

chorused grunts which are commonly given by animals in close proximity with one another.

IV.   PRIMATE HABITAT ACOUSTICS

Background Noise

Marler (1965, 1967, 1968) was one of the first to suggest that habitat differences may have influenced both the modality of choice and the structural complexity of communication signals. Under natural conditions vocalizations must be detected in ongoing and fluctuating background noise. Hence, one key feature of the acoustic environment is the level and spectrum of the background noise. Waser and Brown (1986) conducted measurements of the ambient noise of representative East African primate habitats as a function of time of day. Figure 7.4 shows the ambient noise level of each of the three habitat types measured in third-octave bands from 0600h to 1800h. Overall noise levels were lowest in savanna and highest in riverine forest. In rain forest, noise levels varied strongly with frequency at all times of day; levels were consistently high below 100 Hz, and between 2,000 and 4,000 Hz. Rain forest noise in the 2,000 to 4,000 Hz range, averaged across time of day, exceeded that in riverine and savanna habitats, while noise in the 200 Hz to 1,000 Hz region was as quiet or quieter in rain forest than in the comparison habitats (Fig. 7.5). The sources of noise differed between habitats as did the noise spectra. In savanna, the principal source of noise was wind driven vegetation movement. Biotic sources did not contribute significantly to ambient noise levels except at 0600h where high-frequency insect noise (4,000 Hz) was evident before sunrise and the usual elevation of wind levels. In rain forest, the diurnal increase in noise in the 2,000 to 4,000 Hz band was principally due to the activities of birds and insects, while low-frequency noise was probably due to vegetation movement and dripping condensation. Noise levels were highest in riverine forest at most times of day and at most frequencies. The major source of noise here was the interaction of forest vegetation with wind sweeping off the savanna.

Sound Propagation

Marten and Marler (1977), Marten, Quine, and Marler (1977), and Waser and Waser (1977) were among the first to study sound transmission in respect to its impact on communication in primate habitats. However, these studies as well as others conducted at this time have been criticized (Michelsen, 1978) for failing to measure the amplitude of broadcast signals in an anechoic environment. Hence, the amplitude measurements of broadcast signals were subject to constructive and destructive interference. The problems associated with this measurement situation are discussed later in the section on the measurement of the amplitude of primate calls.

Measurements in primate habitats have been repeated with appropriately calibrated signals (Brown & Waser, 1984; Waser & Brown, 1984, 1986), and the results presented in Fig. 7.6 show that sound propagation differs between habitats and between test frequencies within a habitat. Sound propagation is measured as excess attenuation. Because sound typically radiates spherically in all directions from its origin, the amplitude of the wavefront obeys the inverse square law. Excess attenuation is the extra decrement in signal amplitude that exceeds that predicted by the inverse square law. This excess in attenuation is

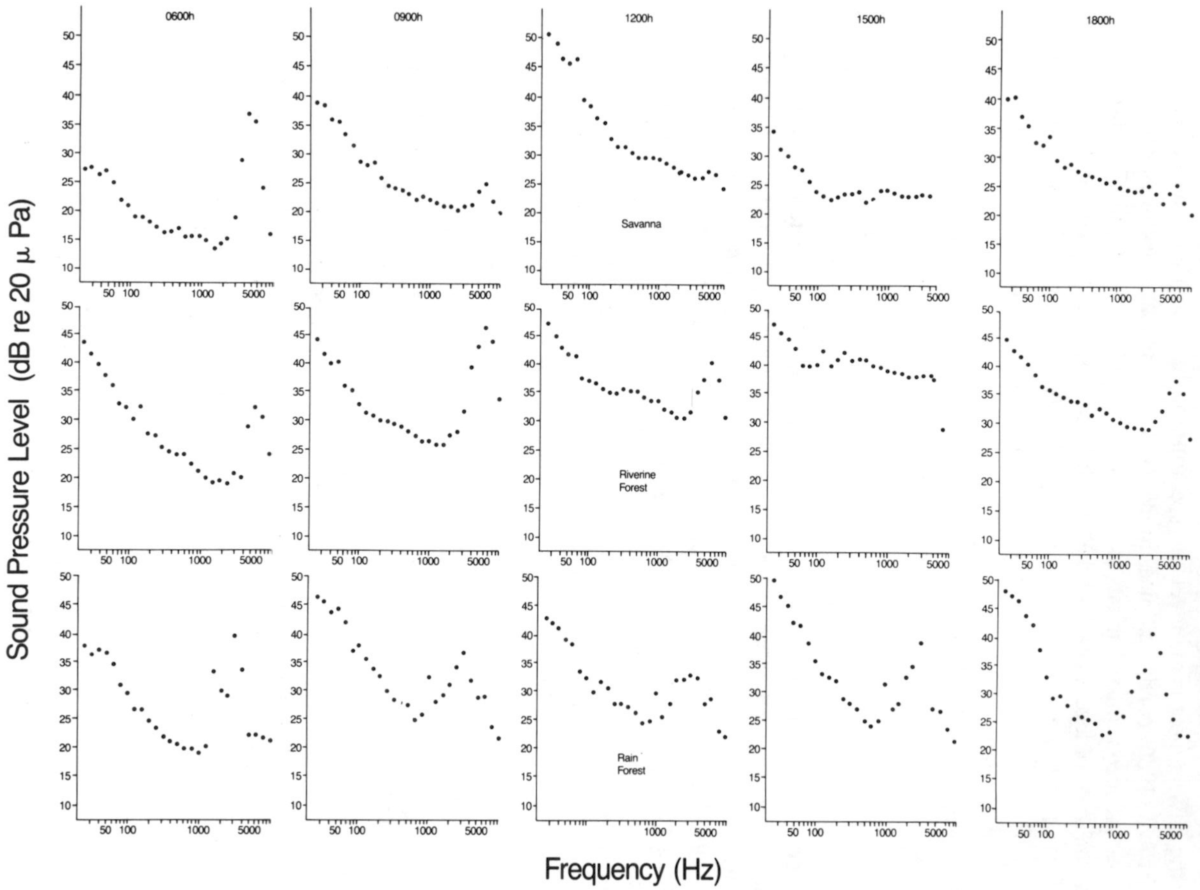

FIG. 7.4. Background noise spectral distribution in each habitat as a function of time of day. Standard deviations for the four 30-second measurements at each frequency and time of day range from 0.5 to 7.9 dB in rain forest, 2.2 to 14.2 dB in riverine forest,

210

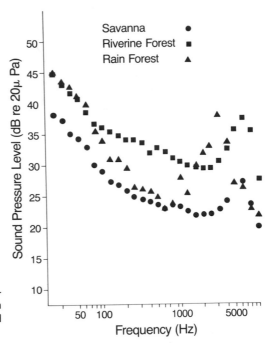

FIG. 7.5. Mean spectral distribution of background noise in each habitat. From Waser and Brown (1986).

principally due to absorption and diffraction of the sound wave with environmental surfaces.

Excess attenuation was more marked in riverine forest and savanna tests than in the rain forest. The differences were particularly evident in the frequency range between 200 and 2,000 Hz. Near the ground in both savanna and riverine forests, excess attenuation tended to increase with an increase in test frequency, and no frequency channel was propagated very favorably. Furthermore, excess attenuation values in these habitats were more variable than those in rain forest. In rain forest, at 200 Hz, the attenuation rate was less than that expected by the inverse square law. Thus a "sound window" for superior long-range propagation was present. This phenomenon was likely due to an inversion-like thermal gradient acting to alter the ray characteristics of the direction of propagation of the wave front such that rays directed towards the upper canopy are bent back into the lower strata occupied by primates (Brown, 1986b). Sound is most favorably propagated in this frequency "window" because it is channeled back into the strata occupied by primates. Channeling of sound in the rain forest is reminiscent of sound channeling in the sofar zone in the ocean (Webb & Tucker, 1970). In both cases long-range acoustic communication signals may have evolved to take advantage of this characteristic of the environment.

In all habitats, the increase in excess attenuation with increasing propagation distances was approximately logarithmic; that is, excess attenuation increased

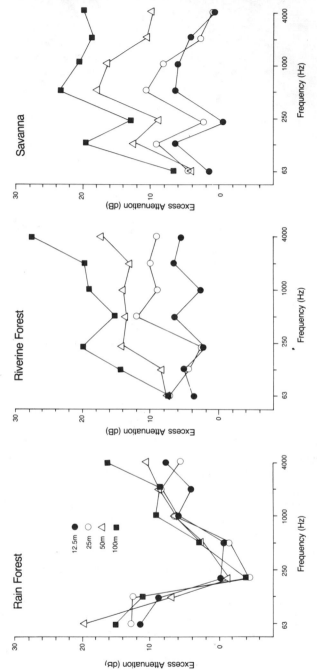

FIG. 7.6. Excess attenuation as a function of tone frequency for source-receiver dis-tances of 12.5, 25, 50 and 100 m. Standard deviations for the six measurements at each frequency and distance range from 1.1–5.8 dB in rain forest, 3.2–10.0 dB in riverine forest, and 1.1–13.9 dB in savanna. From Waser and Brown (1986).

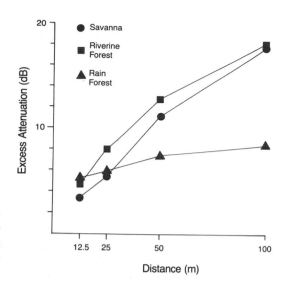

FIG. 7.7. Excess attenuation averaged across broadcast frequencies in each habitat, as a function of broadcast distance. From Waser and Brown (1986).

approximately a constant amount per doubling of distance. The logarithmic relationship between excess attenuation and propagation distance is shown in Fig. 7.7.

The three classes of primate habitats differ both in the background noise and sound propagation characteristics; these differences have consequences for vocal communication over both short and long distances. Over short distances, signals propagate equally well in all habitats (Fig. 7.7). Thus, near the source, signal-to-noise ratios are influenced more by habitat differences in background noise than by habitat differences in propagation rates. Consequently, it is likely that the form of short-range signals should more closely reflect a habitat's background noise characteristics than its attenuation properties. Furthermore, relatively loud short-range signals, those with a large signal-to-noise ratio, should be free to exhibit a form which is independent of the constraints imposed by habitat acoustics. In converse, signals designed to function at the limits of audibility should exhibit a form reflecting habitat-specific constraints.

At distances of 50–100 m, habitat-specific differences in sound transmission become prominent, and equal or outweigh differences in background noise (Fig. 7.7). At these distances, the details of excess attenuation vary complexly with frequency and distance (Fig. 7.6), and this complexity may make it possible for natural selection to have favored calls with certain features for transmission over specific distances. In riverine forest, for example, signals 200 Hz in frequency propagate well to 25 m, but are not propagated well beyond that. This complexity in attenuation characteristics makes it difficult to specify what call structures would be favored for communication over these intermediate distances. One way to circumvent this problem is to broadcast calls and call variants in "appropriate'' and ''inappropriate'' habitats and to conduct measurements of the growth of distortion of the call with transmission distance in each habitat. Relative distortion measurements linking call structure to habitat acoustics have been conducted with bird songs by Gish and Morton (1981), and measurements of this type are under way for primates (Brown & Waser, 1988).

At transmission distances of 100 m or more, habitat differences in attenuation are prominent, and are great enough to outweigh habitat differences in background noise (Waser & Brown, 1986). Hence, the form of long-range signals should more closely reflect the attenuation characteristics of the habitat than its background noise characteristics.

Other Impediments to Vocal Communication

Background noise and attenuation are not the only limiting factors constraining acoustic communication. A call may remain audible after information coded by temporal or frequency modulation has been obscured by environmental variables. Wiley and Richards (1978, 1982; also see Richards & Wiley, 1980) have focused on two critical signal-degrading processes: amplitude fluctuations and reverberation. Amplitude fluctuations are apt to occur when sound is scattered from moving objects, such as turbulent air, and would be expected to be more prominent in open habitats. However, empirical measurements of amplitude fluctuations of broadcast tones (Waser & Brown, 1986) indicate that fluctuations in the rain forest are potentially as troublesome as those in savanna and riverine habitats. In all cases, these fluctuations have the capacity to seriously degrade the transmission of information coded by amplitude modulation, especially at higher carrier frequencies and transmission distances. Under these conditions, like a distant radio station, the information-bearing feature of a signal may fade in and out of reception.

Reverberation is the decay of abrupt signal onsets and offsets due to the scattering and reflection of sound from multiple surfaces in the habitat. Brief pauses or silent intervals in vocal signals are common, and may become obscured by echoes that are present during the silent intervals. Waser and Brown (1986) employed RT60 to measure reverberation because it is a standardized index widely used in architectural acoustics. RT60 is the time it would take for a signal to decay 60 dB from its peak value following its offset. Using this index, reverberation was found to be prominent in both rain forest and riverine forest, but not in savanna. Forest reverberation times were strongly influenced by both transmission distance and carrier frequency. Reverberation time in forested habitats for low-frequency tones (125 Hz) was nearly as short as that in the savanna. Evidently, sounds at this wavelength are not scattered much more in closed than in open habitats.

Environmental impediments to acoustic communication increase with propagation distance. Amplitude fluctuations and reverberation time increase with transmission distance in a way similar to that for attenuation. Hence, ecological constraints on the structure of communication sounds are uniformly more severe for long-range signals. All primate habitat types pose difficulties for amplitude and temporal modulation of signals, yet no studies quantitatively measure difficulties for frequency modulation. Future research should address the relative fidelity of frequency modulation as a function of transmission distance.

Altogether these results suggest that the elaboration of the fine structure of signals is likely restricted to short-range signals for species in all three habitat types. However, because the savanna habitat is free from problems created by reverberation, more elaboration and variation in fine structure may be expected in the signals used in this habitat. The availability of redundant information through the visual modality (Marler, 1965) may supplement the perception of acoustic variants in open habitats. Thus, one may expect finer structural variation both between and within call classes in open country primates relative to those seen in the vocal repertoire of closed habitat primates. Though no quantitative cross-species data are available yet, the vocal patterns of the open country vervets and baboons are suggestive. Vervet monkeys have a more diverse repertoire of short-range signals than do most of the forest *Cercopithecus* species (Gautier & Gautier, 1977; Seyfarth & Cheney, 1982), and baboons, though not quantitatively studied, have one of the richest and most variable vocal repertoires, a repertoire which may be particularly well suited for revealing vocal tract configuration (Andrew, 1963).

V.   PERCEPTION OF ACOUSTIC SIGNALS BY PRIMATES

If the acoustical ecology of the habitat is strong enough to influence the form of vocal signals, is it also strong enough to influence characteristics of the perceptual system? Under laboratory conditions it is possible to quantitatively measure the sensitivity of the auditory system of a wide variety of organisms. Figure 7.8 shows a blue monkey trained by positive reinforcement operant conditioning procedures (Stebbins et al., 1984) to maintain hand contact with a touch sensitive disk until a sound is presented. Upon hearing the presentation of a sound stimulus, the monkey removes its hand from the response disk, and this results in the delivery of food in the food cup. The amplitude of the test sound is controlled by a computer, and standard audiometric procedures are used to measure the subject's sensitivity to a wide variety of sounds presented either in the quiet or in the presence of an ongoing background noise.

Audibility of tones

The audibility of pure tones has been studied in both blue monkeys (Brown & Waser, 1984) and mangabeys (Brown, 1986a), as well as in a variety of open

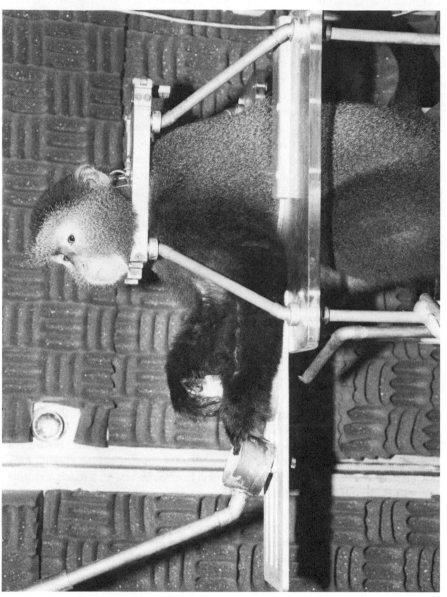

FIG. 7.8. Blue monkey positioned in the test apparatus. The monkey's right hand is

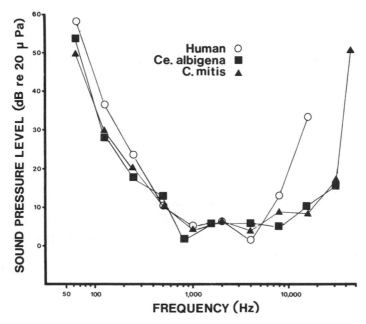

FIG. 7.9. Audiograms for blue monkeys (from Brown and Waser, 1984) and grey-cheeked mangabeys (from Brown, 1986a), and human listeners (from Brown & Waser, 1984).

country primates (Stebbins, 1973). The two rain forest species tested, mangabeys and blue monkeys, exhibit audibility curves that conform to the general U-shaped pattern seen in humans, nonhuman primates, and most birds and mammals (Masterton, Heffner, & Ravissa, 1969; Stebbins, 1973, 1983). These monkeys display superior high-frequency and superior low-frequency hearing relative to human listeners (Fig. 7.9). Though all nonhuman primates tested to date have high-frequency hearing that is superior to that of humans, enhanced low-frequency hearing has only been reported for these two rain forest monkeys. Brown and Waser (1984) noted that at low-frequencies blue monkeys may be as much as 20 dB more sensitive than the comparably sized open country rhesus monkey. Primates which occupy rain forested habitats, and which are arboreal, may capitalize on the low-frequency window for superior signal transmission by developing adaptations for low-frequency sound production and sound reception. What form might such adaptations take? Though studies on the anatomy of the auditory system of blue monkeys and mangabeys are lacking, it has been shown that the relatively enlarged middle ear cavity of kangaroo rats improves their low-frequency hearing compared to that for Norway rats (Webster & Webster, 1972). It is possible that hypertrophied middle ear chambers may aid low-frequency perception in some species of forest primates as well.

In primates, mechanisms underlying low-frequency sound production have received more study than those underlying low-frequency sound reception. In an experimental study, Gautier (1971) has shown that the extralaryngeal vocal sac must be inflated to produce loud low-frequency calls. The inflated sac is believed to act as a resonator, enhancing the amplitude of the low-frequencies to which it is tuned. Gautier (1971) has also shown that many rain forest species have greater development of these extralaryngeal structures relative to species which lack these specialized low-frequency loud calls in their vocal repertoire.

Detection of Complex Signals in Noise

The above results suggest that gross morphological features of a species' audibility function and the frequency range of the vocal repertoire have been influenced by acoustical characteristics of the habitat; in principal it is also possible that details of the structure of communication systems may similarly be specialized to promote communication in the natural environment. Under natural conditions vocal signals are always embedded in ongoing, temporally fluctuating background noise, and Brown (1986a) simulated the ambient noise of rain forests in the laboratory to compare the relative audibility of monkey vocalizations and human speech in a natural acoustic background. Sound spectograms of the monkey test vocalizations were shown in Fig. 7.3. The human speech signals were the stop consonant vowels: *ba, da, ga, pa, ta, ka*, the spondee words: *baseball, lifeguard, vessel, leisure*, and the sentence: *Can you hear me?* Sound spectrograms for these 11 speech signals are presented in Fig. 7.10. Audibility of signals was tested in conspecific listeners: blue monkeys were tested with blue monkey calls, mangabeys were tested with mangabey calls, and human listeners were tested with the speech samples.

In nature, vocal signals of biological significance may occur unpredictably in time, in an ongoing temporally fluctuating acoustic background. This situation creates complex detection problems for the listener, which are illustrated in Figure 11. The top panel of Fig. 7.11 shows a 1.0 s segment of the spectrum by time plot of rain forest background noise. Each frame on the time axis displays the spectrum for a time window of 20 ms. The frequency range for the spectrum is from 0 Hz to 5,000 Hz. The amplitude and spectrum of the noise fluctuates over time. In the middle and bottom panels the spectrum of the blue monkey *chirp* vocalization is superimposed on the forest noise. In the middle panel the signal level is about 30 dB above threshold. At this level signals are easily detected 100% of the time. In the bottom panel the signal is about 3 dB above threshold. It is just visible in the noise, yet it is still detected on about 70% of the trials. At threshold levels, the signals are embedded in the noise and may not be visually perceptible. This figure depicts the basic issues involved in the perception of vocalizations in noise. The detectability of calls in noise may be expressed by the signal-to-noise ratio:

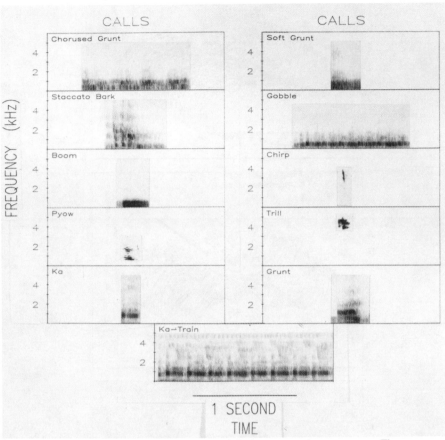

FIG. 7.10. Sound spectrograms of human speech utterances. The horizontal bar indicates 1 second. From Brown (1986a).

$$S/N = 20 \log (\text{level of signal/level of noise}) \qquad (1)$$

Equation (1) shows that if the level of the just detected signal is equal to that for the noise, then the signal-to-noise ratio is equal to 0 dB. If the level of the signal exceeds that for the noise, the ratio will be positive, and if the level of the signal is less than that for the noise, the resulting ratio will be negative.

Figure 7.12 shows the signal-to-noise ratio for the detection of the 22 monkey call and human speech test signals. The least detectable signal was the human utterance *ka,* which was just audible at a signal-to-noise ratio of −8.5 dB. In contrast, the most detectable signal was the blue monkey *boom* (S/N = −30.3 dB). The average signal-to-noise ratios of detection of the monkey calls was

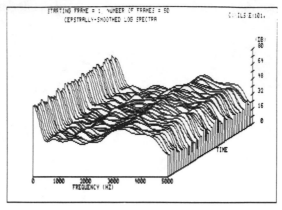

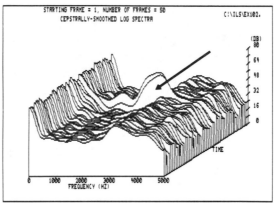

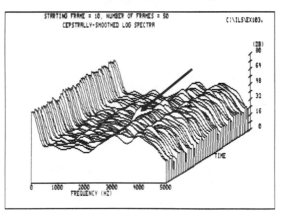

FIG. 7.11.   Spectra by time plots of forest background noise only (top panel); *chirp* vocalization (arrow) superimposed on background noise at a level 30 dB above masked threshold (middle panel); background noise with a *chirp* vocalization at a level 3 dB above masked threshold. Each frame on the time axis represents a duration of 20 ms. Signal amplitude is represented in relative values. From Brown (1986a).

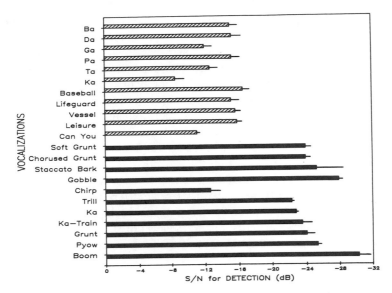

FIG. 7.12.   Signal-to-noise ratios for the detection of 11 human utterances (open bars) and 11 monkey calls (solid bars). The standard error of the mean is denoted by the fine horizontal line. From Brown (1986a).

−23.8 dB, while that for the speech signals was −13.9 dB. The monkey calls were nearly 10 dB more audible in forest noise than were speech signals. It is noteworthy that classic measurements of human speech in noise yielded signal-to-noise ratios of about −16 dB (Hawkins & Stevens, 1950; Miller, 1947). This result is close to that obtained here (−13.9 dB) for human listeners even though the spectral features of the masking noise, the vocal stimuli, and the experimental methods differ. It is also interesting to note that the speech stimuli varied little in regard to their audibility in noise: The sentence *Can you hear me?* was about as detectable in noise as were the two-syllable words, or the single consonant-vowel syllables. The same pattern of results was noted in the classic studies of the audibility of speech in noise: words, phrases, and sentences were audible at similar signal-to-noise ratios. Of the monkey calls studied here, all were more audible in noise than were any of the speech signals except for the blue monkey *chirp* call. These highly audible monkey calls do not sound like speech, and with the exception of the *chirp* call these vocalizations are difficult for a human speaker to mimic. These vocal signals possess structural features that the human speech production apparatus cannot readily reproduce. On the other hand the *chirp* call sounds like an ingressive lateral click as used in Zulu, Xhosa, and some other languages (Ladefoged, 1975).

The nearly identical performance of blue monkeys and mangabeys supports the idea that forest monkeys in general may have developed specializations in the form of their vocal repertoire to promote the audibility of their signals in noise. As shown by measurements of habitat acoustics presented earlier, forest primates reside in relatively noisy environments, and specializations in features of the communication system may have evolved to promote communication in this habitat. Specializations for the heightened audibility of calls in noise could occur in the form of the signals themselves, in the structure of the auditory system, or in both. One key difference between forest monkey calls and human speech is that many forest monkey utterances are discrete signals, whereas human speech sounds would be classified as a graded repertoire (Marler, 1975). Thus, can the graded-discrete dichotomy account for the superior audibility of primate calls in noise? Brown (1986a) reported that the mean signal-to-noise ratio for six discrete primate calls was -23.8 dB, while that for five graded primate calls was -23.9 dB. Consequently, the superior audibility of monkey calls in forest noise, compared to that for speech, cannot be due to the level of stereotypy of the signals, but rather must be due to other features of the form of the utterances or alternatively be due to receptive specializations.

Receptive Specializations

The idea that speech perception was governed by a nonlinear processing, presumably species-specific, subsystem of the brain took root with the early work of Liberman and his colleagues at Haskins Laboratories (Liberman, Cooper, Shankweiler, & Studdert-Kennedy, 1967). One nonlinear phenomenon, that of categorial perception (see Kuhl, 1986, this volume), was once regarded as the hallmark of the speech mode of perception, but it has been found to occur for some visual stimuli (Pastore, Friedman, Baffuto, & Fink, 1976), and for some nonspeech sounds (Cutting, 1982; Cutting, Rossner, & Foard, 1976; Miller et al., 1976; Pisoni, 1977). Furthermore, Kuhl and her colleagues have directly challenged the idea of species-specific perceptual abilities for an organism's own communication sounds (Kuhl, 1986; Kuhl & Miller, 1975, 1978; Kuhl & Padden, 1982; this volume). Kuhl and her associates found that Japanese monkeys, as well as chinchillas, perceived some human speech continua in the same nonlinear discontinuous fashion as human listeners. Hence, some perceptual phenomena thought to reflect the action of speech mode processing did not depend on species-specific capabilities, and hence must reflect the general perceptual tendencies of related vertebrates (see Kuhl, this volume). Specialization for communication would accordingly not depend on exclusive species-specific mechanisms, but rather would depend on the emergence of specializations to produce signals that exploit perceptual characteristics shared by a wide variety of organisms. Some comparative research using nonhuman vocal signals, however, has supported the idea of species-specific perceptual specializations. Petersen and his associates have found that Japanese monkeys exhibit specialized, nonlinear perceptual processing of some of their vocal continua, while discriminat-

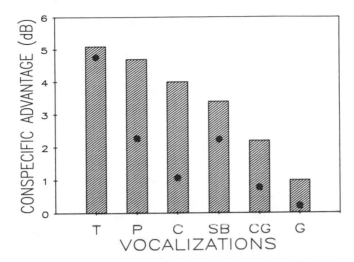

FIG. 7.13.   Relative advantage for detection by conspecific listeners tested with a forest noise masker. Vocalizations: *trill* (T), *pyow* (P), *chirp* (C), *staccato bark* (SB), *chorused grunt* (CG), *gobble* (G). The difference between the worst conspecific subject and the best sympatric subject is given by the solid circle. The positive scores shown here indicate that there was no overlap in the range of the two species. From Brown (1986a).

ing communicatively relevant stimuli (Zoloth et al., 1979). When the same stimuli are used in a noncommunicatively relevant task, linear, unspecialized, processing of the stimulus dimension occurs, similar to that seen for either task by monkey species other than Japanese macaques. The idea of a species-specific subsystem of the brain underlying the perception of vocalizations by Japanese macaques is buttressed by brain lesion studies (Heffner & Heffner, 1984). The Heffners found that the ability of Japanese monkeys to discriminate their own vocalizations on the same communicative dimension as employed by Petersen and his associates (Zoloth et al., 1979) was abolished following controlled damage to the left temporal lobe in a region corresponding to the classical human language areas.

More recently, Brown (1986a) found that blue monkeys and grey-cheeked mangabeys were best able to detect their own species-specific communication signals presented in forest noise relative to their ability to hear the calls of other species of monkeys (Fig. 7.13). When testing was conducted in the absence of a competing background noise, no differences were found in the ability of the two species to hear any of the calls. This result suggests that there is some species-specific perceptual specialization for the detection of signals biologically relevant to forest primates under test conditions simulating the natural situation. The small average difference of the conspecific advantage, 3.4 dB, compared to the

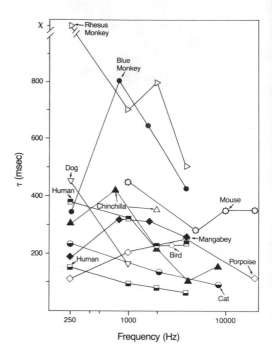

FIG. 7.14. Temporal integration time (tau), measured in msec, as a function of test frequency. Data from blue monkeys and mangabeys (Brown & Maloney, 1986) are compared with that from rhesus monkey (Clack, 1966), porpoise (Johnson, 1968), mouse (Ehret, 1976), chinchilla [open triangle (Henderson, 1969); filled triangle (Clark, 1986)], dog (Baru, 1971), cat (Costalupes, 1983), song bird (Dooling, 1979), and human subjects [top half of square filled (Plomp & Bouman, 1959); bottom half of square filled (Watson & Gengel, 1969).] The X on the ordinate represents values of tau that exceed 1000 ms.

10 dB difference between the audibility of speech and monkey calls in noise (Fig. 7.12) suggests that this difference is due more to differences in the acoustical form of the signal rather than due to differences in the attributes of each species' perceptual system.

Brown and Maloney (1986) compared temporal integration in blue monkeys and mangabeys. Because defects in temporal integration are believed to be involved in a variety of communication disorders in human listeners (Collins & Cullen, 1978; Hall & Fernandez, 1983; Irwin & Purdey, 1982; Nabelek, 1978; Tyler, Summerfield, Wood, & Fernandes, 1982) Brown and Maloney reasoned that differences in temporal integration may underlie differences in call perception in these species. The results displayed in Fig. 7.14 show that the temporal integration times of these two species differed, but the direction of the difference is not readily related to global features of the vocal repertoires. Blue monkeys which characteristically produce brief signals exhibited long temporal integration times, while mangabeys with longer duration calls, produced comparatively short temporal integration times. Brown and Maloney (1986) noted, however, that the "appropriate" relationship between acoustic temporal processing and the form of the vocal communication system has yet to be established. These results do show that species differences occur in the temporal processing abilities of primate auditory systems, as well as in their ability to hear biologically relevant signals in noise. The finding that monkeys differ in their temporal integration function is reminiscent of the finding that birds may differ in their critical bandwidths (Dooling, 1986, this volume). The discovery of an aberrant critical bandwidth was initially mystifying and had no meaning, yet on subsequent analysis it contributed to a new appreciation regarding how birds may exhibit superior processing of species-specific song. It is possible that future research will demonstrate a powerful relationship between temporal integration functions and the perception of vocalizations. Together these findings support the idea that an ensemble of subtle differences may individualize the perception of sound by each species.

How can the results of these studies be so discrepant, where one area of research finds no support for species-specific perceptual abilities, while the other does? It is odd that the studies cited above which favor the idea of species-specific perceptual abilities employ primate calls as stimuli, while those challenging this idea use speech sounds for test signals. One key possibility is that the two opposing outcomes are associated with tests conducted at different levels of processing. Interestingly, those studies supporting the idea of species-specific processing employ signals that are believed to function individually as a complete biologically significant utterance, while those supporting generalized processing abilities employ elements of speech as stimuli which have no functional meaning. For example, both voice-onset-time and place-of-articulation phonetic contrasts studied by a number of investigators (Kuhl & Miller, 1975, 1978; Kuhl & Padden, 1982; Morse & Snowdon, 1975; Waters & Wilson, 1976) focus on the processing of brief sounds such as *ba* or *pa*. These sounds evoke no meaningful referent, and likely require a different level of processing than that underlying the discrimination of the Japanese macaque smooth-early-high and smooth-late-high coo utterances studied by Petersen and his associates (Petersen et al., 1978, 1984; Zoloth et al., 1979). The latter stimuli vocally identify very different situations regarding the reproductive and social relationships of the interactants (Green, 1975). To date, there are no studies using both human and monkey listeners in which primate utterances are used as stimuli, or in which more global speech units, such as words or phrases are used as stimuli. Kuhl (1986) persuasively argues that animal tests with human speech signals are critical for distinguishing those perceptual skills which are dependent upon auditory-level processing from those which require more specialized phonetic-level processing. Though this is true, species-differences and perceptual specializations certainly occur at levels other than that of the auditory and phonetic levels; species differences in temporal integration (Brown & Maloney, 1986) or critical bandwidth (Dooling, 1986) insure that this must be true, and the development of an appreciation of these differences is central for understanding the mechanisms that give rise to language. From this perspective, the results showing species-specific abilities and those not showing such specializations are not in disagreement; the different results reflect the presence or absence of species-specific capabilities at different levels of processing. Furthermore, this perceptive suggests that specializations between species may not be confined to "higher cognitive" processes. Critical differences may be exhibited in characteristics as mundane as temporal summation and critical bandwidths. Additional research in the next decade will certainly address these questions in much more detail.

VI. SOCIAL REGULATION AND THE AUDIBLE RANGE OF VOCALIZATIONS

Though ancestral primates as well as the more recent progenitors of blue monkeys and mangabeys evolved in forested habitats, early man and presumably his communication system evolved in a more open grassland or savanna habitat. Here at least close-range communication is unimpeded by noise, reverberation, or attenuation. As noted above, though open habitats permit vocal signals to be accompanied by corollary visual displays, such habitats are less suitable for long-range acoustic communication. One key parameter of a communication system then, may be the active space, or communicative range, over which it is intended to function. Limits may be imposed by the habitat, and these limits may influence the way the communication system is apt to be used to regulate social exchanges. This consideration is addressed in this section.

The linear audible distance of a signal is governed by five factors, which include characteristics of the signal, characteristics of the environment, and characteristics of the recipient. These factors are: (1) signal amplitude and spectrum at its source, (2) transmission characteristics of signals within the natural environment, (3) degradation of signal structure as a result of transmission within the natural environment, (4) amplitude and spectra of background noise within the environment, and (5) masked auditory threshold of the signal embedded in environmental background noise. In the calculations of audible distance Brown (1989a) used measurements of vocal amplitude conducted by the substitution method described below, and measurements of sound transmission and background noise described above (Brown & Waser, 1984; Waser & Brown, 1984, 1986).

Measurement of Vocal Amplitude

Unless a signal is generated and received in an echo free environment, the level of the signal measured will reflect both the amplitude of the signal at production and the interaction of the signal with environmental structures. Standing waves produced by reflections of on-going signals with environmental surfaces may give rise to both destructive and constructive interference at the point of measurement. Because sound pressure level measurements are the sum of direct and reflected waves, such measurements in most environments are likely to be poor indices of the amplitude of the direct wave. In the case of complex signals composed of many frequencies, interference characteristics at the point of mea-

TABLE 7.1
Sound Pressure Level at 2 m (re 20 uPa) and Sound Power (re 1 pW) of
Test Vocalizations

Species	Vocalization	Frequency	Pressure	Power
Blue	Chirp	4 kHz	87	93
Monkey	Trill	4 kHz	83	87
	Grunt	500 Hz	69	80
	Boom	250 Hz	88	96
	Pyow	2 kHz	100	109
	Ka*	1 kHz	95	
	Ka-train*	1 kHz	95	
Mangabey	Gobble	250 Hz	87	97
	Staccato bark	2 kHz	95	104
	Soft grunt	250 Hz	62	72
	Chorused grunt	250 Hz	87	97
Human	Hey modal	1 kHz	96	110
	Hey maximal	1 kHz	106	120

Peak frequency is measured in the nearest octave corresponding to the measurement bands used for the sound pressure and power measurements.

*Pressure measurements were estimated from those given in Waser and Waser (1977).

surement will differ for the various frequency components. As a result, the relative representation of each frequency component will be determined not only by the composition of the call, but also by the interference characteristics of each frequency component at that point in the environment. The obvious solution is to conduct measurements of signals only in anechoic environments. However, most nonhuman organisms are extraordinarily uncooperative, and will emit only a restricted subset of their vocalizations in an anechoic room. As a result most measurements of animal vocalizations are made under either field conditions, or colony room conditions, and investigators ignore the problems of environmental influences on their measurements. Brown (1989a) has noted that measurements of sound power are more resistant to environmental influences than are sound pressure measurements. Under colony room conditions, sound pressure measurements of monkey calls may be greater than 20 dB in error relative to the actual level of the signal. In contrast, the average error of comparable sound power measurements is less than 1 dB (Brown, 1989a). Table 7.1 presents measurements of the sound power of some primate vocalizations, and corresponding measurements of the sound pressure level of the call conducted in an anechoic room.

Audible Distance

Using the above measurements of vocal amplitude the audible distance of 11 representative forest monkey vocalizations is compared with the human yell *hey*

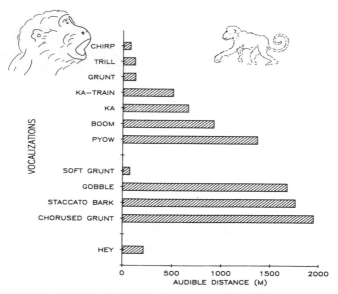

FIG. 7.15.   Audible distance for 12 test vocalizations. Calculations for forest monkey signals were made for an elevation of 8 m, that for the human utterance was made at 1.5 m. From Brown (1989b).

in Fig. 7.15. The audible distance of signals ranged from 79 m for the *chirp* call to 1951 m for the *chorused grunt* vocalization. Vocalizations clustered into two categories: short-range calls with an audible distance of about 100 m, and long-range calls with an audible distance often exceeding 1000 m. The audible distance of the three mangabey long-range calls averaged 1800 m, a value about twice as great as the mean audible distance (890 m) of the four blue monkey long-range calls. The audible range of these forest monkey calls is contrasted with that for the utterance *hey* used by humans; the modal distance for 12 human vocalizers for this signal was 217 m. The loudest *hey* recorded yielded an audible distance of 434 m emitted at ground level in the rain forest. The modal yell was audible only about one ninth as far as the modal *chorused grunt*.

The Active Space of Primate Calls

The active space of a vocal signal is the area surrounding the vocalizer over which the signal is audible; as such it is a fundamental parameter of a signal, and influences the function of the signal in the communication system (Brenowitz, 1982). Though Brenowitz (1982) calculated active space as only a one-dimensional linear distance, Brown (1989b) evaluates active space as the area on a two-dimensional plane over which a signal is audible because arboreal as well as terrestrial primates frequently occupy the same strata at any point in time. In marine organisms traveling in schools which occupy three-dimensional space, the active space of signals may more appropriately be visualized as a volume. Though the active space of primate vocal signals is given by a two-dimensional surface over which the call is audible, the signal may not radiate at equal amplitudes in all directions from the source.

Brown (1989a) has measured vocal radiation patterns in blue monkeys and mangabeys, and has reported that sound radiates from the monkey's mouth in a manner similar to that of typical audio speakers. Table 7.2 shows that sound radiation from the mouth is frequency dependent, with high-frequency sounds being emitted more directionally, while low-frequency sounds are radiated in a more omni-directional pattern. Table 7.2 also shows sound radiation patterns for human speakers (Dunn & Farnsworth, 1939), and for a Kudelski DH loud speaker (Brown & Waser, 1984). From knowing the amplitude of the signal, its pattern of radiation from the source, and the attenuation characteristics of the environment, it is possible to construct equal amplitude contours for signals of a particular dominant frequency on a plane around the source. Calculations of area may be symplified by idealizing the active space as the area of two semicircles

TABLE 7.2
Radiation Patterns of Vocal Signals. Signal Level Is
Measured (dBA) Relative to That Directly in Front of
the Vocalizer's Mouth (0° azinuth, +/−15°).

Signal	0°	90°	180°
Octave band	Data for monkeys		
125 Hz	0	−1.1	0.0
250 Hz	0	−3.0	−1.5
500 Hz	0	−4.1	−1.0
1000 Hz	0	−3.7	−6.0
2000 Hz	0	−5.3	−8.3
4000 Hz	0	−6.9	−7.5
Band pass	Data for human subjects*		
62.5–125 Hz	0	−0.2	−0.6
125–250 Hz	0	−0.3	−4.6
250–500 Hz	0	−1.2	−5.3
700–1000 Hz	0	+1.4	−3.8
1400–2000 Hz	0	−4.1	−12.4
2800–4000 Hz	0	−2.5	−17.2
Pure tone	Kudelski DH loud speaker**		
200 Hz	0	−4.4	+1.1
500 Hz	0	−3.8	−6.0
1000 Hz	0	−9.2	−8.4
2000 Hz	0	−12.4	−5.4
4000 Hz	0	−16.9	−11.7

*Data from Dunn and Farnsworth (1939).
**Data from Waser and Brown (1986).

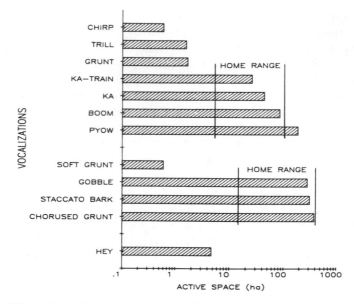

FIG. 7.16.   Active space in hectares for 12 test vocalizations. Calculations were made in reference to the vocal radiation patterns given in
Table 7.2 (see text). From Brown (1989b).

sharing a common base, where the radius of one semicircle is given by the
audible distance of the signal along the vocal axis, and the radius of the second
semicircle corresponds to the audible distance of the signal reduced by the loss in
signal amplitude at 180° for the call's dominant frequency band (Table 7.2). The
active space given in hectares of the 12 test signals is presented in Fig. 7.16.
Estimates of the home range or core area utilized by mangabey and blue monkey
social groups are also presented (Wolfheim, 1983).

Population Density, Distribution and Communication

Given knowledge of population densities, it is possible to plot the expected
number of recipients of a signal assuming a random distribution of potential
recipients around a vocalizer, and assuming that the vocalizer is unaware of the
proximity of any potential recipients or that vocalizations are emitted spontaneously. Though these assumptions may hold for some long-range signals,
they almost certainly do not hold for the production of short-range calls which
likely are not emitted unless visual contact has been established. Figure 7.17
shows calculations of the expected number of recipients using Wolfheim's
(1983) upper value of the densities of blue monkeys and grey-cheeked mangabeys. Lower population densities would necessarily result in decrements in the

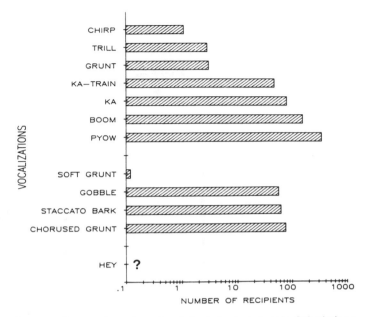

FIG. 7.17. Expected number of recipients for test signals. Calculations were based on the highest natural densities (0.2 mangabeys per ha; 1.834 blue monkeys per ha) reported by Wolfheim (1983). Modified from Brown (1989b).

expected number of recipients over the value given here. The results show that the expected number of recipients cluster into two categories: "private calls" heard by 9 or fewer listeners, and "public signals" audible to 100 or more recipients.

Mangabeys and blue monkeys differ in respect to their home range size, population densities, and audible distances of their long-range calls. The home range of blue monkeys varies from 5.2 to 100 ha, with a median value of 47.4 ha; the home range of mangabeys varies from 13 to 400 ha, with a median value of 193.5 ha (Wolfheim, 1983). The typical mangabey home range at 200 ha is four times that (50 ha) for the blue monkey. The mangabey home range may be idealized as a circle 900 m in diameter (the circle with an area of 200 ha), and the blue monkey home range would correspond to a circle with a diameter of 450 m. The audible range of loud calls differs between species and corresponds well with home range dimensions. The four blue monkey loud calls: *boom, pyow, ka,* and *ka-train* have a mean audible distance of 870 m. The three mangabey long-range calls: gobble, staccato bark and chorused grunt have an average audible distance of 1,800 m. As shown in Fig. 7.18 the audible distance of the typical long-range call of each species may be examined in respect to the dimensions of the home range. The results are striking; the typical blue monkey long-range call

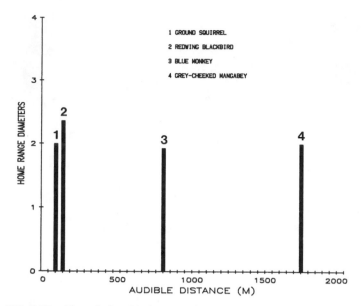

FIG. 7.18. The relationship between long-range call audible distance and home range diameter (see text). The ground squirrel data is adopted from Brown and Schwagmeyer (1984). The red-winged blackbird data is from Brenowitz (1982). The mangabey and blue monkey data is from Brown (1989b).

is audible for 1.95 home range diameters, while that for mangabeys is audible for 2.0 home range diameters. These values are close to those calculated for thirteen-lined ground squirrels (Brown & Schwagmeyer, 1984) and red-winged black-birds (Brenowitz, 1982). Brenowitz (1982), in the first determination of active space, noted that red-winged blackbird territorial calls were audible for about two home range diameters. Brenowitz (1982) hypothesized that the 2:1 ratio of audible distance to home range diameters may be wide spread for it would permit a vocalizer to signal from any position in its home range and have the signal be audible to its neighbor listening from any point in his home range. Brown's (1989b) data agree with this hypothesis, and add support to the idea that social structures, population densities and territorial dimensions have coevolved with features of the communication system permitting the regulation and spacing of individuals by voice.

VII.   ECOLOGICAL ACOUSTICS AND COMMUNICATION

Through integration of perceptual and ecological investigations a detailed appre-ciation of the factors involved in the organization and evolution of primate communication begins to emerge. Though it has been proposed that the discrete, punctate class of utterances may be superior for long-range communication in forests (Gautier & Gautier, 1977; Marler, 1965, 1973, 1975; Waser & Waser, 1977) measurements of audible distance and active space have been lacking. Of the seven long-range calls shown in Fig. 7.16, six are stereotype, discrete signals (*ka-train, ka, boom, pyow, gobble,* and *staccato bark*). Of the long-range calls, only the chorused grunt is a graded utterance. Of the four short-range calls shown in Fig. 7.16 (*chirp, trill, grunt,* and *soft-grunt*), only the *chirp* call is discrete, and the others are all graded signals. The graded-discrete dimension then, is associated with the functional range of the signal. Waser and Brown (1986) suggested that elaboration of fine structure was associated with short-range signals. The graded-discrete dimension and its association with audible range is congruent with this view. Graded signals which permit communicatively significant variation in fine structure are strongly associated with short audible distances in the rain forest, and this trend is likely upheld in riverine and savanna habitats as well.

The terms "long-range calls" and "loud-calls" are often used synonymously (Gautier & Gautier, 1977; Waser & Waser, 1977). Yet it is possible for a call to be loud, and exhibit only a modest audible range. How well does the amplitude of a signal at production predict its audible range? Less than 29% of the variance in audible range of the monkey vocalizations shown in Fig. 7.15 is attributable to the amplitude of the signal at production (Brown, 1989b). Thus, while amplitude is a significant contributor to audible range, so are other factors including signal frequency, background noise and so forth. The simple identification of a signal as a loud call does not ensure its function as a long-range communication signal.

Waser and Brown (1986) argued that the form of long-range calls should be governed more closely by attenuation properties of the habitat than by background noise. The rain forest habitat exhibits a "sound window" for superior propagation for frequencies near 200 Hz. Of the seven long-range calls in Fig. 7.15, three signals, the *boom, gobble,* and *chorused grunt,* utilize the sound window for long-range propagation, while the remaining four calls do not. The form of long-range calls then is not strictly governed by the propagation characteristics of the habitat. A loss in audible distance resulting from the utilization of a dominant frequency outside the sound window may be compensated for by an increase in sound amplitude at production. The four long-range calls not utilizing the sound window exhibit a mean amplitude at production about 10 dB greater than those which do use the sound window.

The form of the four short-range calls shown in Fig. 7.15 showed no consistent relationship with frequency. Waser and Brown (1986) expected that short-range signals would tend to reflect a habitat's background noise characteristics with the dominant frequency concentrated into quiet regions of the ambient noise spectra. In rain forests, background noise (Fig. 7.5) is low—between 500 and 800 Hz, and above 10,000 Hz. There is no evidence that adult Old World monkeys communicate with frequencies above 10,000 Hz, though they may hear to 40,000 Hz or beyond and the background noise above 10,000 Hz is low. Of the four short-range calls shown in Fig. 7.15, only the blue monkey's *grunt* and some *soft grunt* variants given by mangabeys would fall in the 500–800 Hz zone. In contrast the *trill* and *chirp* calls, with dominant energy near 3,000 Hz, clearly fall into a region of high background noise. It is interesting to note that the *chirp* and *trill* calls are relatively loud short-range calls with an average amplitude at 1.25 m of 87 dB and 83 dB respectively (see Table 7.1). The blue monkey and mangabey *grunt* calls are much quieter signals, and are given at levels of 69 dB and 62 dB respectively (Table 7.1). Thus the two loud short-range calls are given at a level about 20 dB greater than the two quiet short-range calls. This 20 dB difference in signal level is nearly matched by a 15 dB difference in the background noise level at the dominant frequencies of the loud and quiet classes of short-range signals. These observations support the idea that loud short-range signals, those with a high signal-to-noise ratio at production, may be free to exhibit a dominant frequency free from environmental constraints. Furthermore, it should be noted that some short-range calls, such as the *trills* and *chirps,* are less commonly emitted than others, and it is possible that the most typical or commonly produced short-range utterances are approximately 500–800 Hz in frequency matching the quiet zone in the ambient noise. In summation, the quiet class of short-range calls appears to be constrained by the spectrum of background noise in rain forest as predicted by Waser and Brown (1986), while loud short-range signals, like loud long-range signals, are not constrained by environmental acoustics.

These observations are consistent with the idea that the form of vocal signals is frequently a compromise reflecting selection for an ensemble of attributes (Brown, 1982b). Often the optimal specification for one characteristic of a signal may be contradictory with that for another. For example, the optimal frequency for sound propagation may differ from the optimal frequency for obscuring the location of the vocalizer, and selection for ventroloquial attributes of a signal (Brown, 1982a, 1982b; Marler, 1955) may be at odds with selection for the maximal audible range. The form of most signals then, may be an acoustic compromise in which selection for the composite qualities of the signal result in a form which departs from the optimal specification for any isolated attribute. Some features of the structure of many primate vocalizations may be resistant to modification because of the stability of the physical and acoustical atributes of the habitat. It is self-evident that sophisticated communication systems do not evolve in a solitary species. Communication systems are involved in the social regulation of communal living species and, presumably, have evolved to individually and collectively reduce the costs and increase the benefits of living in groups. Long-range calls have been shown to regulate the spacing of individuals both within and between groups (Waser, 1975; Whitehead, 1987). The relationship between the audible range of long-range calls and home range dimensions shown in Fig. 7.18 underscores the fact that the "need" for social regulation by voice (or the benefit derived by such a system) must be one of the principal driving forces in the evolution of acoustic communication systems. The point here is that the questions investigators most commonly ask regarding the evolution of speech and communication systems are focused singularly on the origin (or distribution) of physiological, perceptual, or cognitive mechanisms, without consideration of the behavioral ecology of the species in question. Yet, it is the behavioral ecology of organisms, the habitat and social milieu, which determined the form of both the perceptual and productive components of the communication system, and it is in this natural context in which the "success" of the design of the components of the system is ultimately determined. The behavioral ecology of vocal exchanges is probably the most understudied area in communication, and breakthroughs in the understanding of the "speech code" may be dependent on understanding the role of speech-like mechanisms in the communicative behavior of nonhuman organisms.

ACKNOWLEDGMENTS

I thank J. Hart, P. Phillips, R. Kunze, and P. Waser who commented on an earlier version of this manuscript. The research reviewed in this chapter was supported by NIH grants R01 NS16632-09 and K04 NS00880-05.

REFERENCES

Andrew, R. A. (1963). Trends apparent in the evolution of vocalizations in the Old World monkeys and apes. *Symposium of the Zoological Society of London, 10,* 89–101.
Baru, A. V. (1971). Absolute thresholds and frequency difference limen as a function of sound duration in dogs deprived of the auditory cortex. In G. V. Gersuni (Ed.), *Sensory processes at the neuronal and behavioral levels* (pp. 265–285). New York: Academic Press.
Brenowitz, E. A. (1982). The active space of red-winged blackbird song. *Journal of Comparative Physiology, 147,* 511–522.
Brown, C. H. (1982a). Ventroloquial and locatable vocalizations in birds. *Zeitschrift für Tierpsychologie, 59,* 338–350.
Brown, C. H. (1982b). Auditory localization and primate vocal behavior. In C. T. Snowdon, C. H. Brown, & M. R. Petersen (Eds.), *Primate communication* (pp. 144–164). Cambridge, England: Cambridge University Press.
Brown, C. H. (1986a). The perception of vocal signals by blue monkeys and grey-cheeked mangabeys. *Experimental Biology, 45,* 145–165.
Brown, C. H. (1986b). Forest noise and sound transmission in East African primate habitats. In M. J. M. Martens (Ed.), *Proceedings of the workshop on sound propagation in forested areas and shelterbelts* (pp. 185–196). Nijmegen, Netherlands: Faculty of Sciences Catholic University of Nijmegen.
Brown, C. H. (1989a). The measurement of vocal amplitude and vocal radiation pattern in blue monkeys and grey-cheeked mangabeys. *Bioacoustics,* in press.
Brown, C. H. (1989b). The active space of blue monkey and grey-cheeked mangabey vocalizations. *Animal Behaviour,* in press.

Brown, C. H., & Maloney, C. G. (1986). Temporal integration in two species of Old World monkeys: Blue monkeys (*Cercopithecus mitis*) and grey-cheeked mangabeys (*Cercocebus albigena*), *Journal of the Acoustical Society of America, 79,* 1058–1064.

Brown, C. H., & Schwagmeyer, P. L. (1984). The vocal range of alarm calls in thirteen-lined ground squirrels. *Zeitschrift für Tierpsychologie, 65,* 273–288.

Brown, C. H., & Waser, P. M. (1984). Hearing and communication in blue monkeys (*Cercopithecus mitis*). *Animal Behaviour, 32,* 66–75.

Brown, C. H., & Waser, P. M. (1988). Environmental influences on the structure of primate vocalizations. In D. Todt, P. Goedeking, & D. Symmes (Eds.), *Primate vocal communication* (pp. 51–66). Berlin: Springer-Verlag.

Capranica, R. R. (1974). Why auditory neurophysiologists should be more interested in animal sound communication. *The Physiologist, 15,* 55–60.

Chalmers, N. R. (1968). The visual and vocal communication of free-living mangabeys in Uganda. *Folia Primatologia, 9,* 258–280.

Clack, T. D. (1966). Effect of signal duration on the auditory sensitivity of humans and monkeys (*Macaca mulatta*). *Journal of the Acoustical Society of America, 40,* 1140–1146.

Clark, W. W. (1986). Cochlear damage: Audiometric correlates? In T. Glattke (Ed.), *Sensorineural hearing loss: Mechanisms, diagnosis, and treatment* (pp. 59–82). Iowa City: University of Iowa Press.

Collins, M. J., & Cullen, J. K. (1978). Temporal integration of tone glides. *Journal of the Acoustical Society of America, 63,* 469–473.

Costaloupes, J. A. (1983). Temporal integration of pure tones in the cat. *Hearing Research, 9,* 42–54.

Cutting, J. E. (1982). Plucks and bows are categorically perceived, sometimes. *Perception and Psychophysics, 31,* 462–476.

Cutting, J., Rosner, B., & Foard, C. (1976). Perceptual categories for music-like sounds: Implications for theories of speech perception. *Quarterly Journal of Experimental Psychology, 28,* 1–18.

Dooling, R. J. (1979). Temporal summation for pure tones in birds. *Journal of the Acoustical Society of America, 65,* 1058–1060.

Dooling, R. (1986). Perception of vocal signals by budgerigars (*Melopsittacus undulatus*). *Experimental Biology, 45,* 193–216.

Dunn, H. K., & Farnsworth, D. W. (1939). Exploration of the pressure field around the human head during speech. *Journal of the Acoustical Society of America, 10,* 184–199.

Ehret, G. (1976). Temporal auditory summation for pure tones and white noise in the house mouse (*Mus musculus*). *Journal of the Acoustical Society of America, 59,* 1421–1427.

Gautier, J.-P. (1971). Étude morphologique et fonctionnelle des annexes extra-laryngées des Cercepithecine; liaison avec les cris d'espacement. *Biol Gabon, 7,* 229–267.

Gautier, J.-P, & Gautier, A. (1977). Communication in Old World monkeys. In T. A. Sebeok (Ed.), *How animals communicate* (pp. 890–964). Bloomington: Indiana University Press.

Gish, S. L., & Morton, E. S. (1981). Structural adaptations to local habitat acoustics in Carolina wren songs. *Zeitschrift für Tierpsychologie, 56,* 74–84.

Green, S. (1975). Variation of vocal pattern with social situation in the Japanese monkey (*Macaca fuscata*): A field study. In L. A. Rosenblum (Ed.), *Primate Behavior* (Vol. 4). New York: Academic Press.

Green, S., & Marler, P. (1979). The analysis of animal communication. In P. Marler & J. G. Vanderberg (Eds.), *Social behavior and communication* (pp. 73–158). New York: Plenum Press.

Hall, J. W., & Fernandes, M. A. (1983). Temporal integration, frequency resolution, and off-frequency listening in normal-hearing and cochlear-impaired listeners. *Journal of the Acoustical Society of America, 74,* 1172–1177.

Hawkins, J. E. Jr., & Stevens, S. S. (1950). Masking of pure tones and speech by noise. *Journal of the Acoustical Society of America, 22,* 6–13.

Heffner, H. E., & Heffner, R. S. (1984). Temporal lobe lesions and perception of species-specific vocalizations by macaques. *Science, 226,* 75–76.

Henderson, D. (1969). Temporal summation of acoustic signals by the chinchilla. *Journal of the Acoustical Society of America, 46,* 474–476.

Irwin, R. J., & Purdey, S. C. (1982). The minimum detectable duration of auditory signals for normal and hearing-impaired listeners. *Journal of the Acoustical Society of America, 71,* 967–974.

Johnson, C. S. (1968). Relation between absolute threshold and duration-of-tone pulses in the bottle nosed porpose. *Journal of the Acoustical Society of America, 43,* 757–763.

Kortlandt, A. (1986, July). Studying the treescape. In J. G. Else & P. C. Lee (Eds.) *10th Congress of the International Primatological Society, Nairobi, Kenya. Primate Ecology and Conservation* (pp. 263–276). Cambridge, England: Cambridge University Press.

Kuhl, P. K. (1986). Theoretical contributions of tests on animals to the special-mechanism debate in speech. *Experimental Biology, 45,* 231–263.

Kuhl, P. K., & Miller, J. D. (1975). Speech perception by the chinchilla: Voiced-voiceless distinction in alveolar plosive consonants, *Science, 190,* 69–72.

Kuhl, P. K., & Miller, J. D. (1978). Speech perception by the chinchilla: identification functions for synthetic VOT stimuli. *Journal of the Acoustical Society of America, 63,* 905–917.

Kuhl, P. K., & Padden, D. M. (1982). Enhanced discriminability at the phonetic boundaries for the voicing feature in macaques. *Perception and Psychophysics, 32,* 542–550.

Ladefoged, P. (1975). *A Course in Phonetics.* New York: Hartcourt Brace Jovanovitch.

Liberman, A. M. (1982). On finding that speech is special. *American Psychologist, 37,* 148–167.

Liberman, A., Cooper, F., Shankweiler, D., & Studdert-Kennedy, M. (1967). Perception of the speech code. *Psychological Review, 74,* 431–461.

Lind, E. M., & Morrison, M. E. S. (1974). *East African Vegetation.* London: Longman.

Marler, P. (1955). Characteristics of some animal calls. *Nature, 176,* 6–8.

Marler, P. (1965). Communication in monkeys and apes. In I. DeVore (Ed.), *Primate behavior: Field studies of monkeys and apes* (pp. 544–584). New York: Holt, Rinehardt and Winston.

Marler, P. (1973). A comparison of vocalizations of red-tailed monkeys and blue monkeys, *Cercopithecus ascanius* and *C. mitis* in Uganda. *Zeitschrift für Tierpsychologie, 33,* 233–247.

Marler, P. (1975). On the origin of speech from animal sounds. In J. R. Kavanagh, & J. E. Cutting (Eds.), *The role of speech in language* (pp. 11–40). Cambridge, MA: MIT Press.

Marten, K., & Marler, P. (1977). Sound transmission and its significance for animal vocalizations. I. Temperate habitats. *Behavioral Ecology and Sociobiology, 2,* 272–290.

Marten, K., Quine, D., & Marler, P. (1977). Sound transmission and its significance for animal vocalizations. II. Tropical forest habitats. *Behavioral Ecology and Sociobiology, 2,* 291–302.

Masterton, R. B., Heffner, H., & Ravizza, R. (1969). The evolution of human hearing. *Journal of the Acoustical Society of America, 45,* 966–985.

Michelsen, A. (1978). Sound reception in different environments. In B. A. Ali (Ed.), *Perspectives in sensory ecology* (pp. 345–373). New York: Plenum.

Miller, G. A. (1947). The masking of speech. *Psychological Bulletin, 44,* 105–129.

Miller, J., Wier, C., Pastore, R., Kelly, W., & Dooling, R. (1976). Discrimination and labeling of noise-buzz sequences with varying noise-lead times: An example of categorical perception. *Journal of the Acoustical Society of America, 60,* 410–417.

Morse, P. A., & Snowdon, C. T. (1975). An investigation of categorical speech discrimination by rhesus monkeys. *Perception and Psychophysics, 17,* 9–16.

Nabelek, I. V. (1978). Temporal summation of constant and gliding tones at masked auditory threshold. *Journal of the Acoustical Society of America, 64,* 751–763.

Pastore, P. E., Freidman, C., Baffuto, K. J., & Fink, E. A. (1976). Categorical perception of both simple auditory and visual stimuli. *Journal of the Acoustical Society of America, 59,* 524S.

Petersen, M. R., Beecher, M. D., Zoloth, S. R., Moody, D. B., & Stebbins, W. C. (1978). Neural lateralization of species-specific vocalizations by Japanese macaques (*Macaca fuscata*). *Science, 202,* 324–327.

Petersen, M. R., Beecher, M. D., Zoloth, S. R., Green, S., Marler, P. R., Moody, D. B., & Stebbins, W. C. (1984). Neural lateralization of vocalizations by Japanese macaques: Communicative significance is more important than acoustic structure. *Behavioral Neuroscience, 98,* 779–790.

Pisoni, D. (1977). Identification and discrimination of the relative on-set time of two-component tones: Implications for voicing perception in stops. *Journal of the Acoustical Society of America, 61,* 1352–1361.

Plomp, R., & Bouman, M. A. (1959). Relation between hearing threshold and duration for tone pulses. *Journal of the Acoustical Society of America, 31,* 749–758.

Richards, D. G., & Wiley, R. H. (1980). Reverberations and amplitude fluctuations in the propagation of sound in a forest: Implications for animal communication. *American Naturalist, 115,* 381–399.

Rowell, T. E., & Hinde, R. A. (1962). Vocal communication by rhesus monkey (*Macaca mulatta*). *Symposium of the Zoological Society of London, 138,* 279–294.

Seyfarth, R. M., & Cheney, D. L. (1982). How monkeys see the world: A review of recent research on East African vervet monkeys. In C. T. Snowdon, C. H. Brown, & M. R. Petersen (Eds.), *Primate communication* (pp. 239–252). Cambridge, England: Cambridge University Press.

Stebbins, W. C. (1973). Hearing of Old World monkeys (*Cercopithecinae*). *American Journal of Physical Anthropology, 63,* 357–364.

Stebbins, W. C. (1983). *The acoustic sense of animals.* Cambridge, MA: Harvard University Press.

Stebbins, W. C., Brown, C. H., & Petersen, M. (1984). Sensory function in animals. In I. Darian-Smith (Ed.), *Handbook of physiology, Volume 3, Section 1: The nervous system* (pp. 123–148) Washington, D. C.: American Physiological Society.

Tyler, R. S., Summerfield, O., Wood, E. J., & Fernandes, M. A. (1982). Psychoacoustic and phonetic temporal processing in normal and hearing-impaired listeners. *Journal of the Acoustical Society of America, 72,* 740–752.

Waser, P. M. (1975). Experimental playbacks show vocal mediation of intergroup avoidance in forest monkeys. *Nature, 255,* 56–58.

Waser, P. M. (1976). *Cercocebus albigena:* Site attachment, avoidance, and intergroup spacing. *American Naturalist, 110,* 911–935.

Waser, P. M., & Brown, C. H. (1984). Is there a "sound window" for primate communication? *Behavioral Ecology and Sociobiology, 15,* 73–76.

Waser, P. M., & Brown, C. H. (1986). Habitat acoustics and primate communication. *American Journal of Primatology, 10,* 135–154.

Waser, P. M., & Waser, M. S. (1977). Experimental studies of primate vocalizations: Specializations for long-distance propagation. *Zeitschrift für Tierpsychologie, 43,* 239–263.

Waters, R. S., & Wilson, W. A. (1976). Speech perception by rhesus monkeys: The voicing distinction in synthesized labial and velar stop consonants. *Perception and Psychophysics, 19,* 285–289.

Watson, C. S., & Gengel, R. W. (1969). Signal duration and signal frequency in relation to auditory sensitivity. *Journal of the Acoustical Society of America, 46,* 989–997.

Webb, D. C., & Tucker, M. J. (1970). Transmission characteristics of the sofar channel. *Journal of the Acoustical Society of America, 48,* 767–769.

Webster, D. B., & Webster, M. (1972). Kangaroo rat auditory thresholds before and after middle ear reduction. *Brain, Behavior and Evolution, 5,* 41–53.

Wiley, R. H., & Richards, D. G. (1978). Physical constraints on acoustic communication in the atmosphere: Implications for the evolution of animal vocalization. *Behavioral Ecology and Sociobiology, 3,* 69–94.

Wiley, R. H., & Richards, D. G. (1982). Adaptations for acoustic communication in birds: Sound transmission and signal detection. In D. E. Kroodsma & E. H. Miller (Eds.), *Acoustic communication in birds* (pp. 131–181). New York: Academic Press.

Whitehead, J. (1987). Vocally mediated reciprocity between neighboring groups of mantled howing monkeys, *Aloutta palliata palliata. Animal Behaviour, 35,* 1615–1627.

Wolfheim, J. H. (1983). *Primates of the world: Distribution, abundance and conservation.* Seattle, WA: University of Washington Press.

Zoloth, S. R., Petersen, M. R., Beecher, M. D., Green, S., Marler, P., Moody, D. B., & Stebbins, W. (1979). Species-specific perceptual processing of vocal sounds by Old World monkeys. *Science, 204,* 870–873.

Editor's Comments on Marler and Peters

There are no adequate mammalian models for studying the relation between auditory perception and the ontogeny of a learned vocal repertoire. Oscine songbirds remain the best model for investigating many of these processes that at one time seemed to be uniquely human. Indeed, over the years, the comparative approach to the study of vocal ontogeny in birds has provided a disproportionate number of insights into the development of complex behavior including acoustic communication. This approach is best exemplified by the work of Marler and his colleagues on two congeneric species of sparrow—the swamp sparrow and the song sparrow.

In this chapter, Marler and Peters describe the differences in the songs of swamp and song sparrows and examine the case for early perceptual preferences versus motor contraints in guiding the vocal learning process. Marler and Peters demonstrate on the one hand that there are learning preferences in these sparrows for conspecific song elements and, on the other hand, that much of the complex temporal organization seen in normal song also develops in birds reared in isolation but not in birds deafened as young. These data rally support for the notion that the major factors shaping learning preferences in these two species are perceptual rather than motor and probably involve rather complex, central auditory specifications for song rather than simple differences in audibility.

8

Species Differences in Auditory Responsiveness in Early Vocal Learning

Peter Marler
Susan Peters
The Rockefeller University

INTRODUCTION

Every oscine bird studied thus far has proved to have a learned song. With almost 300 species of songbird now investigated (Kroodsma, 1982) it seems probable that, in all 4000 or so oscines, natural patterns of male singing behavior are transmitted as learned cultural traditions from generation to generation. In many cases, birds brought into captivity and reared out of hearing of song of their own kind but in the company of other species have acquired the songs of those other species, either in part, or in their entirety. The acquisition of the song of another species (i.e., heterospecific song) has been recorded, not only in birds that are natural mimics such as mockingbirds, starlings, marsh warblers, and lyrebirds, but also in birds that rarely mimic species other than their own in the wild (Scott, 1901, 1902, 1904a,b,c; Daines Barrington, 1773; Baptista & Petrinovich, 1986). In nature, it is estimated that less than 12% of oscines commonly mimic species other than their own. In the hands of aviculturalists, however, many species render heterospecific songs with precision. Evidently the vocal apparatus of songbirds is capable of a wider range of sounds than that typically produced under natural conditions. What, then, is responsible for imposing this limitation on vocal production?

Here we explore the question of whether, given a choice of learning either heterospecific song or conspecific song (i.e., song of the bird's own species), there is a tendency for birds to favor sounds of their own kind. Evidence is reviewed for the existence of such learning preferences in two songbirds, and then consideration is given to the acoustic features upon which the preferences are based.

The subjects are two closely related songbirds, members of the same genus, living in sympatry and often breeding within earshot. That the song sparrow,

Melospiza melodia, and the swamp sparrow, *Melospiza georgiana* are indeed genetically close is implied by the occasional survival of natural hybrids, and by the results of electrophoretic analyses of blood serum proteins (Dickerman, 1961; Paynter, 1964; Zink, 1982). Despite this close relationship, their songs are quite distinct, one having a much simpler song than the other.

I. NATURAL SONG PATTERNS OF SWAMP AND SONG SPARROWS

Normal song duration is approximately similar in the two species, about 2.5 s, but song sparrow songs tend to average slightly longer. Swamp sparrow song consists of a simple trill of identical, multinote syllables, delivered at a regular tempo (Fig. 8.1). Typically it thus comprises a single phrase, although two-phrased songs occasionally occur. In contrast, song sparrow songs are always multipartite, consisting of several phrases (Fig. 8.1). The terms "phrase" and "segment" are used interchangeably in this chapter, as one aspect of "song syntax." The term "phonology" will refer to song structure at the level of individual elements or "notes."

The syntax of song sparrow song is invariably more complex than that of the swamp sparrow. Two distinct phrase types are present in every song sparrow song, termed "trills" and "note complexes" (Mulligan, 1963). Sequences of consecutively repeated multinote syllables form trills, comparable in syntactical structure to the single trill of the one-segmented swamp sparrow song. Groups of unrepeated notes form note complexes, which have no equivalent in swamp sparrow song. These tend to alternate with trills in song sparrow song. Table 8.1 summarizes the syntax of a sample of song sparrow songs, illustrating the variety of forms they can take, and Fig. 8.2 displays sound spectrograms of several exemplars.

In addition to syntactical differences, songs of the two species also differ in tempo. That of swamp sparrow songs is always regular, whereas in song sparrow song syllable delivery rates vary, often accelerating in the first introductory trill (Fig. 8.1B). Internote intervals within note complexes are irregular.

The two species also differ in phonology, although only swamp sparrow phonology has been worked out in detail. All known swamp sparrow songs are constructed from a relatively simple set of phonological units or notes, as summarized in Fig. 8.3. The same note types recur in different populations, with the same relative frequencies. However the arrangement of note types into syllables varies from one swamp sparrow population to another so that it is possible to define dialects in swamp sparrow song by the local rules for syllabic construction. We term this phenomenon "syllabic syntax," as contrasted with the larger scale "segmental syntax" of the entire song. Balaban (1988) has demonstrated that both male and female swamp sparrows are responsive to these local variations in rules for syllabic syntax.

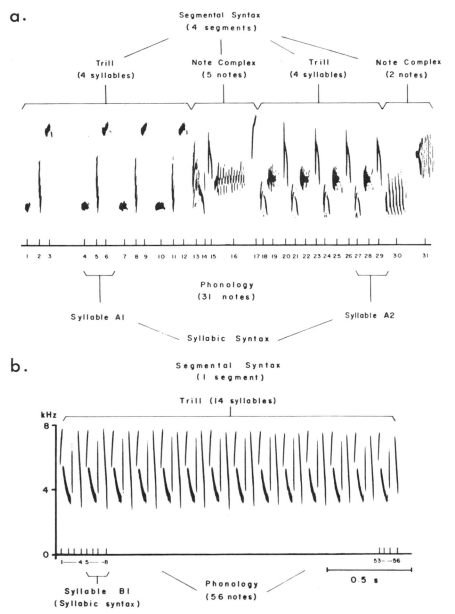

FIG. 8.1. An illustration of the way in which sound spectrograms of birdsong can be broken down into basic "phonological" units, or notes, in song sparrow (a) and swamp sparrow song (b). This particular song sparrow song comprises 31 notes arranged in four segments, two trills and two note complexes. The two trills both consist of four repeated syllables (A1 for the first, and A2 for the second). Usually there are fewer syllables in the first trill than in later ones. The swamp sparrow song shown contains 56 notes. Typically there are twice as many notes as in a song sparrow song, arranged in a trill. Fourteen identical repetitions of the 4-note syllable (B1) make up the song.

245

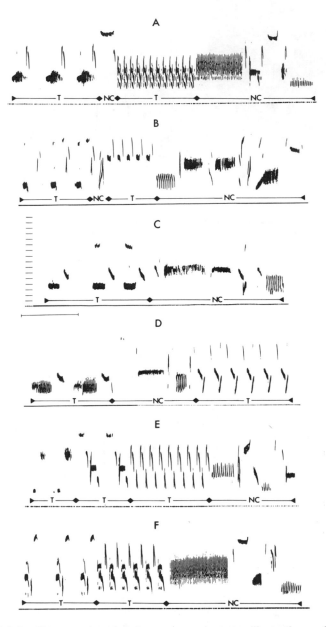

FIG. 8.2. Six examples of male song sparrow song, illustrating variation in the arrangement and number of trills (T) and note complexes
(NC). A & B illustrate the most common song form, with four segments, and trills and note-complexes alternating. The time marker
indicates half a second. Frequency markers are in 500 Hz intervals.

246

TABLE 8.1
Syntax of Song Sparrow Song

Segmental Pattern (T = Trill; NC = Note complex)						Number of Songs (N = 72)
T	NC	T	NC			33
T	NC	T				8
T	T	NC				5
T	T	NC	T	NC		5
T	T	T	NC			4
T	NC	T	NC	T	NC	4
NC	T	NC				4
T	NC					3
NC	T	T	NC			2
NC	T	NC	T	NC		2
T	NC	T	T	NC		1
NC	T	NC	T			1

*The segmental syntax of a sample of 72 song sparrow songs, 38 in New York State, and 34 in Ontario, Canada. The pattern of alternating trills and note complexes clearly predominates. Trills introduce songs in a majority of cases.

Song sparrow songs are constructed from note types significantly different from those of the swamp sparrow, although with some overlap. Song sparrow phonology has yet to be fully investigated, but it appears that, as in the swamp sparrow, there is a universal set of phonological units from which the majority if not all song sparrow songs are constructed. Preliminary investigation of geographical variation in how the notes are assembled into songs suggests that song structure in separate populations differ at several levels. These include: the frequency with which different note types are represented; the ways in which they are assembled into trill syllables and note complexes; and the predominant patterns of segmental syntax.

Finally, the two species differ in song repertoire size. In the eastern United States, for example, swamp sparrows have about three song types per male, whereas song sparrow repertoires average three times larger. There are thus numerous auditory cues upon which a sparrow could reliably base a learning preference in favor of songs of its own species, and against songs of the other. Those actually employed are explored in a later section. First the evidence is reviewed on whether sparrows, given a choice between natural songs of their own species and another, display a learning preference.

II. PREFERENCES IN LEARNING FROM TAPE-RECORDED SONGS: THE SONG SPARROW

How do young male song sparrows behave when presented with the opportunity to learn from a variety of tape recorded songs, some of their own species, and

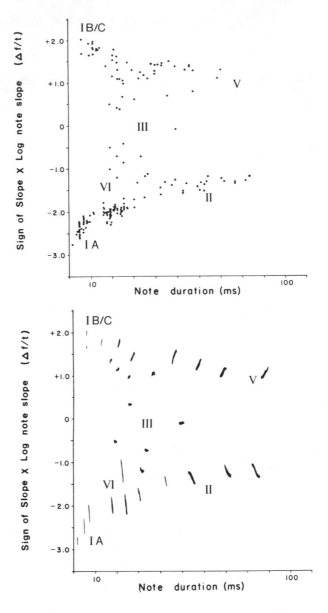

FIG. 8.3. Song phonology in the male swamp sparrow. By breaking sound spectrograms of many swamp sparrow songs down into their constituent notes, and classifying them, all are found to be constructed from the same, relatively simple system of phonological units. *A* shows a scatter plot of 192 swamp sparrow notes with a measure of note slope on one axis and duration on the other. The location of note types from I to VI is indicated, and *B* shows vignettes of sound spectrograms of 29 of the same notes. From Marler and Pickert (1984) and Clark, Marler, and Beeman (1987).

Normal Swamp Sparrow Songs   Normal   Song Sparrow Songs

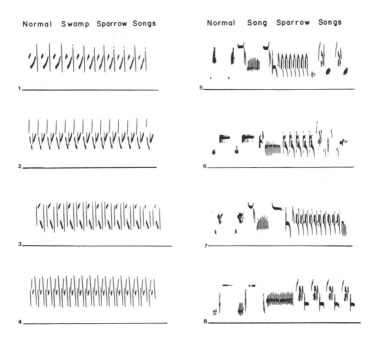

FIG. 8.4.   Examples of the normal song sparrow and swamp sparrow songs played as tape-recordings to young male song sparrows. Conspecific songs were clearly favored in the acquisition process. From Marler and Peters (1988b).

some of another? By playing tape recorded songs to young male song sparrows early in life, a typical experiment sought to establish whether they would favor conspecific songs over swamp sparrow songs, whether the behavior would vary with early and late exposure in the juvenile period, and whether they had any inclination to favor songs of the father and other males in the immediate neighborhood of the birthplace as learning stimuli, having experienced them as nestlings (Marler & Peters, 1988b).

Three song sparrow nests were located and songs of the fathers and of neighboring males were recorded. The nestlings were taken between 6- and 10-days-of-age. Two broods were from adjacent territories, and the third was from a separate area. For the purposes of this experiment it was assumed that effective experience of song stimulation began on the day of hatching (this was before we knew that the sensitive period does not begin until 20 days after hatching: Marler & Peters, 1987). Immediately on being brought into the laboratory to be reared by hand, the birds were exposed to playback of tape recordings of songs of the father and male neighbors, 19 songs altogether. An equal number of swamp sparrow songs was also played. Examples of stimulus songs are illustrated in Fig. 8.4.

Because the nests came from two areas, it was necessary to prepare two separate sets of tapes using different song sparrow songs for each, one for the two adjacent broods (yielding four male nestlings), and another for the third brood (yielding one male nestling). The same set of heterospecific songs was used for all five birds. The songs were arranged in bouts of a single song type, as they are delivered in nature, each repeated once per 10 sec for a 3 min bout, matching a normal rate of delivery. After 1 min of silence, a bout of another song type would ensue. Each training tape, including bouts of all 38 songs types, in a random order, were played to the birds twice a day. The birds were exposed to this stimulus regime for 20–24 days, and it was assumed that they had experienced something similar as nestlings, adding up to 30 days exposure altogether for each subject.

At about 4 weeks young song sparrows become independent of their parents and disperse. Thus at 30-days-of-age, a new set of training tapes was substituted for the previous one, consisting of the same number of song and swamp sparrow songs, but now using songs recorded 5 kilometers away—an estimate of the distance to which birds might have moved from the birthplace by 1-month-of-age. Thus by the end of the 60-day-period of training each bird had heard—in the laboratory at least—a total of 76 normal tape recorded songs, half conspecific, half heterospecific.

When the crystallized song repertoires of the five males were recorded in the following spring, they had learned all or part of 25 of the songs to which they had been exposed. These songs were drawn in equal proportions from the first and second training periods, suggesting that they are ready to learn both after dispersal from the birthplace and before.

Of the 25 songs learned, 23 (92%) were song sparrow songs. This figure actually underrepresents the preference, because some of the stimulus songs were imitated by more than one male. Collectively, the group of five subjects experienced 380 song types (5 × 76). Taken as a group, they learned from 37 of these, 35 of which (95%) were song sparrow songs.

It could be argued that the apparent preference is a reflection of the greater complexity of song sparrow song as compared with swamp sparrow song. Because of the multisegmented structure of song sparrow song, subjects were in fact exposed to almost four times as many song sparrow *phrases* as they were phrases of swamp sparrow song. As a group, we calculated that the birds were exposed to a total of 934 song phrases, 200 from swamp sparrow songs and 734 from song sparrow songs. Even with this correction, the tendency to favor conspecific songs remains statistically significant. They reproduced 50 song sparrow, and only 2 swamp sparrow phrases.

We conclude that young male song sparrows strongly favor conspecific songs when they are learning to sing. Despite exposure to songs of the father as nestlings for 6–10 days before being brought into the laboratory, we could detect no bias in favor or against learning of the father's songs.

III. LEARNING FROM LIVE TUTORS: THE SWAMP SPARROW

In view of the emphasis of recent research on social influences on song learning in birds (Baptista & Petrinovich, 1984, 1986; Payne, 1983; Pepperberg, 1985), one may question whether a conspecific preference in learning would persist if live tutors were substituted for tape recordings. An experiment was conducted therefore to compare responses of young male swamp sparrows to swamp and song sparrow song delivered as tape recordings on the one hand, and by live, socially interactive tutors on the other (Marler & Peters, 1988a).

One aim of the study, which does not concern us here, was to define sensitive periods for song acquisition under these two conditions. To this end, live tutors and tape-recorded songs were changed regularly, some every 6 weeks, and some, with tape-recorded stimulation, every week. Exposure began at 2- to 4-weeks-of-age. Each cohort of live tutors consisted of four birds, two swamp sparrows (conspecific) and two song sparrows (heterospecific), all kept in song by implants of testosterone. The tutors were separately caged at the focus of an arc of open-sided boxes from which pupils could see and interact with the tutors, but not with one another. Similarly with tape-recorded stimulation, birds heard equal numbers of song sparrow songs (heterospecific) and swamp sparrow songs (conspecific). There were 16 subjects in the live tutoring experiment and 15 in the tape-tutoring experiment.

Of the birds that learned from tape recordings (N = 12) 21 songs were learned in part or in their entirety. Without exception, every one was a swamp sparrow song. There was no heterospecific song learning whatsoever. Thus both song and swamp sparrows are selective in acquiring songs from tape recordings.

The results of the live tutoring experiment were similar. All but two of the 14 songs learned were acquired from swamp sparrow tutors. Of the two that were learned from a male song sparrow, both were unusual. Each pair of conspecific tutors in a cohort consisted of one wild male, and one laboratory-reared male that had been tutored with song, and thus had relatively normal song patterns. One of the hand-reared song sparrow tutors, however, had acquired some swamp sparrow song material, and it was from this male that two songs were learned by one of the swamp sparrow subjects, one consisting of a single song sparrow syllable, and the other of a swamp sparrow syllable that this tutor had learned previously.

The results of this experiment show that, when given a choice, male swamp sparrows will favor a conspecific live tutor over a heterospecific one. This is not to say that, if they were given access only to heterospecific songs, and more especially if these songs were provided by a live, socially interactive tutor rather than a tape recorder, heterospecific songs would not be acquired. This has in fact been demonstrated convincingly by Baptista and Petrinovich (1984, 1986) with male white-crowned sparrows, *Zonotrichia leucophrys,* another species that will favor its own species song when given a choice between conspecific and hetero-specific tape recordings (Marler, 1970).

It should be noted that we have focused on only one of many song discrimination problems that confront these sparrows in nature. The geographical range of the song sparrow is extensive, and the swamp sparrow is one of many species that are sympatric with it. Others whose presence may exert selection pressures on the emergence of learning preferences include species of *Junco, Zonotrichia,* and *Passerella,* the vesper sparrow (*Pooecetes gramineus*) (Kroodsma, 1972; Ritchison, 1981), in addition to the congeneric Lincoln's sparrow (*Melospiza lincolnii*) (Martin, 1977; Zink, 1982).

IV. SONG TEMPO, SEGMENTAL SYNTAX AND LEARNING PREFERENCES: THE SWAMP SPARROW

What are the acoustical cues upon which preferences in favor of conspecific song and against heterospecific song are based? Most conspicuous to our ears are the differences in segmental syntax—the fact that swamp sparrow song is unisegmental, and song sparrow song is multisegmental. The differences in tempo are also striking. Swamp sparrow syllables are always delivered at a constant rate.

TABLE 8.2
The Design Plan for the First Set of Synthesized Songs

Overall Pattern	Song Type	Tempo	Syllable Types (No.)
Swamp sparrow-like (one-part)	A	Steady, fast	1
	B	Steady, slow*	1
	C	Accelerated	1
	D	Decelerated	1
Song sparrow-like (two-part)	E	Fast/slow*	2
	F	Slow/fast	2
	G	Decelerated/slow	2
	H	Decelerated/fast	2
	I	Accelerated/slow	2
	J	Accelerated/fast*	2

All songs were about 2 seconds in duration. The ten artificial songs of one set were created from 16 different song sparrow syllables. Another set was created of the same song patterns, but with 16 different swamp sparrow syllables. Examples of the patterns marked with asterisks are shown in Fig. 6. Five complete sets were created, all based on the same set of 32 different syllable types, but with each syllable type placed in a different pattern in each of the five sets. A given bird heard one set only, thus experiencing 32 natural syllable types, 16 of each species.

SYNTHETIC SONGS PRESENTED TO
YOUNG MALE SWAMP SPARROWS

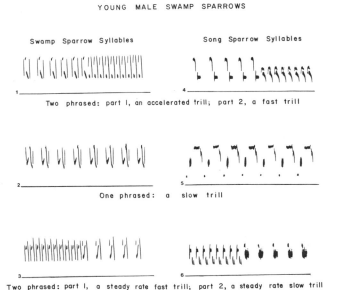

FIG. 8.5. Examples of songs synthesized from natural syllables of swamp and song sparrow song and presented as learning stimuli to young male swamp sparrows. Songs 2 and 5 match normal swamp sparrow syntax closely. The others have some simple syntactical features of song sparrow song.

The rate of song sparrow syllable delivery varies considerably, and song sparrows are especially prone to accelerate the tempo of syllables in the first trill in the song.

To explore the contributions of these two factors to learning preferences, young swamp sparrows were brought into the laboratory as nestlings, and reared out of hearing of adult conspecific song (Marler & Peters, 1977). During the sensitive period (defined precisely in Marler & Peters, 1988a) they were exposed to a range of computer-modified, tape recorded songs with these features systematically varied (Zoloth, Dooling, Miller, & Peters, 1980). Normal trill syllables were edited out from tape recordings of normal local songs of each species. These were spliced together in a variety of simple temporal patterns of normal, standardized duration, as summarized in Table 8.2. Examples are illustrated in Fig. 8.5.

Some patterns were "swamp sparrow-like" (e.g., one-phrased, constant tempo songs, either slow or fast) (see Fig. 8.5, songs 2 and 5), some had mixed attributes (e.g., one-phrased songs [swamp sparrow-like] with an accelerating or decelerating tempo [song sparrow-like]). Some were even more "song sparrow-like" (e.g., accelerating or decelerating tempo in the first of two phrases, or two consecutive trills, one slow and the other fast). The most song sparrow-like pattern consisted of two trills, the first with a slow, accelerating tempo, the second with a constant fast rate (Fig. 8.5, songs 1 and 4). Normal song sparrow songs usually consist of three or more segments (see Table 8.1), but we hypothesized that the contrast between one- and two-phrased songs might suffice for discrimination to occur, especially since two-phrased swamp sparrow songs are found in nature, but at a low rate (<5%).

Each set of 10 song patterns was created in duplicate, once with 16 different swamp sparrow syllables and a second time with 16 different song sparrow syllables. Each syllable type was used only once in a set. The syllable types were chosen to be sufficiently distinct that, if an imitation occurred, it would be possible to determine from which temporal pattern it was selected.

Anticipating that some conspecific syllables might be favored over others, five different sets of training tapes were prepared from the same 32 syllables, but with each pattern assembled from a different syllable type in each set. A given bird heard only one of these five sets.

Eight young male swamp sparrows were exposed to tape-recordings of these artificial songs, twice per day, from 20–50 days-of-age. When they came into song some months later, on a typical time schedule (see Fig. 8.6), they had clearly imitated significant amounts of material from the training tapes. Altogether the group of 8 subjects produced 19 syllable types. As in nature, each male sang several songs, ranging from one to three types. Upon spectrographic analysis, 12 of the 19 songs were judged to be good quality imitations of training songs. Every one of them consisted of swamp sparrow syllables.

Thus all subjects displayed a strong learning preference, favoring conspecific song syllables for imitation, and rejecting song sparrow syllables, even when presented in swamp sparrow-like patterns. The choice was clearly made, therefore, at the level of syllabic structure, and was uninfluenced by the experimental variations in tempo and segmental syntax. For example, while four of the 12

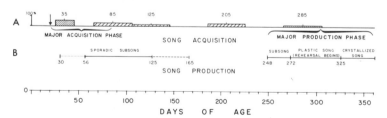

FIG. 8.6. The pattern of male swamp sparrow song development in the first year of life. The sensitive period for song acquisition from live tutors (A) begins at 20 days of age (arrow) and peaks at about 35 days. The first production of imitations occurs much later, with the onset of plastic song, at about 270 days. Subsong involves no rehearsal of memorized songs. From Marler, Peters, and Wingfield (1987).

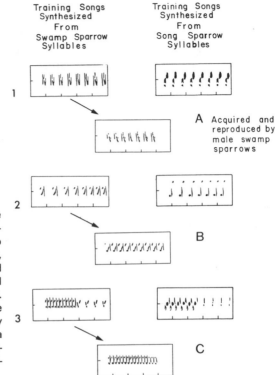

FIG. 8.7. Examples of three pairs of synthetic songs presented as learning stimuli to young male swamp sparrows, and the three imitations based on them. A is a relatively faithful rendition of the model imitated. In B and C syllables of the model are rendered accurately but the syntax is modified to a normal swamp sparrow pattern. Only swamp sparrow syllables were acquired.

learned syllables were extracted from one-phrased songs, which is the normal swamp sparrow pattern, eight were taken from two-phrased models, which are closer in segmental syntax to the song sparrow pattern. Two-segment songs are still within the range of natural variation in swamp sparrow songs, but occur rarely (<5%). Five of the imitated syllables came from sequences with a constant rate (the normal swamp sparrow pattern) and seven from accelerated or decelerated sequences (a song sparrow trait). Young male swamp sparrows evidently make their choice without reference to variations in tempo or segmental syntax (Marler & Peters, 1980).

Nor did the syntactical patterns in which learned syllables were reproduced necessarily match the syntax of the model. Thus syllables presented in artificial two-phrased songs, or with variable syllable rates, were usually transposed into one-phrased patterns with a constant rate, as is typical of this species. Evidently swamp sparrows have an innate ability (see Marler & Sherman, 1985) to gain access to information about the normal temporal organization of the song of their species (Fig. 8.7).

A similar focus of attentional processing on the phonology of song is also seen in the responsiveness of males to song stimulation in adulthood. Use of the aggressive approach of wild males on their territories, in response to tape-recorded songs played through a loudspeaker, as an index of the effectiveness of synthetic songs like those used in the present experiment, revealed once again that adults are more responsive to the structure of notes and syllables than to the temporal patterns into which they are organized (Peters, Searcy, & Marler, 1980).

V. SEGMENTAL SYNTAX AND LEARNING
PREFERENCES: THE SONG SPARROW

The unresponsiveness of young male swamp sparrows to song syntax correlates with the syntactical simplicity of their natural song, and the degree to which information about species-specificity, dialects, and individual identity is bound up in the fine structure of song syllables. The temporal organization of song sparrow song is more complex, and one should be prepared for the possibility of differences in the song features upon which learning preferences are based.

To explore this question, five young male song sparrows were taken as nestlings and reared in the laboratory. They were exposed during the sensitive period (see Marler & Peters, 1988b) to the same sets of tape recorded song stimuli used previously, consisting of 10 different one- or two-segmented song patterns created in duplicate, either with swamp sparrow syllables, or with song sparrow syllables. The variables manipulated were the tempo of syllable delivery, and the number of song segments, either one or two as shown in Table 8.2, and illustrated in Fig. 8.5. The birds were trained with these songs, twice per day, for 30 or 40 days, beginning between the ages of 18 and 31 days-of-age.

Analysis of crystallized songs produced some 8 months later revealed that in response to the same set of tape-recorded songs, they had responded very differently from the swamp sparrows. Four of the five subjects produced good quality imitations. Three of the four copied both song and swamp sparrow syllables; and the fourth learned conspecific syllables only. As a group, the birds drew imitations from nine song sparrow and ten swamp sparrow songs, thus displaying no overall learning preference one way or the other, a striking contrast with the behavior of swamp sparrows.

When the data were rearranged by reference to temporal organization, however, evidence of preferences emerged. The nine conspecific songs imitated were almost evenly divided between one-phrased and two-phrased songs. The ten swamp sparrow songs imitated, however, were mostly derived from two-phrased songs. This suggests that song sparrows are more ready to accept alien song syllables when presented in a two-phrased, trilled song than in a one-phrased trill. In other words, they appear to be less prone to reject heterospecific syllables when they are couched in "song sparrow-like" syntax. This hypothesis was explored further in another experiment.

VI.   SYLLABIC PREFERENCES IN THREE- AND FOUR-SEGMENTED SONGS: THE SONG SPARROW

Songs consisting of two segments occur occasionally in the song sparrow, usually consisting of a trill and a note complex. More commonly they consist of three to five segments (Table 8.1). Thus a two-phrased pattern can hardly be viewed as a case of normal song sparrow syntax. Taking a further step in this direction, a continuum of synthetic songs was created consisting of one, two, three, and four segments (Marler & Peters, 1988b). All incorporated trills. One phrased songs consisted either of a single trill, or one long note complex. The three- and four-segmented songs also included note complexes. The songs were created from notes and syllables from field recordings of normal songs, one set from conspecific phonological material, the other from swamp sparrow material. In the course of synthesis, the duration and position of note complexes, trill type position, syllable number within trills, and note number within note complexes were all standardized. Because note complexes do not occur in swamp sparrow song (see Fig. 8.1), those with swamp sparrow phonology had to be created by combining notes from trill syllables. In all, 11 synthetic song patterns were created, one set with song sparrow phonology, the other with swamp sparrow phonology, yielding a total of 22 synthetic songs (examples in Fig. 8.8). Tape-recordings of these songs were played for 30 days to seven males taken as nestlings and reared in the laboratory, starting between 24 and 28 days-of-age. Analysis of crystallized songs recorded some 8 months later revealed that all individuals had imitated some of the tape-recorded material. Both song and swamp sparrows songs were imitated by six subjects, and the seventh imitated song sparrow songs only. Considering the subjects as a group, 40 imitations were derived from conspecific syllable models, and 13 from swamp sparrow syllable models. There was thus an overall preference for song sparrow syllables.

Presentation of the one-phrased songs again revealed strong responsiveness to syllabic phonology. In such cases, the birds clearly preferred conspecific over heterospecific syllable songs. All 13 of the imitations were derived from songs with conspecific phonology. Included in this result are imitations of both trills and note complexes, a point to be taken up again later.

In addition to this overall preference for learning songs with conspecific phonology, patterns of segmental syntax also had an influence. With two phrased models the preference disappeared, as in the previous experiment. Fourteen models were copied, 8 of which were conspecific (57%). With three- and four-segmented songs the birds tended to favor songs with conspecific phonology,

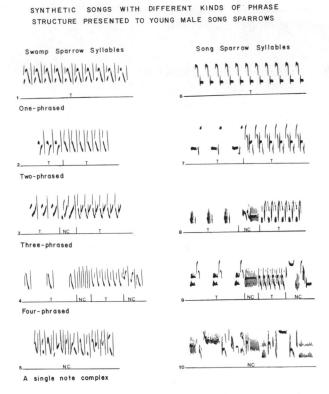

SYNTHETIC SONGS WITH DIFFERENT KINDS OF PHRASE
STRUCTURE PRESENTED TO YOUNG MALE SONG SPARROWS

Swamp Sparrow Syllables   Song Sparrow Syllables

1   T   6   T

One-phrased

2   T | T   7   T   T

Two-phrased

3   T |NC| T   8   T |NC| T

Three-phrased

4   T |NC| T |NC   9   T |NC| T |NC

Four-phrased

5   NC   10   NC

A single note complex

FIG. 8.8. Examples of synthetic songs with varying numbers of segments presented to young male song sparrows as learning stimuli.
One-phrased songs consisted either of a trill (1, 6) or a note complex
(5, 10). Two-phrased songs consisted of two trills. Three- and four-
phrased songs incorporated both trills and note complexes, as illustrated. From Marler and Peters (1988b).

although the numbers imitated were small, and the trend was not statistically
significant. Seventeen of the 23 three-phrased models copied were conspecific,
and 2 of the 3 four-phrased models copied were conspecific.

As another way of viewing the results, we can consider the relative accept-
ability of swamp sparrow syllables in the context of one-segmented versus multisegmented songs. Previous indications that alien song syllables are more readily
learned from multisegmented than from one-segmented songs were borne out.
This trend was not, however, a simple function of progression from one-segmented to more complex, increasingly song sparrow-like patterns. The proportion of songs learned with heterospecific phonology dropped from 50% with two
segments to 25% with three, and the proportion was even smaller with four-
segmented songs (two trills, two note complexes). The three- and four-seg-

mented models were the most song sparrow-like in segment number of all of those presented. Even more significantly, as indicated below, the three- and four-segmented songs all included note complexes.

Thus in contrast with the swamp sparrow, song syntax makes a contribution to vocal learning preferences in the song sparrow. The effects are complex, however, and the experiments reported on thus far do not establish the precise nature of the syntactical contribution to the learning preference.

VII. INTERNAL PHRASE STRUCTURE AND SYLLABIC LEARNING PREFERENCES: THE SONG SPARROW

The successive segments of a typical song sparrow song have a particular internal substructure. The first phrase is always a trill, consisting of two or three relatively long syllables, with intersyllable intervals that are also relatively long, usually decreasing as the phrase progresses (Kroodsma, 1977; Mulligan, 1963). The second segment is typically, though not invariably, a note complex, followed by a second trill of five or six relatively short syllables, with intersyllable intervals that are constant in duration and short. The terminal segment is usually a note complex, although there is much variation (Table 8.1).

To explore the contribution of variations in structure of the introductory trill and subsequent trills on learning preferences, eight different four-segmented song patterns were synthesized, with various permutations of syllable duration, syllable number, and tempo (accelerating or constant) (see Table 8.3). Trills of

TABLE 8.3
The Design Plan for Eight Synthesized Four-Segment Songs
Played to Young Male Song Sparrows

Features of Trill Syntax	Song Types A–H. Number 1 & 2 Indicate Trill in Which Feature Appears							
	A	B	C	D	E	F	G	H
Accelerated tempo	1	1	1	1	2	2	2	2
3 syllables	1	1	2	2	1	1	2	2
Long duration	1	2	1	2	1	2	1	2
Regular tempo	2	2	2	2	1	1	1	1
6 syllables	2	2	1	1	2	2	1	1
Short duration	2	1	2	1	2	1	2	1

*There were trills in first and third positions, and note complexes in second and fourth positions. Note complex structure was not systematically varied. Trills varied in tempo, number and duration, as indicated. We judged song type A to be most song sparrow-like, and song type H the least, on the basis that an accelerated tempo seemed the most salient feature, to our ears. Syllable number was ranked next in salience, then syllable duration.

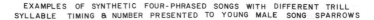

EXAMPLES OF SYNTHETIC FOUR-PHRASED SONGS WITH DIFFERENT TRILL
SYLLABLE TIMING & NUMBER PRESENTED TO YOUNG MALE SONG SPARROWS

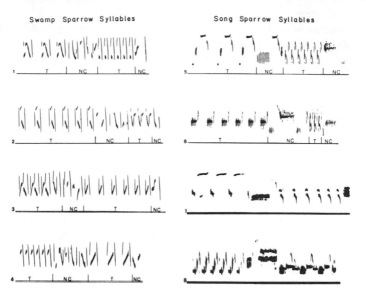

FIG. 8.9. Examples of four-segmented synthetic songs presented to
young male song sparrows as learning stimuli. The trill syntax varies
from most song sparrow-like (1, 5) to least song sparrow-like (4, 8) in
syllable number, duration and timing. From Marler and Peters (1988b).

three or six syllables were placed either in first or third position, alternating with
note complexes in second and fourth positions. Once more, all song types were
created in duplicate, from song and swamp sparrow syllables (Fig. 8.9). In the
former case, long syllables were always taken from natural introductory trills,
and short syllables from third segment trills. Intersyllable and interphrase intervals were standardized on the basis of measurements from a sample of natural
song sparrow songs. Note complexes were created from swamp sparrow material
by combining elements from trill syllables, the notes being arranged with the
same timing as in the song sparrow songs.

In addition to these 16 four-segmented songs, three pairs of one-segmented
songs were also created, all consisting of uniform-rate trills. One had long
syllables and one short syllables. Finally two other songs synthesized for special
purposes were included that do not concern us here (see Marler & Peters,
1988b). Tape-recordings of all of these songs were played twice a day to 13
young male song sparrows for 30 days, beginning at 25–32 days of age.

Eight of the subjects produced good quality imitations of the models, six
imitating both song and swamp sparrow material. One learned only from songs
with song sparrow phonology, and one from songs with swamp sparrow pho-

nology. As a group, they drew one or more imitations from 36 models, of which 23 had conspecific phonology and 13 heterospecific phonology.

Three one-segmented models were imitated, each by two males, but, although conspecific syllables were favored, numbers were small. This was the same trend as found previously.

Of the four-segmented songs presented, those constructed from song sparrow syllables were favored. Two thirds of the 30 songs imitated consisted of song sparrow syllables, following a trend found previously. Again, numbers were small, and the difference failed to reach significance. The general trend was clear, however. The proportion of learned phrases that were heterospecific dropped from 33% with one-segmented models to 22% with four-segmented models. The trend is complicated, however, by the special contribution of note complexes, two of which were present in every four-segmented song.

Here and elsewhere, it is evident that note complexes make a special contribution to the rejection of swamp sparrow material by song sparrows. Whereas the 8 birds favored neither trills nor note complexes when selecting conspecific imitations, when learning swamp sparrow syllables, 85% were acquired from trills, and only 15% from note complexes (Fig. 8.10). Thus there is a significant reduction in the readiness to accept heterospecific syllables, even when presented in multisegmented songs, if they are placed in note complexes rather than trills.

Viewing the data from the aspect of segmental syntax, the subjects showed no preference for first or second trills, or first or second note complexes when imitating conspecific material. With swamp sparrow material, however, they strongly favored introductory trills. Of 11 syllables imitated from four-segmented songs, nine were in the first trill, and only two in the second (i.e., in the

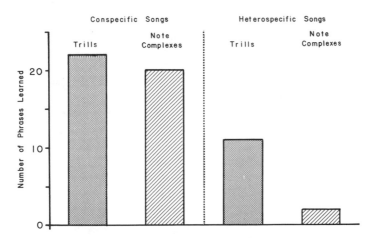

FIG. 8.10.   Numbers of song phrases learned by male song sparrows from trills and from note complexes in songs made up of either conspecific or heterospecific phrases.

third segment). Thus in the imitation of heterospecific syllables, the song sparrow subjects displayed a preference for trills over note complexes, and for the first trill of four-segmented songs.

In addition to song segmentation, this experiment also appraised the importance of number, duration and tempo of syllables in relation to phrase position in the song. The four-segmented synthetic songs were designed as a ranked series from one to eight, with one having the most song sparrow-like attributes, and eight the least (Table 8.3).

When constructed from conspecific syllables, there was a significant positive relationship between the popularity of a song type, as reflected in the number of males that used it as a model, and its position on the scale from most to least song sparrow-like. Evidently, within a series of songs that all have song sparrow phonology, young male song sparrows display preferences according to the degree to which the internal structure of segments conforms to the species typical pattern. This is a striking contrast with young male swamp sparrows, which, as far as is known, are quite unresponsive to such syntactical details.

VIII. CONCLUSIONS ON RESPONSIVENESS TO SUPRA-SYLLABIC SONG STRUCTURE: THE SONG SPARROW

In learning to sing, young male song sparrows are clearly responsive to the structure of the minimal acoustic units or notes from which song patterns are constructed—the phonology—and to the ways in which they are assembled into syllables—the syllabic syntax. By using matched pairs of song stimuli with equivalent patterns of temporal organization constructed either from conspecific or from heterospecific elements, the contributions to learning preferences of notes and syllables were separated from those of other acoustic properties of song. When other cues are eliminated, male song sparrows display a clear learning preference, favoring conspecific songs, based on phonological and syllabic cues alone.

On the other hand, supra-syllabic aspects of song structure also influence learning preferences in the song sparrow. Alien syllables are more likely to be learned when presented in multisegmented songs than in one-segmented songs. Furthermore, intrasegmental temporal organization influences learning preferences. Heterospecific (swamp sparrow) notes and syllables are less likely to be acquired from note complexes than from trills.

Finally, there appear to be order effects, such that changes in trill structures as a song sparrow song proceeds, with a few long syllables in the first trill, and more, shorter syllables in the second trill, also influences the choice of models for song learning. Young male song sparrows are thus responsive to aspects of song organization that have no influence on song learning preferences in the swamp sparrow.

IX. SONG LEARNING PREFERENCES ARE INNATE: SONG AND SWAMP SPARROWS

In the experiments reported so far, subjects were all taken in the wild as nestlings at ages ranging from 4–10 days-of-age. Thus they had had the opportunity to learn from songs audible at the nest for as much as 10 days in some cases prior to acoustic isolation in the laboratory. Might they have learned something of natural song stimuli during that period that would then influence subsequent responsiveness to song?

To explore this possibility we first reared 6 male swamp sparrows in isolation. Eggs were taken from wild nests early in incubation, fostered and, with the aid of supplemental feeding, reared under canaries in the laboratory. These six males were placed in individual isolation and exposed from 20 to 50 days-of-age to tape-recorded songs that were synthesized in a variety of syntactical patterns, some swamp sparrow-like and others song sparrow-like. One half of the songs were made up from normal swamp sparrow song syllables; the other half from song sparrow syllables that were either normal (two males) or subjected to a 13% upward transposition in frequency (four males). The methods for frequency transposition are described in Zoloth et al. (1980). This transposition matched a tendency for normal song sparrow syllables to be pitched 13% lower than those of swamp sparrows, although nevertheless overlapping greatly in frequency range. Of the ten song types that subjects developed, six of them matched models closely. Without exception, all were derived from swamp sparrow syllables. Thus the learning preference of young male swamp sparrows is innate (Marler & Peters, 1977).

In a second experiment, 7 male song sparrows were raised from the egg and trained with tape recorded songs of swamp and song sparrows in a similar fashion. Each week, the song sparrow heard 8 new songs, 4 swamp sparrow and 4 song sparrow, up to a total of 80 song types for the 10-week training period. Altogether the birds learned from 31 song sparrow tape recordings and 6 swamp sparrow recordings. Thus there was a highly significant bias in favor of conspecific songs ($X^2 = 14.55$, $p < 0.001$). The results of these two experiments on song learning in birds reared from the egg are summarized in Figure 5, together with data on birds of both species reared from the nestling phase and trained with tape recordings. An interesting species difference is revealed in the degree of conspecific preference. The preference is more extreme in swamp sparrows than in song sparrows. The same contrast was found in birds of the two species reared as nestlings as in those reared from the egg (Fig. 8.11).

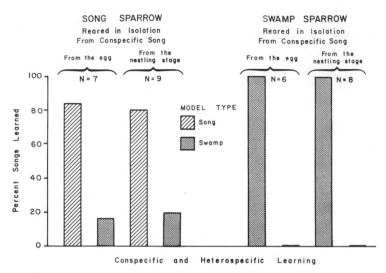

FIG. 8.11. Learning preferences of male song and swamp sparrows raised from the egg and from the nestling phase. Information on training of the egg-reared subjects is given in the text. The song sparrow nestlings were taken at 2–10 days of age and exposed to tape recorded swamp and song sparrow songs for the first year of life beginning at 11 days of age. Song types were changed every 1–6 weeks. Nestling swamp sparrows were collected from wild nests at 4–8 days. They heard tape-recorded swamp and song sparrow songs, changed every 1–6 weeks, for the first year of life, beginning at 17 days of age (see Marler & Peters, 1987, 1988a for more details on the nestling experiments).

There is evidently some discrepancy between the experimental test situation and that which occurs in nature. In the wild, song sparrows do not imitate swamp sparrows, despite the fact that they often live within earshot. Presumably some aspect of natural experience that is lacking from the highly simplified tape-recorded song paradigm is responsible for this disparity. It may be that social factors of other kinds, involving perhaps specific visual responsiveness, or social exchanges of an interactive nature also have potential effects on learning preferences, and that these factors have more of an influence upon song acquisition in song sparrows than in swamp sparrows. In swamp sparrows, tape-recording and live tutor training paradigms have yielded very similar results (Marler & Peters, 1987), but a direct comparison has yet to be made in song sparrows. Using a quite different approach, employing cardiac responses as an index of responsiveness of young male song and swamp sparrows to song stimulation, Dooling and Searcy (1980) also found responsiveness of male swamp sparrows to tape-recorded conspecific song to be more selective than that of song sparrows.

Unlike precocial species such as chickens and ducks, which are hatched at a much later developmental age than altricial species such as these sparrows, and are responsive to vocal sounds even prior to hatching (e.g., Gottlieb, 1971), these and other experiments have confirmed that oscines do not learn anything specific from song stimulation as nestlings (review in Slater, 1983). In fact, the sensitive period for song acquisition in the song sparrow, the only species for which an accurate determination has been made (Marler & Peters, 1987), does not begin until about 20-days-of-age, more than a week after fledging occurs. The timing of onset in swamp sparrows is probably similar (Marler & Peters, 1988a). Thus the indications are that all of the preference behavior described here, involving subjects that were isolated from natural song stimulation as nestlings, is innate.

X. SPECIES DIFFERENCES IN THE ACOUSTIC BASIS OF LEARNING PREFERENCES: A SUMMARY

Conspecific and heterospecific songs are not equipotent as learning stimuli for either swamp sparrows or song sparrows. Using song production as an index of what has been learned, a clear and unequivocal bias is revealed in favor of learning conspecific songs. The two species differ, however, in the cues upon which the preferences are based. In young male swamp sparrows the preference for learning conspecific song over song sparrow song appears to be based entirely on phonology and syllabic syntax. Song sparrows also favor conspecific phonology and syllabic syntax over that of the swamp sparrow (Fig. 8.12B). In addition, however, song sparrows are responsive to other attributes of song. These include: (1) The number of segments—heterospecific phonology is more likely to be learned when presented in multisegmental songs, as compared with uni-segmental songs (Fig. 8.12B & C). (2) Internal phrase structure—they are less likely to learn heterospecific phonology when presented as a note complex than as a trill. (3) Tempo and numbers of trill syllables—young male song sparrows are more receptive to an accelerated introductory trill with few, long syllables than to one with a constant tempo and more, shorter syllables. There is no evidence that young male swamp sparrows are responsive to any of these syntactical features.

The precise contribution of some of these factors has yet to be fully isolated. The role of an accelerated introduction cannot yet be separated from effects of other covarying features such as the longer duration and smaller number of syllables in an introductory trill as compared with subsequent trills in the song. The contribution of syllabic syntax has yet to be fully disentangled from that of pure note phonology. Details of song phonology, and the ways in which notes are arranged into syllables have yet to be completely worked out in the song sparrow.

In the swamp sparrow song phonology has been analyzed by two different

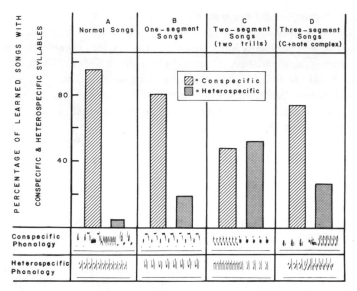

FIG. 8.12.   Song learning preferences of young male song sparrows presented with tape recordings of normal songs and synthetic song with one, two or three segments. In every case a choice was given between conspecific and heterospecific (swamp sparrow) syllables. A illustrates the conspecific preference with normal song. B shows a significant preference based on phonology and syllable structure alone. C illustrates loss of the conspecific preference with two-phrased songs. D shows reinstatement of a conspecific syllable preference by addition of a note complex to C. The data are summarized from several experiments in Marler and Peters (1988b).

techniques. Both indicate that all swamp sparrow songs are constructed from a surprisingly limited set of phonological units (Clark, Marler, & Beeman, 1987; Marler & Pickert, 1984). Marler and Pickert divided song phonology into six basic units or "note types." Subsequent work has shown that at least two of the categorical boundaries were probably arbitrary (Clark et al., 1987), and that there may be only three or four basic note types, two with relatively limited within-category variation, a third with extensive variation, and a fourth that is rare.

The arrangement of swamp sparrow note types into syllables conforms to certain rules. The rules of syllable syntax adhered to by an individual are a function of early experience, and can be used to define what appear to be dialects in swamp sparrow song. The number of possible dialects appears to be limited, however, by a strong tendency for two of the three note types to occur in boundary positions in a syllable, either introducing the syllable, or terminating it. The most variable note category typically falls in middle positions within a syllable. These rules are probabilistic rather than completely determinate, but they are sufficiently regular that they could provide cues for species identification, in addition to the cues provided by basic note phonology. Thus in both species, it remains to be seen whether, aside from syllabic syntax, phonology alone is a sufficient basis for the maintenance of song learning preferences.

XI.   PERCEPTION, PRODUCTION AND LEARNING PREFERENCES

Several developmental steps intervene between the acquisition of a song, and the production of a crystallized imitation (Fig. 8.7). Might the vocal tracts of these two sparrow species be sufficiently different in construction that it is easier for them to produce conspecific than heterospecific song? Such a hypothesis could suffice as an explanation for learning preferences, at least at the phonological level. Although this hypothesis is difficult to exclude entirely until we achieve a better understanding of how the oscine syrinx operates, and a fuller appreciation of the contributions made by supra-syringeal components of the vocal tract to song production (Nowicki, 1987; Nowicki & Capranica, 1986), at the present state of knowledge this interpretation of learning preferences seems unlikely. The anatomical structure of the oscine syrinx is highly conservative. Far from diverging in structure and function between close relatives, it varies remarkably little, and this uniformity explains its uses as one of the traits upon which higher levels of oscine taxonomy are based (Ames, 1971; Gaunt & Gaunt, 1985; Greenewalt, 1968).

The potential ability of many birds to produce sounds of other species, even when they rarely do so under normal conditions, also argues against any strict limitations imposed on phonation by interspecies variations in vocal tract structure. Not only are heterospecific songs occasionally learned and reproduced in nature (e.g., Eberhardt & Baptista, 1977), but birds can also be readily persuaded to reproduce them in the laboratory (e.g., Baptista & Petrinovich, 1986).

We have already indicated many cases of song sparrows imitating swamp sparrow syllables when presented in the appropriate song sparrow-like syntax. In other experiments we have also found that swamp sparrows can also be persuaded to imitate song sparrow phonology by embedding single notes within normal swamp sparrow phonological units (Fig. 8.13). The vocal tract of each species is thus capable of producing the phonology of the other.

Species may nevertheless differ in the ease with which conspecific and heterospecific songs can be produced. Aside from differences in the peripheral effectors, the possibility of species differences in central neuromotor mechanisms cannot be excluded. The gross abnormality of song phonology in early-deafened sparrows (Konishi, 1965; Marler & Sherman, 1983) and the absence of most normal phonology in the songs of sparrows reared in isolation implies that, if

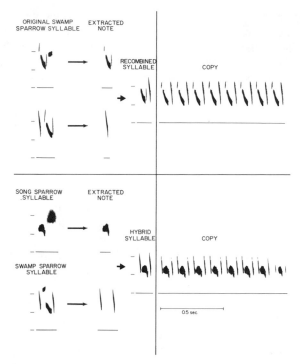

FIG. 8.13. Male swamp sparrows will accept song sparrow notes as learning stimuli if they are embedded in swamp sparrow syllables. The bottom panel shows the creation of such a hybrid syllable, and its imitation by a male swamp sparrow, on the right. The top panel illustrates the control procedure, in which only swamp sparrow notes are used. From Zoloth et al. (1980).

species-specific neuromotor mechanisms are involved in production, their development is sensitive to effects of auditory feedback and conspecific song stimulation. It is nevertheless the case that, although the phonology of isolation-reared sparrows is abnormal, certain species differences persist (Marler & Sherman, 1985), perhaps as a direct reflection of contrasting patterns of neural organization in relatively peripheral motor mechanisms.

For example, data presented in this review all derive from crystallized song production. In the swamp sparrow, transitions through subsong, plastic song and crystallized song have been documented in detail (Marler & Peters, 1982a, 1982b). Extensive overproduction of songs has been found in plastic song. The excess of songs is then subjected to a process of attrition as development proceeds towards crystallization (Fig. 8.14). Crystallized song thus fails to reveal all that has been learned earlier in life. Detailed study of the attrition process has revealed that if male swamp sparrows are persuaded to incorporate heterospecific

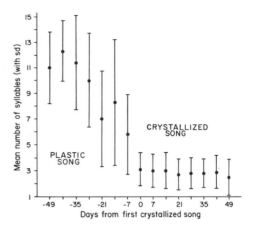

FIG. 8.14. Data showing the overproduction of song types by male swamp sparrows in the plastic song stage of development. The repertoire is reduced drastically as the time for song crystallization approaches (Day 0). A typical, mature swamp sparrow song repertoire consists of three song types. From Marler and Peters (1982a).

imitations in their plastic song (Fig. 8.13), these are more likely to be rejected as candidates for crystallized songs than conspecific imitations (Fig. 8.15). Species-specific differences in neuromotor organization might well contribute to this process of selective attrition in late stages of motor development. Although yet to be investigated in detail, similar processes may operate in song sparrow development.

The major factors shaping learning preferences are probably perceptual, however, rather than motor. Young sparrows possess perceptual mechanisms that can

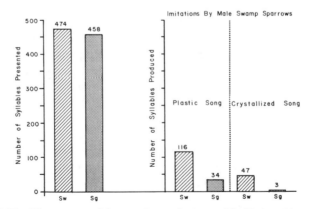

FIG. 8.15. Histograms of the numbers of conspecific (Sw) and heterospecific (Sg) syllables in songs presented to young male swamp sparrows as learning stimuli. Imitations in plastic song clearly favor conspecific songs. In the transition from plastic to crystallized song the balance favors conspecific songs even more strongly. There is a significant tendency to reject previously learned heterospecific songs in the crystallization process. Data from Marler and Peters (1982a).

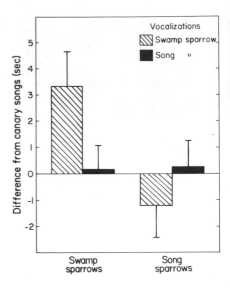

FIG. 8.16. Cardiac orienting responses of young song and swamp sparrows to tape recordings of their own and each other's song, relative to the response of each species to the neutral auditory stimulus of canary song. From Dooling and Searcy (1980).

sustain discrimination of conspecific from heterospecific songs, as is indicated by the experiments of Dooling and Searcy (1980). They used heart rate changes to measure the relative salience of songs as auditory stimuli presented to recently fledged sparrows, prior to any song production (Fig. 8.16). Swamp sparrows of both sexes displayed preferential responsiveness to conspecific song as early as three weeks of age, the time when the sensitive period for song acquisition begins (Marler & Peters, 1987, 1988a).

Another line of evidence also points towards innate, species-specific auditory responsiveness to song. Much of the normal temporal organization of song sparrow song develops in birds reared in social isolation, as long as their hearing is intact. This is true both at the level of segmentation and also in details of syntactical organization (Marler & Sherman, 1985). Aside from some basic aspects of segmentation, most of this structure fails to develop in birds that are unable to hear their own voice during development because they are deaf (Marler & Sherman, 1983). This finding provides direct support for the concept of innate species-specific auditory template mechanisms (Konishi, 1965; Marler, 1976). Swamp and song sparrows evidently possess different central auditory specifications for song (Marler, 1984).

With the auditory feedback loop intact these sparrows develop some of the same syntactical song features that provide the sensory basis for learning preferences (Marler & Sherman, 1985). As templates guiding motor development, they operate late in ontogeny, in the production of plastic and crystallized song. If they also exist and can operate earlier in life, during song acquisition, prior to the onset of any singing, the same innate auditory mechanisms may serve both functions, sustaining conspecific learning preferences and serving, template fashion, to shape song production as well.

ACKNOWLEDGMENTS

This project was supported in part by BRSG S07 RR07065 awarded by the Biomedical Research Support Grant Program, Division of Research Resources, National Institutes of Health, and by grant number MH 14651 to Peter Marler. Esther Arruza prepared the figures and typed the manuscript. We thank Judith and Cathy Marler and Eileen McCue for rearing the birds. We are indebted to Drs. Douglas Nelson and Stephen Nowicki for discussion and criticism, and to the New York Botanical Garden Institute of Ecosystem Studies at the Mary Flagler Cary Arboretum for access to study areas.

REFERENCES

Ames, P. L. (1971). The morphology of the syrinx in passerine birds. *Peabody Museum of Natural History Bulletin, 37,* 1–194.

Balaban, E. (1988). Cultural and genetic variation in swamp sparrows (*Melospiza georgiana*). II. Behavioral salience of geographic song variants. *Behaviour, 105,* 292–322.

Baptista, L. F., & Petrinovich, L. (1984). Social interaction, sensitive phases and the song template hypothesis in the white-crowned sparrow. *Animal Behaviour, 32,* 172–181.

Baptista, L. F., & Petrinovich, L. (1986). Song development in the white-crowned sparrow: social factors and sex differences. *Animal Behaviour, 34,* 1359–1371.

Barrington, D. (1773). Experiments and observations on the singing of birds. *Philisophical Transactions Royal Society, 63,* 249–291.

Clark, C. W., Marler, P., & Beeman, K. (1987). Quantitative analysis of animal vocal phonology: An application to swamp sparrow song. *Ethology,* 76: 101–115.

Dickerman, R. W. (1961). Hybrids among the fringillid genera *Junco, Zonotrichia* and *Melospiza. Auk, 78,* 627–632.

Dooling, R. J., & Searcy, M. H. (1980). Early perceptual selectivity in the swamp sparrow. *Developmental Psychobiology, 13,* 499–506.

Eberhardt, C., & Baptista, L. (1977). Intra- and inter-specific song mimesis in the song sparrow, *Melospiza melodia. Bird Banding, 48,* 193–205.

Gaunt, A. S., & Gaunt, S. L L. (1985). Syringeal structure and avian phonation. In R. F. Johnston (Ed.), *Current Ornithology,* (Vol. 2, pp. 213–245). New York: Plenum Press.

Gottlieb, G. (1971). *Development of species identification in birds.* Chicago: University of Chicago Press.

Greenewalt, C. H. (1968). *Bird song: acoustics and physiology.* Washington, D.C.: Smithsonian Institute.

Konishi, M. (1965). The role of auditory feedback in the control of vocalization in the white-crowned sparrow. *Zeitschrift für Tierpsychologie, 22,* 770–783.

Kroodsma, D. (1972). Variations in songs of vesper sparrows in Oregon. *Wilson Bulletin, 84,* 173–178.

Kroodsma, D. (1977). A reevaluation of song development in the song sparrow. *Animal Behaviour, 25,* 390–399.

Kroodsma, D. (1982). Learning and the ontogeny of sound signals in birds. In D. E. Kroodsma & E. H. Miller (Eds.), *Acoustic communication in birds* (Vol. 2, pp. 1–23). New York: Academic Press.

Marler, P. (1970). A comparative approach to vocal learning: song development in white-crowned sparrows. *Journal of Comparative and Physiological Psychology, 71*:2 (Monog.), 1–25.

Marler, P. (1976). Sensory templates in species-specific behavior. In J. Fentress (Ed.), *Simpler networks and behavior* (pp. 314–329). Sunderland, MA: Sinauer Associates.

Marler, P. (1984). Song learning: innate species differences in the learning process. In P. Marler & H. S. Terrace (Eds.), *The biology of learning* (pp. 289–309). Berlin: Springer-Verlag.

Marler, P., & Peters, S. (1977). Selective vocal learning in a sparrow. *Science, 198,* 519–521.

Marler, P., & Peters, S. (1980). Birdsong and speech: Evidence for special processing. In P. Eimas & J. Miller (Eds.), *Perspectives on the study of speech* (pp. 75–112). Hillsdale, NJ: Lawrence Erlbaum Associates.

Marler, P., & Peters, S. (1982a). Developmental overproduction and selective attrition: new processes in the epigenesis of birdsong. *Devel. Psychobiol., 15,* 369–378.

Marler, P., & Peters, S. (1982b). Structural changes in song ontogeny in the swamp sparrow, *Melospiza georgiana. Auk, 99,* 446–458.

Marler, P., & Peters, S. (1987). A sensitive period for song acquisition in the song sparrow, *Melospiza melodia:* A case of age-limited learning. *Ethology, 76:* 89–100.

Marler, P., & Peters, S. (1988a). Sensitive periods for song acquisition from tape recordings and live tutors in the swamp sparrow, *Melospiza georgiana. Ethology, 77,* 76–84.

Marler, P., & Peters, S. (1988b). The role of song phonology and syntax in vocal learning preferences in the song sparrow, *Melospiza melodia. Ethology, 77,* 125–149.

Marler, P., Peters, S., & Wingfield, J. (1987). Correlations between song acquisition, song production and plasma levels of testosterone and estradiol in sparrows. *Journal of Neurobiology, 18,* 531–548.

Marler, P., & Pickert, R. (1984). Species-universal microstructure in the learned song of the swamp sparrow (*Melospiza georgiana*). *Animal Behaviour, 32,* 673–689.

Marler, P., & Sherman, V. (1983). Song structure without auditory feedback: Emendations of the auditory template hypothesis. *Journal of Neuroscience, 3,* 517–531.

Marler, P., & Sherman, V. (1985). Innate differences in singing behaviour of sparrows reared in isolation from adult conspecific song. *Animal Behaviour, 33,* 57–71.

Martin, D. J. (1977). Songs of the fox sparrow. I. Structure of song and its comparison with song in other emberizidae. *Condor, 79,* 209–221.

Mulligan, J. A. (1963). A description of song sparrow song based on instrumental analysis. *Proceedings XIII International Ornithological Congress,* 272–284.

Nowicki, S. (1987). Vocal tract resonance in oscine bird sound production: Evidence from birdsongs in a helium atmosphere. *Nature, 325,* 53–55.

Nowicki, S., & Capranica, R. (1986). Bilateral syringeal coupling during phonation of a songbird. *Journal of Neuroscience, 6,* 3595–3610.

Payne, R. B. (1983). The social context of song mimicry: song-matching dialects in indigo buntings (*Passerina cyanea*). *Animal Behaviour, 31,* 788–805.

Paynter, R. A. Jr. (1964). Generic limits of Zonotrichia. *Condor, 66,* 277–281.

Pepperberg, I. M. (1985). Social modeling theory: a possible framework for understanding avian vocal learning. *Auk, 102,* 854–864.

Peters, S. S., Searcy, W. A., & Marler, P. (1980). Species song discrimination in choice experiments with territorial male swamp and song sparrows. *Animal Behaviour, 28,* 393–404.

Ritchison, G. (1981). Variation in the songs of vesper sparrows *Poecetes gramineus. American Midland Naturalist, 106*(2), 392–398.

Scott, W. E. D. (1901). Data on songbirds: Observations on the song of Baltimore orioles in captivity. *Science, 14,* 522–526.

Scott, W. E. D. (1902). Data on song in birds: The acquisition of new songs. *Science, 15*, 178–181.

Scott, W. E. D. (1904a). The inheritance of song in passerine birds. Remarks and observations on the song of hand-reared bobolinks and red-winged blackbirds (*Dolichonyx oryzivorus* and *Agelaius phoeniceus*). *Science, 19*, 154–155.

Scott, W. E. D. (1904b). The inheritance of song in passerine birds. Remarks on the development of song in the rose-breasted grosbeak, *Zamelodia ludoviciana* (Linnaeus) and the meadowlark, *Sturnella magna* (Linnaeus). *Science, 19*, 947–959.

Scott, W. E. D. (1904c). The inheritance of song in passerine birds. Further observations on the development of song and nest-building in hand-reared rose-breasted grosbeaks, *Zamelodia ludoviciana* (Linnaeus). *Science, 20*, 282–283.

Slater, P. J. B. (1983). Bird song learning: theme and variations. In G. H. Brush & G. A. Clark Jr. (Eds.), *Perspectives in ornithology* (pp. 475–511). Cambridge, England: Cambridge University Press.

Zink, R. M. (1982). Patterns of genic and morphologic variation among sparrows in the genera *Zonotrichia, Melospiza, Junco* and *Passerella*. *Auk, 99*, 632–649.

Zoloth, S. R., Dooling, R., Miller, R., & Peters, S. (1980). A minicomputer system for the synthesis of animal vocalizations. *Zeitschrift für Tierpsychologie, 54*, 151–162.

Editorial Comments on Beecher, Loesche, Stoddard, and Medvin

How do songbirds distinguish their offspring? In species where nests are isolated, the problem may not be so difficult, but in colonial species such as the cliff swallow, the problem must be very difficult indeed. In this chapter the authors argue that identification depends potentially on cues that the young provide through their calls, through differences in the way the calls are perceived by the parent, and in the decision rules the parents may follow given the signal and the perceptual processing the signal has undergone.

An analysis of the natural calls of noncolonial barn swallows and colonial cliff swallows reveals that there is much more potential discriminative information carried in the calls of the cliff swallows. That is, there is much more individual variation among calls. In a laboratory experiment comparing the ability of the two species of swallows to discriminate calls of their own and of the other species, cliff swallow calls were easier to discriminate than barn swallow calls, but that was equally so for both species. Hence, there was no evidence for any specialized perceptual capacities on the part of cliff swallows for their own calls.

This research joins that of Kuhl and others in this book which is trying to untangle the issue of specificity in acoustic communication. Does "language," whether animal or human, have some specialized status in the perceptual world? The answer to that question may turn out to be neither simple nor general, but for cliff as compared with barn swallows at least, the problem of individual recognition seems to have been solved by increasing the complexity of the call rather than modifying in some special way the perceptual apparatus designed to detect and process it.

9

Individual Recognition by Voice in Swallows: Signal or Perceptual Adaptation?

Michael D. Beecher
Patricia Loesche
Philip K. Stoddard
Mandy B. Medvin
University of Washington

INTRODUCTION

Comparative studies have shown that individual recognition is present or well developed only in those species in which there is a strong pressure for this ability, such as occurs in most colonial species (e.g., Beecher, 1982; Jouventin, 1982). For example, we have found that in the colonial cliff swallow (*Hirundo pyrrhonota*), parents recognize their young, yet in the closely related but non-colonial barn swallow (*Hirundo rustica*), parents show no evidence of recognition (summarized in Beecher, Medvin, Stoddard, & Loesche 1986). The comparative evidence thus contradicts the common, intuitive view that individual recognition is the inevitable consequence of ubiquitous phenotypic variation and well-developed perceptual systems. In our work on individual recognition by voice in birds, we have asked to what extent have traits been directly molded by selection for individual recognition, and to what extent have they evolved in other contexts and been secondarily exploited for this purpose.

We will define "individual recognition" as the differential treatment of an individual or class of individuals (e.g., offspring) based on individually distinctive cues. Here and throughout, we are considering only the interesting case where discrimination of one individual from another (or one class from another) cannot be accomplished solely on the basis of circumstantial evidence. Individual recognition is clearly required by a parent attempting to find its offspring in a creche of hundreds of similar-aged young, whereas a parent returning to its nest can be certain (in most species) that the young there are its own.

Although it is often convenient to speak of "individual recognition" as if it were a simple trait, it is in fact an *outcome* or a *composite* of several separate

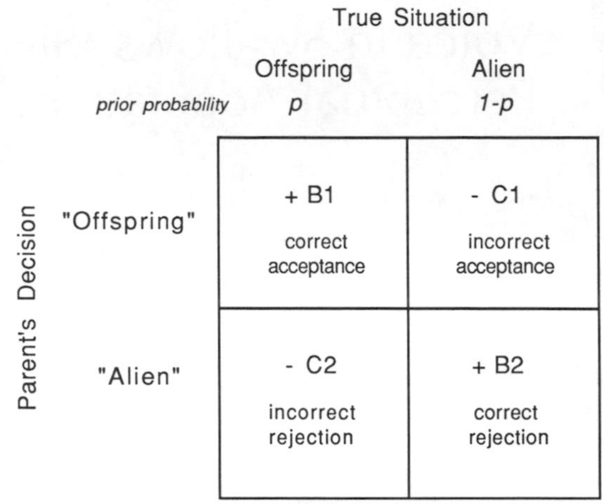

True Situation

	prior probability	Offspring p	Alien 1-p
"Offspring"		+ B1 correct acceptance	- C1 incorrect acceptance
"Alien"		- C2 incorrect rejection	+ B2 correct rejection

Parent's Decision

FIG. 9.1.   Key features of the general recognition problem, presented in the context of a parent seeking its offspring. The parent (the receiver) must decide whether a particular individual it encounters (the sender) is in fact its offspring or an unrelated ("alien") individual. There are four possible outcomes. The parent can correctly decide that the sender is its offspring or correctly decide that the sender is not. It receives a benefit (payoff) B1 or B2 respectively. The parent can make two types of error, rejecting its offspring or accepting an alien young. These errors carry costs C2 and C1 respectively. Given the prior probability of encountering offspring and alien young in this situation and the values of the various benefits and costs, an optimal decision rule can be arrived at via decision theory.

traits. This is easily seen by considering the generalized recognition problem. One animal (the receiver) seeking another individual (the target individual, e.g., its mate or its offspring) is confronted by an individual (the sender) that may or may not be the target individual. The recognition process consists of three logically independent components. First, the sender must provide *cues* as to its identity ("signature" cues). Although we should not necessarily expect that the sender will always signal "honestly," it is clear that the receiver requires such cues if it is to have any basis for a decision (assuming circumstantial evidence is inadequate). Second, the receiver must process these cues in order to *perceive* the difference between target and nontarget individuals. Finally, the receiver must *decide* whether the sender is the target individual. The receiver's decision problem is represented in Fig. 9.1 (in the context of parent seeking offspring). In theory, the receiver's decision rule should be based in part on the *a priori* probability of the receiver being the target individual, the costs of the two types of error and the benefits of the two types of correct decisions. The key point is that natural selection can promote individual recognition by acting appropriately on any of the *signal*, *perceptual* and *decision* components of recognition. Among the possible actions, three stand out. Selection can (1) increase signature variation among individuals and/or decrease it within individuals, thus making individuals more distinctive; (2) increase perceptual sensitivity to the signature traits, thus allowing receivers to more readily discriminate among senders; (3) modify the decision rule so as to lead to the optimal solution of the problem posed in Fig. 9.1. Within the second class of adaptation, we must distinguish *special* from *general* perceptual adaptations. In the first case, the perceptual sharpening is restricted to the specific signature cues, whereas in the latter case, discrimination is enhanced to a broad range of stimuli beyond the signature cues. In this chapter we concentrate on signal and perceptual adaptations.

We present data from two studies bearing on acoustic specializations for individual recognition in cliff swallows (*Hirundo pyrrhonota*) and barn swallows (*Hirundo rustica*). First, we present an information analysis of the calls of cliff swallow and barn swallow chicks (Beecher, Medvin, Stoddard, & Loesche 1986; Medvin, Stoddard, & Beecher, in prep). This analysis supports the signal adaptation hypothesis, as the measured information capacity of cliff swallow calls is considerably higher than that of barn swallow calls. Second, we present a preliminary analysis of data from a perceptual experiment in which we compared the ability of cliff swallows and barn swallows to discriminate among the calls of different chicks of both species (Loesche, Stoddard, Higgins, & Beecher, in prep). These data likewise support the signal adaptation hypothesis, as cliff swallows and barn swallows alike found the cliff swallow calls more discriminable than the barn swallow calls. They do not support the perceptual adaptation hypothesis, at least not the special adaptation version of this hypothesis, as there was no general perceptual advantage for conspecific calls.

I. BACKGROUND FIELD STUDIES

In this paper we will focus on the comparison between cliff swallows and barn swallows. We have done parallel studies and obtained comparable results on another pair of swallow species, the colonial bank swallow (*Riparia riparia*) and noncolonial rough-winged swallow (*Stelgidopteryx serripennis*) (Beecher & Beecher, in prep; Beecher, Beecher, & Hahn 1981; Beecher, Beecher, & Lumpkin, 1981). We chose to do our perceptual studies on the cliff swallow–barn swallow pair, however, for a variety of reasons, the chief one being that they are so closely related (congenerics). The primary difference between cliff swallows and barn swallows is that the cliff swallow is colonial. The implication for individual recognition in general, and parent-offspring recognition in particular, is that intermingling will generally be much more common and more extensive in the colonial species. Needless to say, this correlation is not inevitable—witness the much-cited example of the colonial but cliff-nesting kittiwake, where there is no intermingling of chicks (Cullen, 1957)—but must be evaluated by careful studies of the "natural history" of recognition. Occasionally, one may find barn swallows in small "colonies" or cliff swallows in small groups or even solitarily, yet cliff swallows show many adaptations for coloniality which barn swallows do not. Cliff swallow colonies are usually larger (generally much larger); reproduction within cliff swallow colonies is synchronized while that within barn swallow colonies is not; cliff swallow nests are aggregated (abutting) while barn swallow nests are maximally dispersed over the "colony," and cliff swallows, but not barn swallows, routinely forage together (e.g., Bent, 1942; Brown, 1986; Emlen, 1955; Medvin & Beecher, unpublished data; Shields, 1984; Snapp, 1976). Thus, it is fair to describe the selective background of cliff swallows as colonial, and of barn swallows as noncolonial.

We summarize our field studies on cliff swallows and barn swallows later (Beecher, Stoddard, & Loesche, 1985; Medvin & Beecher, 1986; Stoddard & Beecher, 1983). In this chapter we consider only recognition of offspring by parents, although our results on recognition of parents by offspring are similar.

1. Chick intermingling is a characteristic feature of cliff swallow colonies. In fact, fledgling chicks are often left in large groups (creches) away from the nest while the parents forage. Chick intermingling is uncommon in barn swallows, however, even when the birds are found in loose colonies. In fact, barn swallow parents make special efforts to keep their fledglings apart from other unrelated chicks, particularly in the first few days after fledging when they are still providing much of the chick's food.

2. Cross-fostering experiments and call playback studies, both done with chicks of fledging age, give no evidence that barn swallow parents can recognize their offspring. This is true whether the parents are tested in colonial or solitary nesting circumstances. On the other hand, playback studies clearly show that cliff swallow parents can recognize their chicks by voice. In addition, cliff swallow chicks show marked individual variation in face color pattern, while barn swallow chicks show no such variation. We have not investigated the significance of this visual variation, however, and we are concerned here only with the call variation.

Thus the need for and the extent of parental recognition is greater in cliff swallows than in barn swallows. Our evidence suggests that one focus of selection in cliff swallows has been on parental recognition of the chick "signature call." We can unambiguously identify the homologous call in barn swallows, for it is given in precisely the same circumstances (e.g., begging for food, chasing the parent). Barn swallow parents, however, do not discriminate among the calls of different chicks. This failure may occur because the calls are not individually distinctive (in which case "signature call" is a misnomer), or because the parents do not have the perceptual capability to discriminate among calls, or because the parents choose not to do so, i.e., use a rule such as "always accept" when faced with a recognition decision. Needless to say, the true reason could be some weighted combination of these three possibilities. Because this chapter focuses on acoustic adaptations (of signal or perception), we will pass over evidence bearing on "decision rules" at this point (but see General Discussion section).

We cannot really distinguish between signature and perceptual adaptations with field experiments. The problem is that in any field comparison of the two species, the relative powers of parental discrimination are confounded with the relative discriminability of chick calls. Thus, we have taken two alternative approaches to evaluating and contrasting the signal adaptation and perceptual adaptation hypotheses. In the first approach, described in the next section, we measured the information capacity of the calls used in recognition. In the second approach, described in the section following, we took cliff swallows and barn swallows into the laboratory and measured their ability to discriminate among the calls of both species.

II. INFORMATION ANALYSIS OF SIGNATURE CALLS

Problem

The calls of 4 cliff swallow chicks and 4 barn swallow chicks are shown in Fig. 9.2. The most obvious way to test the signature adaptation hypothesis is to analyze a representative set of such calls. Although this method is direct and objective, it neglects the effects of the receiver's perceptual system, a significant problem if the receiver's perceptual analysis is very different from our analysis of the sonagrams. We discuss this problem in the next section. In this section we outline the logic and assumptions of our information analysis of the sonagrams (described in detail in Beecher, 1982; in press) and present some of our results (a full description is in Medvin, Stoddard, & Beecher, in prep).

Method

The signature call system is conceived of as the set of individual signature calls. This set contains both between-individual variation, and within-individual variation. Clearly the information capacity of this system—its capacity to reliably identify individuals—increases with the between-individual variation, and decreases with the within-individual variation. We quantify the information capacity by measuring variance between and within individuals on each of several measured call parameters.

The information analysis begins with extraction of measurements from sonagrams of calls. Call parameters are chosen so as to describe the call as completely as possible with the fewest number of parameters. The measurements derived from the sonagrams are next subjected to a principal components analysis. This analysis conserves the total non-redundant variance in the original set of measurements. Simple ANOVAS are carried out on the principal components and between-individual, within-individual and total variance estimates obtained according to the Model II (Random Effects) model. The total information is

$$H = \Sigma \log \sqrt{\sigma^2_{Ti}/\sigma^2_{wi}}$$

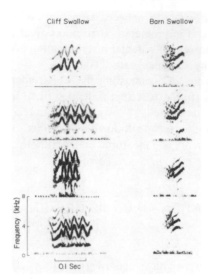

FIG. 9.2.   Left: Calls of 4 cliff swallow chicks. Right: Calls of 4 barn swallow chicks. Effective bandwidth of sonagrams is 180 Hz. Five parameters (four in the barn swallows) were extracted for the information analysis. (*1*) Duration of the call (T), measured from the first major frequency peak of cliff swallow calls, from the onset of the call for barn swallow calls. (*2*) Peak frequency (f), of the lower voice. (*3*) Frequency difference between the upper and lower voices (Δv), measured at the first frequency peak. (*4*) Frequency modulation range of the lower voice (Δf), measured between the first frequency peak and first frequency trough (cliff swallows) or between the highest frequency and the frequency 24 msec earlier (barn swallows). (*5*) The period of frequency modulation (P). This last parameter pertains to cliff swallows only.

where $\sigma^2_{T_i}$ and $\sigma^2_{w_i}$ are the total and within-individual variance estimates for the ith principle component.

Several assumptions are implicit in this analysis. First, we assume that we have extracted all (or most of) the relevant information from the calls. In fact, in our present data set we can reconstruct fair replicas of the original calls from our measurements (Medvin et al., in prep). While the replicas are relatively crude, they are better for the barn swallow calls. Thus given our hypothesis, this is a conservative error, since it means that our method underestimates the information capacity of the cliff swallow calls more than that of the barn swallow calls. Second, our method weights all parameters equally. Third, the method provides a measure of information capacity of the calls, not information extracted by the receiver. In a sense it presumes an ideal receiver. It should be clear that all of these assumptions relate to the perceptual issue mentioned above. Ideally, we would put our question about the relative information capacity of these two sets of calls to the birds themselves, and skip the call measurement step. In reality, however, call measurements are much more feasible and cost-effective than the comparable perceptual measurements from the birds. Thus comparisons between the two methods, such as the preliminary comparison we have in this paper, are potentially quite valuable.

Results and Discussion

The call analysis is summarized in Table 9.1, in terms of the original measurements (means, standard deviations based on variance estimates, and between-individual parameter intercorrelations). The measured information capacity is 8.74 bits for cliff swallow calls and 4.57 bits for barn swallow calls. This finding of a greater information capacity for the signature calls of the colonial species parallels the difference found between the colonial bank swallow and non-colonial rough-winged swallow in an earlier study using a preliminary version of this method (Beecher, 1982). The difference between cliff swallows and barn swallows of 4.17 bits can be roughly translated to say that approximately 20 times more individuals can be identified, to the same degree of precision, with the cliff swallow signature system.

TABLE 9.1
Means, Standard Deviations and Correlation Coefficients
for Information Analysis.

	Cliff Swallows					Barn Swallows			
	T	f	Δ v	Δ f	P	T	f	Δ v	Δ f
Mean	74.4	3.71	1.53	1.25	29.0	67.0	3.84	1.14	0.797
SD among	31.8	0.395	0.404	0.304	5.12	7.76	0.359	0.183	0.261
SD within	8.88	0.084	0.142	0.141	0.662	3.62	0.083	0.107	0.151
T	.	−0.42	−0.39	−0.16	+0.37	.	−0.28	−0.53	+0.04
f	.	.	+0.23	+0.58	−0.32	.	.	−0.44	+0.02
Δv	.	.	.	−0.23	+0.50	.	.	.	−0.30
Δf	.	.	.	.	+0.20	.	.	.	.

Parameters are as identified in Fig. 9.2. Numbers in the bottom half of the table are correlation coefficients based on the among-individual data. The descriptive information in this table is based on the original measurements, not the principal components used for the information analysis.

III. PERCEPTUAL STUDIES

Problem

The information analysis has two shortcomings with respect to our goal of disentangling the two sorts of acoustic adaptations, signal and perceptual. First and most obvious, it does not evaluate the perceptual adaptation hypothesis at all. Second and more subtle, it may be misleading. The argument is as follows. The essence of the information analysis just described can be captured informally by asking human observers to sort these sonagrams into piles corresponding to individuals. It turns out that the observers, whether naive or experienced, find it easier to do this for cliff swallow sonagrams than barn swallow sonagrams. A disquieting observation, however, is that at least on casual listening, these same humans find it quite difficult to reliably identify individuals by the calls themselves, for *either* species. Although we have not yet rigorously tested this discrepancy, it cautions us that our sonagram analysis could be misleading. Among the possible sources of error, two stand out. First, measurements taken from visual representations of the calls may give quite different results from those obtainable via direct perception of these calls. Differences include modality (visual vs. auditory) and duration (prolonged inspection of the sonagram vs. brief percept of the call). Second, there may be significant differences between humans and birds in their perception of complex acoustic signals (see Dooling and Hulse chapters, this volume). The major point is that the signal adaptation hypothesis, as well as the perceptual adaptation hypothesis, must be tested at the level of the birds' perception of these signals. This was our goal in the experiments to be described now.

We tested the hypothesis that the cliff swallow calls are more discriminable than barn swallow calls by training lab-reared birds of both species to discriminate among the calls of different individuals of each species. We used the methods of "animal psychophysics" (Stebbins, 1970), training birds to discriminate among calls for food reward. The reward contingencies (for example, responses to the call of cliff swallow A are rewarded, and responses to the call of cliff swallow B are not) allow us to circumvent confounding natural contexts and natural decision rules and focus in on signal and perceptual adaptations. Figure 9.3 presents the basic design of the experiment and several possible outcomes. In Case A (*signal adaptation* only), we hypothesize a single action of selection: that it has made the calls of cliff swallow chicks more discriminable. Thus in our experiment we would expect individuals of *both* species to discriminate more easily among cliff swallow calls than among barn swallow calls. In Case B (*specific perceptual adaptation* only) we hypothesize that selection has acted on both species to allow them to discriminate more finely among conspecific calls. Case C is a simple combination of the two previous types of adaptations. In Case D (*general perceptual adaptation* only) we hypothesize that selection has acted

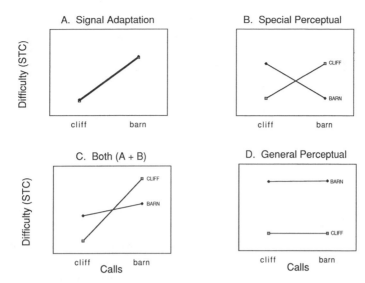

FIG. 9.3.   Design of the experiment and some possible outcomes. Abscissa is type of call discrimination, among cliffs or among barns. Ordinate is task difficulty (measured in sessions to criterion, STC). Parameter is subject, cliff swallow or barn swallow. Four cases shown are ideal cases intended to illustrate the logic of the experimental design. Case A: Selection has acted only on the signal (signature) of cliff swallows. Thus cliff swallow calls are more discriminable (less difficult) than barn swallow calls, and equally so for both species. Case B: Selection has acted on the perceptual systems of both species equally to make conspecific calls more discriminable. Case C: A combination of Cases A and B, i.e., selection has acted symmetrically on the perceptual systems of the two species and asymmetrically on the signature systems (more on cliff swallow calls than barn swallow calls). Case D: Selection has acted primarily on cliff swallow perceptual system but in such a way that cliff swallows find barn swallow calls as well as cliff swallow calls more discriminable. Selection presumed not to have acted on signature system at all in this case.

on cliff swallows to allow them to discriminate more finely among their calls but that this adaptation is sufficiently general that incidentally they can discriminate more finely among barn swallow chick calls as well. Given the similarity of chick calls in the two species (see Fig. 9.2), a general perceptual adaptation may actually be more plausible than a specific perceptual adaptation. We note that outcome *D* can arise in a number of ways other than a true perceptual adaptation for call discrimination. In particular, outcome D could occur if the cliff swallow subjects simply happen to be superior on the general task. We discuss this point in more detail below.

On the basis of our measurements of the calls, we predicted that cliff swallow calls would be more distinctive, or discriminable, than barn swallow calls. On the other hand, we had no compelling reason to predict either specific or general perceptual adaptations. In fact, given the highly developed auditory system of passerine birds, it seemed plausible that such species-specific adaptations were unnecessary. To date we have results for two cliff swallows, two barn swallows, and one European starling (*Sturnus vulgaris*), all hand-raised. As our swallows were taken from the nest at the onset of homeothermy and hand-raised together in an aviary, any species differences we might obtain would not be confounded with experiential differences.

Method

Our birds were trained as adults to discriminate among chick calls. The stimulus file consisted of 14 cliff swallow and 12 barn swallow chick calls. These chick calls were randomly selected from a large call set which had been recorded in the field over several breeding seasons. The calls were digitized at 45K sample/sec on a PDP-11 computer, and high-pass filtered to remove field noise. Each call in the stimulus file was measured on the parameters listed in Fig. 9.2. The means and variances of each parameter in the stimulus file were not significantly different from those of the larger data base, and so we regard them as representative samples. Three birds received discrimination training on five cliff swallow and five barn swallow call pairs and two birds got 10 of each. Pairs were randomly chosen with the restriction that no pair be used more than once.

Birds were trained in a custom-made soundproof booth equipped with loudspeaker, light, fan, feeder, and two pecking keys (Stoddard, 1987). Responses on the left, "observing" key turned on a call. For each pair of calls, one was arbitrarily designated the positive (GO) stimulus and the other the negative (NOGO) stimulus. Keypecks on the right, "report" key within 1 sec of the GO call were reinforced with an opportunity to feed (mealworm bits for the swallows, turkey starter for the starling). A keypeck within 1 sec of a NOGO call, or a failure to respond to a GO call, produced a time-out period during which the houselight was out. A bird received only one pair of calls in a given session, with the two calls always being from different individuals of the same species. The bird remained on a particular call discrimination until it reached a criterion of 85% correct responses in a session. Our measure of the discriminability of a call pair was thus the number of sessions to reach this criterion. Training on a new pair began in the next session. The experiment was terminated when a bird had learned 5 or 20 pairs each of cliff swallow and barn swallow calls (not counting two "training" pairs used in the initial training).

Results and Discussion

All 5 birds took longer, on average, to learn barn swallow call pairs than they did to learn cliff swallow pairs (Fig. 9.4). Pooling all the data, the 5 birds took 106

FIG. 9.4. Mean sessions to criterion for cliff swallow call pairs (dark) and barn swallow call pairs (stippled). Based on 10 pairs for the cliff swallow subjects and barn swallow A, 20 pairs for barn swallow B and the starling.

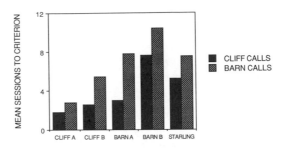

sessions for cliff swallow calls, and 167 sessions for barn swallow calls. When we compare learning of cliff swallow vs. barn swallow pairs at equivalent states of the experiment (e.g., the second cliff swallow pair with the second barn swallow pair) for each bird, then we find that in the 25 cases, the cliff swallow pair was learned sooner in 18 cases, the barn swallow pair in 4 cases and there was no difference in 3 cases. Thus these data are consistent with the information analysis of the preceding section, and support the signal adaptation hypothesis.

The results provide no support for the special perceptual adaptation hypothesis. We can take the ratio of the total number of sessions to criterion on the barn swallow call set to that on the cliff swallow call set as a measure of the relative discriminability of the two species call sets. Then the special perceptual adaptation hypothesis predicts that the conspecific advantage should accentuate the cliff swallow call advantage for cliff swallows but reduce it for barn swallows (see Fig. 9.3C), i.e., the discriminability ratio should be larger for cliff swallows (and the starling should be intermediate). This prediction is not supported, as the two barn swallows (ratios 2.60, 1.12) bracketed the two cliff swallows (2.08, 1.56).

The two cliff swallows learned discriminations more quickly in general than did the two barn swallows: 23 and 40 total sessions to criterion for the cliff swallows vs. 54 and 102 sessions for the two barn swallows. This outcome is consistent with the general perceptual adaptation hypothesis, that is, could be viewed as a combination of outcomes A and D in Fig. 9.3. As suggested earlier, however, the cliff swallow superiority could arise in a number of other ways, such as a general superiority on this type of task. We are currently evaluating this hypothesis further with additional birds and control tasks.

The same line of reasoning that leads to the prediction that cliff swallow calls will be more discriminable than barn swallow calls, can be extended to predict variation in discriminability *within* a species call set. It can be seen in Fig. 9.4 that each bird showed considerable variation in learning speed (sessions to criterion, or STC) across call pairs within a species call set, at least for barn swallow calls. If we express this variation as the range of STC for each bird within each species set, we see that it is large for barn swallow calls (average range 6.6 sessions) and much less for cliff swallow calls (average range 2.6 sessions). We decided to see if performance on a call pair could be predicted by the degree of measured similarity between the two calls. We did this for barn swallow calls

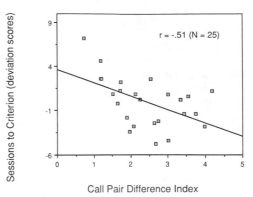

FIG. 9.5. Correlation between call pair difficulty and call pair difference index. The two measures are explained in the text.

only, as there was insufficient variation in our dependent variable (STC) for cliff swallow calls. In the analysis, we modified the dependent variable to account for overall differences among the birds (some birds were faster learners than others) by subtracting each bird's mean STC from its STC on each of the call pairs. With these deviation scores we were able to pool data from all five subjects. Our independent variable, or measure of difference between the two calls in a pair (*difference index*), is similar to the information measure described in the preceding section. For each call, we measured the 4 barn swallow parameters described in Fig. 9.2. We then converted the measurements on each parameter to standard scores (relative to the complete stimulus set). For each call pair, we took the difference between the two values for each parameter, squared the difference, summed these squared differences across the four parameters, and took the square root of the sum. This value represents the Euclidean distance between the two calls on the assumption that the 4 parameters are independent, equally weighted dimensions. While the independence assumption is approximately true (see Table 9.1), the weighting assumption can only be evaluated by perceptual experiments. The obtained correlation between deviation STC and call pair difference index, shown in Fig. 9.5, is moderate but significant ($r = -.51$, $p < .01$). Considering the number of arbitrary assumptions that go into the difference index, this is a relatively strong correlation. As an alternative approach to this problem, and one that is free of assumptions about signal or perception, we are presently replicating our experiment with a second set of animals: if the degree of similarity between the two calls in a pair is a major determinant of discrimination difficulty, we should find a correlation between STC for two animals tested on the same pairs.

IV.   GENERAL DISCUSSION

Signature vs. Perceptual Adaptations

Our results support the hypothesis that selection has acted on signature traits in the colonial cliff swallow. Both sonagram measurements and perceptual judgments by birds of 3 different species indicate that cliff swallow signature calls are more complex and perceptually distinctive than the comparable calls of the closely-related but noncolonial barn swallow. At the same time, we find no evidence for specific perceptual adaptations for discrimination of signature calls in cliff swallows, for our cliff swallows did not find their own calls relatively more discriminable than did the other birds. This negative evidence does not surprise us, for given the highly developed auditory system of passerine birds, it is not obvious why any further specialization should be necessary. We cannot rule out, however, the possibility of a general perceptual adaptation in cliff swallows that permits them to discriminate more readily among both cliff swallow *and* barn swallow calls. Indeed, considering the general similarity of cliff swallow and barn swallow chick calls, it is hard to imagine an adaptation that would affect perception of one but not the other. We are presently collecting data on additional birds and looking at other, more ''neutral'' discriminations, which should allow us to make a fairer evaluation of the general perceptual adaptation hypothesis.

Additional support for the signature adaptation hypothesis comes from two additional sources. First, our earlier measurements of the chick calls of the bank swallows and rough-winged swallows also showed greater information capacity for the colonial species (Beecher, 1982). Second, cliff swallow chicks, but not barn swallow chicks, have conspicuous, individually distinctive facial markings, although we have not yet evaluated their functional significance (Stoddard & Beecher, 1983).

Special Perceptual Mechanisms

There is considerable interest in the idea that animals may possess special perceptual mechanisms for their acoustic communication signals. Generally the term ''special mechanism'' is meant to imply that the mechanism is species-specific and innate. Perhaps the strongest case for such mechanisms comes from studies of song learning in birds. Marler in particular has championed the idea of an innate ''template'' for species-specific song which guides song learning (Marler, 1970; Marler & Peters, 1980). Very few studies, however, have directly investigated such mechanisms. Whether the study uses perceptual experiments or neurophysiological methods, it must answer the following questions.

1. Does the species in question give evidence of special processing mechanisms for its vocal communication signals?

2. Is this a species-specific mechanism, i.e., does the study species show a perceptual advantage for conspecific signals compared to an appropriately-chosen, closely related species? These first two conditions are fulfilled by the experimental design of Fig. 9.3.

3. To what extent does this species difference depend on species-specific developmental histories?

In the simplest case, this question can be addressed by doing the experiment of Fig. 9.3 on both lab-raised and wild-born adults (in some cases it may be possible to simulate the critical features of the species-typical developmental history in the lab, as has been done in song-learning studies).

To date, only three studies using perceptual methods have come close to meeting the conditions for demonstrating special perceptual mechanisms. In our study, we found no conspecific advantage, suggesting no special perceptual adaptations in cliff swallows for their signals. While we did not test subjects with species-typical developmental histories, this omission is not critical in this case since we found no comparative difference in lab-raised birds. Experiments on the perception of "coo" calls by Japanese macaque monkeys reveal a somewhat different pattern of results (Beecher et al., 1979; Heffner & Heffner, 1984; Petersen et al., 1984). These coo calls are highly differentiated in Japanese macaques (Green, 1975). While similar calls are found in other macaque species, it is generally presumed that the communicatory significance of call variants is somewhat different from species to species (unfortunately, there are no field data on vocal signals in these other macaque species). In perceptual experiments, wild-born Japanese macaques show a learning advantage for, and right-ear (left hemisphere) advantage for discriminations among their different coo types, while other macaque species learn these discriminations more slowly and show no ear advantage. Missing in this experiment are lab-raised Japanese macaques and tests of the comparable calls of the control species. Thus, while the observed difference between Japanese macaques and other closely related macaque species suggests a high level of specialization, it is very possible that the observed species difference can be traced to the species-typical developmental history of the wild-born Japanese macaque subjects. Finally, Sinnott (1980) tested the perception of red-winged blackbird and cowbird song by wild-caught adults of both species. Both species showed a learning advantage for conspecific songs, but here we must presume that species-typical experience with conspecific song was critical in this advantage. In conclusion, none of these studies provide evidence for special perceptual mechanisms, at least in the restrictive sense of this term.

Decision Rule Adaptations

As mentioned earlier and summarized in Fig. 9.1, a third possible target of selection for individual recognition is the "decision rule" employed by the receiver in the recognition context. This has not been the focus of this paper, but for completeness we conclude with a few comments on this aspect of the recognition problem. We have some field evidence on differences in parental "decision rules" in bank swallows and rough-winged swallows (Beecher, 1981; Beecher & Beecher, in prep). We have carried out interspecific cross-fostering experiments, where a parent finds its own young plus one heterospecific young in its nest. In this case, the difference between natal and foster young is conspicuous, yet we have found that the colonial bank swallow rejects the heterospecific young while the non-colonial rough-winged swallow accepts them. This difference suggests that parents in the latter species apply the rule "always accept" to young it finds in its nest. In another cross-fostering experiment, we have presented rough-winged swallow parents with a choice between a brood of heterospecific young in their nest, and their own brood in an adjacent nest. In this case, they choose their own young. This finding implies that rough-winged swallow parents can make a discrimination between their own and alien young under some circumstances, at least when the difference to be discriminated is large enough. These studies and others (Shugart, 1977, in press), suggest that the parent's decision rule may vary with the costs and benefits inherent in the test situation and that species with less need for recognition may have more conservative rules (be less likely to reject alien chicks under any circumstances). Thus at least in these cases a change in decision rules or associated behaviors appears to be a factor in the evolution of parental recognition, although it is not sufficient in itself. A second factor, we have shown, is the elaboration of the signature traits of the young. Undoubtedly there are other factors, such as, perhaps, the tendency of parents to play close attention to relevant cues, or to engage in behaviors designed to facilitate recognition, such as searching for young, carefully inspecting dubious young, and the like. Finally, elaboration of the signature traits of the parents is likely as well. For example, reciprocal calling between parents and young is conspicuous in cliff swallows and bank swallows in recognition contexts. Mutual recognition of calls has been demonstrated in both species and preliminary evidence suggests elaboration of the parent call (Beecher, Stoddard, & Loesche, 1985; Sieber, 1985; Stoddard & Beecher, 1983).

ACKNOWLEDGMENTS

We thank B. J. Higgins for heroic efforts in developing the behavioral conditioning procedure. This research was supported by grants from the National Science Foundation.

REFERENCES

Beecher, M. D. (1981). Development of parent-offspring recognition in birds. In R. K. Aslin, J. R. Alberts, & M. R. Petersen (Eds.), *Development of perception* (Vol. 1, pp. 45–66). New York: Academic Press.

Beecher, M. D. (1982). Signature systems and kin recognition. *American Zoologist, 22,* 477–490.

Beecher, M. D. (in press). Signalling systems for individual recognition: An information theory approach. *Animal Behaviour.*

Beecher, M. D., & Beecher, I. M. (in prep). Parent-offspring recognition in the Northern rough-winged swallow.

Beecher, M. D., Beecher, I. M., & Hahn, S. (1981). Parent-offspring recognition in bank swallows. II. Development and acoustic basis. *Animal Behaviour, 29,* 95–101.

Beecher, M. D., Beecher, I. M., & Lumpkin, S. (1981). Parent-offspring recognition in bank swallows. I. Natural history. *Animal Behaviour, 29,* 86–94.

Beecher, M. D., Medvin, M. B., Stoddard, P. K., & Loesche, P. (1986). Acoustic adaptations for parent-offspring recognition in swallows. *Experimental Biology, 45,* 179–193.

Beecher, M. D., Petersen, M. R., Zoloth, S. R., Moody, D. B., & Stebbins, W. C. (1979). Perception of conspecific vocalizations by Japanese macaques: Evidence for selective attention and neural lateralization. *Brain, Behavior and Evolution, 16,* 443–460.

Beecher, M. D., Stoddard, P. K., & Loesche, P. (1985). Recognition of parents' voices by young cliff swallows. *Auk, 102,* 600–605.

Bent, A. C. (1942). Life histories of North American flycatchers, larks, swallows and their allies. *U.S. National Museum Bulletin,* No. 179.

Brown, C. R. (1986). Cliff swallow colonies as information centers. *Science, 234,* 83–85.

Cullen, E. (1957). Adaptations in the kittiwake to cliff nesting. *Ibis, 99,* 275–303.

Emlen, J. T., Jr. (1955). Social behavior in nesting cliff swallows. *Condor, 54,* 177–191.

Green, S. (1975). Communication by a graded vocal system in Japanese macaque monkeys. In J. Rosenblum (Ed.), *Primate behavior* (Vol. 4, pp. 1–102). New York: Academic Press.

Heffner, H. E., & Heffner, R. S. (1984). Temporal lobe lesions and perception of species-specific vocalizations by macaques. *Science, 226,* 75–76.

Jouventin, P. (1982). *Visual and vocal signals in penguins, their evolution and adaptive characters.* Berlin: Verlag Paul Parey.

Loesche, P., Stoddard, P. K., Higgins, B. J., & Beecher, M. D. (in prep). Perception of swallow calls by barn swallows and cliff swallows.

Marler, P. (1970). A comparative approach to vocal learning: Song development in white-crowned sparrows. *Journal of Comparative and Physiological Psychology, 71,* 1–25.

Marler, P., & Peters, S. (1980). Birdsong and speech: evidence for special processing. In P. Eimas (Ed.), *Perspectives on the study of speech.* Hillsdale, NJ: Lawrence Erlbaum Associates.

Medvin, M. B., & Beecher, M. D. (1986). Parent-offspring recognition in the barn swallow (*Hirundo rustica*). *Animal Behaviour, 34,* 1627–1639.

Medvin, M. B., Stoddard, P. K., & Beecher, M. D. (in prep). Information analysis of the calls of cliff swallows and barn swallows.

Petersen, M. R., Beecher, M. D., Zoloth, S. R., Green, S., Marler, P., Moody, D. B., & Stebbins, W. C. (1984). Neural lateralization of vocalizations by Japanese macaques: Communicative significance is more important than acoustic structure. *Behavioral Neuroscience, 98,* 779–790.

Shields, W. M. (1984). Factors affecting nest and site fidelity in Adirondack barn swallows. (*Hirundo rustica*). *Auk, 101,* 780–789.

Shugart, G. W. (1977). The development of chick recognition by adult caspian terns. *Proceedings Colonial Waterbird Group, 1,* 110–117.

Shugart, G. W. (1987). Individual clutch recognition by adult caspian terns. *Animal Behaviour, 35,* 1563–1565.

Sieber, O. J. (1985). Individual recognition of parental calls by bank swallow chicks (Riparia riparia). *Animal Behaviour, 33,* 107–116.

Sinnott, J. M. (1980). Species-specific coding in bird song. *Journal of the Acoustical Society of America, 68,* 494–497.

Snapp, B. D. (1976). Colonial breeding in the barn swallow (*Hirundo rustica*) and its adaptive significance. *Condor, 78,* 471–480.

Stebbins, W. C. (1970). *Animal psychophysics: the design and conduct of sensory experiments.* New York: Appleton-Century-Crofts.

Stoddard, P. K. (1987). Inexpensive solid-state peck key for the operant conditioning of small birds. *Behavior Research Methods, Instruments & Computers, 19,* 446–448.

Stoddard, P. K., & Beecher, M. D. (1983). Parental recognition of offspring in the cliff swallow. *Auk, 100,* 795–799.

Editorial Comments on Ralston and Herman

In this chapter, we turn from animals of the land and air to a highly developed denizen of the sea, the bottlenosed dolphin. Dolphins have long been known for their ability to process acoustic information, and here we learn first about the types of sounds that dolphins produce, and then about how they are sensitive to sound both fundamental psychophysical sense, and then in the perception of complex sounds.

Dolphins produce whistles and burst pulse sounds which are relatively low frequency and are broadcast in all directions simultaneously. They also produce high-frequency signals which are emitted in a highly directed beam. The low frequency sounds are apparently used for communicative purposes while, of course, the high frequency beams are used for echolocation. In general, dolphins hear acutely, as one might imagine. The upper limit for hearing appears to be near 150 khz, and there is an impressive degree of frequency, intensity, and angular resolution.

In experiments with complex sounds, dolphins have demonstrated enormous cognitive skill. There is much evidence for vocal mimicry of both natural and unnatural sounds. In studies of short-term memory capacity, rates of learning have been rapid and sounds can be coded and recalled after delays as long as 120 sec., the longest delay tested. Other memory functions, the coding and recall of lists of sounds for example, and still other higher cognitive tasks such as acoustic concept formation testify further to the remarkable facility of the animal with complex acoustic information. Of perhaps greatest interest, dolphins have been trained to respond to a series of acoustic sounds as if they were words in an artificial language.

This chapter provides but an opening glimpse of the fascinating acoustic world in which dolphins live, but it will lead the reader to rich resources for further study. The dolphin, with its extraordinarily complex brain, offers an exceptionally fertile territory for studies of complex auditory perception.

10 Dolphin Auditory Perception

James V. Ralston
*Kewalo Basin Marine Mammal Laboratory**

Louis M. Herman
Kewalo Basin Marine Mammal Laboratory, and University of Hawaii

INTRODUCTION

The dolphin[1] has been depicted since the days of the ancient Greeks as an acoustically oriented animal. Aristotle noted that these animals squeaked and moaned when taken from their water (Reyesenback de Haan, 1957). The Greek poet-musician Arion was said to have attracted dolphins to his rescue from a mutinous crew by playing a song on a lyre (Bulfinch, 1986). These and other similar stories indicate that humans have been aware of the dolphins' remarkable sound capabilities for some time. Today we know that dolphin vision is also well-developed, which complements the auditory capabilities of these animals (Madsen & Herman, 1980).

Dolphins have evolved highly specialized mechanisms to support sound production and reception (Bullock & Gurevich, 1979; Dormer, 1979; Evans & Maderson, 1973; Lawrence & Schevill, 1956; Mackay, 1980; Morris, 1986; Norris, 1964, 1968, 1969, 1980, 1986; Woods, Ridgway, Carder, & Bullock, 1986). Although the morphology and physiology of the sound production and reception mechanisms are fascinating and sometimes controversial topics, they remain outside the scope of this chapter. Here, we review the functional results of these adaptations on sound production and reception.

---

*now at the Department of Psychology, Indiana University

[1]Aristotle's dolphin was likely *Delphinus delphis*, the common dolphin, found throughout the Mediterranean Sea. In this paper, "dolphin" refers to *Tursiops truncatus*, the bottlenose dolphin. Particular emphasis will be placed on populations found along the east, south, and west coasts of North America.

A correspondence has often been noted between the productive and receptive capacities of a species. By considering dolphin vocalizations as acoustic patterns, we may develop hypotheses about perceptual processing. These hypotheses may then be tested in future experiments to refine an evolving model of audition. In addition, knowledge of the acoustic structure of vocalizations may enhance future attempts to characterize and interface with the dolphins' natural communication system.

I. SOUND PRODUCTION

The sounds produced by the bottlenose dolphin have generally been classified into two broad types: pure-tone whistles and broad-band clicks. The click sounds may be further subdivided into echolocation signals and burst-pulse sounds (Gish, 1979; Herman & Tavolga, 1980; Lang & Smith, 1965; Lilly & Miller, 1961a; Norris, 1969).

Whistles

Whistles are continuous (100–2000 ms duration) in the time domain, have a narrow band of energy, and a number of low-amplitude harmonics. Whistles may be of constant frequency, but are more commonly frequency- and amplitude-modulated. The fundamental frequency of FM whistles are swept between approximately 5 kHz and 15 kHz. The rate of FM may be as great as approximately 10 Hz (personal observation). Rates of amplitude modulation may exceed 500 Hz (Tyack, 1986). Whistles may function as "contact calls," as they are of sufficiently high amplitude (125–140 dB re: 1 μPa/1 m) (Tyack, 1986) and of low enough frequency to propagate in a broad emission pattern for long distances relative to other dolphin sounds (Gish, 1979; Herman & Tavolga, 1980; Lang & Smith, 1965; Norris, 1969).

Dolphin whistles have been almost universally regarded as intraspecies communication signals (Burdin, Reznik, Skornyakov, & Chupakov, 1974; Dreher & Evans, 1964; Evans, 1967; Evans & Dreher, 1962; Gish, 1979; Lang & Smith, 1965; Lilly, 1962; McBride & Hebb, 1948; Schevill & Lawrence, 1956; Wood, 1953). However, the nature of the communication system remains obscure. Part of the difficulty stems from an inability to determine which variations in whistle structure are perceived as meaningful differences by the dolphins, and which are not. Some investigators have attempted to correlate the contour (frequency versus time) of spontaneous whistles to environmental and behavioral events (Dreher, 1966; Dreher & Evans, 1964). Dreher and Evans (1964) observed the behavior of wild dolphins while simultaneously recording their vocalizations with a hydrophone system. They identified 17 whistle contours and tentatively related them to concurrent events. Similarly, Lilly (1963) identified a putative "distress call" in the bottlenose dolphin, the contour of which was reportedly specific to stressful situations (also see Busnel & Dziedzic, 1966 and Dreher & Evans, 1964 for other putative alarm calls). The variability across several reports, however, casts suspicion on the claim of an invariant "distress" whistle contour.

The Caldwells and other investigators have provided statistical evidence for a high degree of stereotypy in the whistle contours of individual dolphins (Caldwell & Caldwell, 1965, 1968, 1971; Caldwell, Caldwell, & Miller, 1973; Tyack, 1986). The Caldwells' analyses of stereotypy were primarily of the number of FM cycles ("loops"), the duration of individual whistles, and presence of frequency transitions. Up to 90% of all whistle contours emitted by bottlenose dolphins may be stereotyped, each "signature whistle" specific to an individual (Caldwell & Caldwell, 1968). Tyack (1986) has suggested that the presence of amplitude modulations may serve a signature function as well. More recently, Gish (1979) has corroborated the existence of signature whistles. Whistles recorded in contexts when dolphins were "searching" for one another were successfully assigned to speaker (dolphin) by a discriminant analysis program.

Dolphins exhibit vocal antiphonic behaviors (Caldwell & Caldwell, 1965, 1968; Gish, 1979; Lang & Smith, 1965; Watkins & Schevill, 1974). When one dolphin vocalizes, other individuals often call in response. Herman and Tavolga (1980) have noted a rough correlation between the gregariousness (in terms of the size of social groups) of odontocete species and the likelihood that the species possesses a whistle sound. These and other data strongly suggest a communicative role for the whistle, and that dolphins may recognize specific whistle patterns. Therefore, a theory of dolphin audition should account for the perception of whistles.

Echolocation Signals

Probably all odontocetes produce clicks, or pulsed sounds (Norris, 1969). Both echolocation clicks and "burst-pulse" sounds are pulsatile signals. Dolphins can *simultaneously* produce whistles and pulsed sounds (Evans & Prescott, 1962; Gish, 1979; Lilly, 1962; Lilly & Miller, 1961a). This capacity may be helpful in executing cooperative behaviors during food gathering, in the case of simultaneous echolocation clicks and whistles (Herman & Tavolga, 1980), or it may carry an additional communicative load, in the case of simultaneous burst-pulse sounds and whistles (Gish, 1979).

In contrast to whistles, echolocation clicks are of short duration (<200 μs), broadband, and are projected in a tightly focused emission beam (Au, Floyd, & Haun, 1978; Au, Penner, & Kadane, 1982; Au, Floyd, Penner, & Murchison, 1974; Diercks, Trochta, Greenlaw, & Evans, 1971; Diercks, Trochta, & Evans, 1973; Evans, 1973). In the time domain, individual echolocation pulses often appear as a few pressure oscillations with a rapid rise-fall envelope. Although spectral analysis reveals a wideband structure for individual clicks, there is usually a distinct peak in energy about 25 kHz (Diercks et al., 1971; Evans, 1973). Sound pressure levels been reported for bottlenose dolphins as great as 228.6 dB re: 1 μPa/1 m (Au et al., 1974). Echolocation clicks are not emitted in isolation, but in a series, or train. The spectral structure of individual clicks is fairly constant within a train, except near the beginning and end of the train, where peak frequency and amplitude tend to fluctuate (Au et al., 1982). The interaction between successive broad-band clicks and their corresponding echoes may produce an interference pattern, or "rippled" frequency-domain spectra, provided the temporal interval between the successive sounds is not excessively large (Au & Hammer, 1980; Floyd, 1980; Johnson & Titlebaum, 1976).

Burst-Pulse Sounds

Burst-pulse sounds appear to be distinct in function from echolocation signals, but similar in physical characteristics. Burst-pulse sounds are trains of clicks that are emitted at relatively high repetition rates. Although little data are available, there is reason to believe the individual clicks may have much lower peak frequencies than echolocation clicks (Watkins, 1967). The perceptual quality (for humans) of these sounds has led investigators to label them qualitatively as "squawks," "quacks," "blats," "barks," "mewings," and "pops" (Caldwell & Caldwell, 1967, 1968; Caldwell, Haugen, & Caldwell, 1962; Evans & Prescott, 1962; Lilly & Miller, 1961a; Wood, 1953). Burst-pulse sounds have spectral energy from less than 250 Hz up to nearly 16 kHz, most energy concentrated in a band below 8 kHz. The pulse-train rate may vary from less than 100 Hz to greater than 500 Hz (Lilly, 1965; Lilly, Miller, & Truby, 1968). The duration of recorded burst-pulse sounds varies from less than 100 ms to greater than 250 ms (Caldwell & Caldwell, 1967; Evans & Prescott, 1962). Burst-pulse sounds are the most similar in structure and percept to human speech sounds, particularly vowels. Due to their banded structure in spectrographic representations, they superficially appear to possess a formant (resonance) structure similar to human voiced segments.

The burst-pulse sounds are generally regarded as social signals with possible communicative significance. They have been recorded in a variety of social contexts and are often projected into the air, as well as underwater (Caldwell & Caldwell, 1967; Evans & Prescott, 1962; Herman & Tavolga, 1980). In contrast to the echolocation clicks, burst-pulse sounds are usually emitted in what have been judged as highly emotional contexts, such as aggressive episodes, before copulatory sequences, and concurrent with the introduction of novel or unexpected environmental objects or events (Caldwell & Caldwell, 1967; Lilly & Miller, 1961a). Burst-pulse sounds have sometimes been recorded in antiphonic exchanges (Gish, 1979; Watkins & Schevill, 1974). The fine structure of these signals are largely unexplored.

Non-vocal sounds.   Dolphins may produce other nonvocal acoustic signals in the wild, including sounds produced by the slapping of body parts on the surface of the water and "jawclaps," or percussive sounds accompanying the rapid closure of the beak (Herman & Tavolga, 1980; McBride & Hebb, 1948; Wood, 1953; Wursig & Wursig, 1980). The jaw clap is generally thought to be a sign of aggression. Leaps, body slaps (on the surface of the water), and other aerial behaviors appear to function as social signals in many cetacean species (Norris & Dohl, 1980a, 1980b; Wursig, 1986; Wursig & Wursig, 1979, 1980). In contrast to the narrow echolocation beam, jumps and leaps generate low-frequency noise of limited duration (<1 s) which propagages omnidirectionally less than one kilometer (Norris & Dohl, 1980a; Wursig & Wursig, 1980).

Conclusion.   In summary, dolphins vocally produce narrow-band whistles and broad-band clicks. Whistles and burst-pulse sounds are of relatively low frequency and are broadcast omnidirectionally. In contrast, echolocation signals are of high frequency and are broadcast in a focused beam. Whistles are amplitude- and frequency-modulated at relatively rapid rates. Pulsed sounds may be modulated to produce a wide range of sounds, including burst-pulse sounds and echolocation clicks. Burst-pulse sounds are similar in structure and function to human speech sounds. Whistles and burst-pulse sounds appear to be primarily communicative, whereas echolocation signals are reflected off underwater objects to derive information about target structure and location. There is also circumstantial evidence that dolphins may possess a "stun beam" which is an evolved form of the echolocation beam (Hult, 1982; Norris & Mohl, 1983). Finally, there are several nonvocal sounds which may convey important information between dolphins. The remainder of this chapter discusses the dolphin's perception of these and other sounds in an attempt to catalog their underlying auditory cues. Investigations of dolphin hearing suggest that perceptual processes may have evolved specifically to detect and recognize those signals which they generate. Increased knowledge about dolphin audition may yield insights into the nature of their cognitive world.

II. AUDITORY PERCEPTION

Auditory perception in the bottlenose dolphin may be divided into two major categories, passive hearing, which probably operates on energy below 20 kHz and echolocation, or active hearing, which probably operates on energy up to 100 kHz. Although these form logically distinct categories, the mechanisms of passive hearing are of course engaged during echoranging. Our emphasis here is on passive hearing. Passive hearing experiments have examined both basic psychophysics and the perception of complex stimuli. Psychophysical studies have investigated the threshold perception of fundamental sound parameters (frequency, amplitude, duration) of isolated pure tones. Other studies have examined the perception of complex sounds that defy simple description, such as signature whistles, or sounds that clearly constitute strings or sequences, such as in imposed language studies (Herman, Richards, & Wolz, 1984).

Basic Psychophysics

Pure-tone thresholds.   Although there have been anecdotal accounts of the dolphin's sensitivity to sounds for some time (Fraser, 1947), only recently have controlled experiments been conducted.

Earlier experiments by Kellogg and Kohler (1952) and Kellogg (1953) first assessed the unconditioned response of captive bottlenose dolphins and spotted dolphins (*Stenella plagiodon*) to sounds ranging from 100 Hz to 200 kHz. The dolphins reliably responded to frequencies between 50 and 80 kHz, but did not respond to higher frequencies. Because the power output of the system was variable above 10 kHz, it was not possible to obtain threshold data.

At nearly the same time as Kellogg was conducting his initial investigations, Schevill and Lawrence (1953a, 1953b) were conducting similar studies with an isolated bottlenose dolphin trained on an operant task. The dolphin almost always responded on trials with sounds ranging from 150 Hz to 120 kHz, responded on about half the trials with sounds near 126 kHz, and on only about 13% of the trials with sounds near 151–153 kHz. Although the sound level of the test sounds was unpredictably variable and the position of the listening dolphin was not fixed, Schevill and Lawrence estimated an upper hearing limit of 126 kHz.

The first well-controlled threshold experiment with a bottlenose dolphin was conducted by C. S. Johnson (1967a). Sufficient data were collected to generate a complete audiometric curve over the complete range of hearing. The results were generally consistent with those of Schevill and Lawrence, indicating sensitivity to an exceptionally broad range of signals, from 75 Hz to 150 kHz. The greatest sensitivity was near 65 kHz (-59.2 dB re: 1 μbar), in a band of heightened sensitivity from 20 to 100 kHz. The roll-off in sensitivity above 65 kHz was quite rapid, nearly 495 dB per octave (C. S. Johnson, 1986). Figure 10.1 displays audiograms from a number of odontocetes.

Frequency perception.   Peripheral auditory processing has been conceptualized as a bank of overlapping band-pass filters, or "critical bands" (Fletcher, 1940; Scharf, 1970). The narrower the bandwidth of these filters ("critical bandwidth"), the finer the possible frequency analysis. Several experiments have been conducted with dolphins in order to better understand the properties of these filters, such as their number, bandwidths, and shapes (Au & Moore, 1983; C. S. Johnson, 1968a, 1968b, 1971; Moore & Au, 1982).

C. S. Johnson (1971) collected thresholds for pure tones in the presence of a

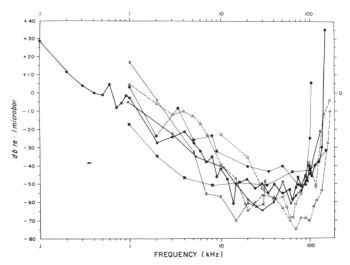

FIG.10.1.   Odontocete auditory sensitivity. Behavioral studies are indicated by a solid line and electrophysiological studies by a broken line.
Symbols: ✱ - *D. leucas* (composite of two animals, White et al., 1978);
✦ - *I. geoffrensis* (Jacobs & Hall, 1972); x - *O. orca* (Hall & Johnson,
1972); ■ - *P. phocoena* (Anderson, 1971); o - *S. coeruleoalba* (Bullock
et al., 1968); △ - *T. gilli* (Bullock et al., 1968); ● - *T. truncatus* (Johnson,
1967a). Reprinted with permission from Popper (1980a).

second, masking tone of 70 kHz. Data were collected for 40 dB and 80 dB SL
masking levels. The obtained thresholds were qualitatively similar to human data
(Egan & Hake, 1950; Wegel & Lane, 1924):

(a) there was greater masking of signals above the masking frequency than
below ("upward spread of masking");

(b) masking generally decreased with increasing frequency difference between signal and masker; and

(c) there was a local decrease in masking for test tones near the masker. The
results suggest that the dolphin's auditory system acts as a bank of filters with
asymmetrically shaped skirts in the frequency domain, much like that of the
human auditory system (Green, 1976; Scharf, 1970).

C. S. Johnson (1968a, 1968b) conducted two threshold studies which gave
estimates of critical bandwidths. The first (C. S. Johnson, 1968a) was a threshold task with tones of variable duration. For each test frequency, a time constant
was determined, which was the point at which thresholds stopped decreasing
with increasing stimulus duration. The resulting measurements were similar to
those for human subjects for those test frequencies also used with human subjects

(Hamilton, 1957; Plomp & Bouman, 1959). Computations using the time constants produced critical bandwidth estimates of 3.5 kHz and 8 kHz for 20 kHz and 40 kHz center frequencies, respectively.

In a masked threshold experiment, C. S. Johnson (1968b) determined critical ratios in a bottlenose dolphin for 15 frequencies from 5 to 100 kHz. The critical ratio was first proposed by Fletcher (1940) as an index of critical bandwidth. The value, expressed in dB, is defined as the ratio of the signal power to noise spectrum level at masked threshold. Johnson's computed critical bandwidths were equal to about 800 Hz at 10 kHz and were near 10 kHz at 100 kHz. Johnson estimated that dolphins have about 40 critical bands, whereas humans have approximately 24 (Zwicker, 1961).

More recently, Moore and Au (1982) and Au and Moore (1983) have measured critical ratios and bandwidths in a bottlenose dolphin at a number of test frequencies. Whereas Johnson assumed that the relationship between the critical ratio and critical band was constant at a factor of 2.5 (Scharf, 1970), Au and Moore (1983) empirically determined that the relationship is more complex, changing from a factor of 10 at 30 kHz to a factor of 1 at 120 kHz. The results indicate that the critical ratio may not be a reliable index of critical bandwidth for dolphin audition, consistent with previous suspicions and data for other species (Green, 1976; Seaton & Trahiotis, 1975). However, the data of Moore and Au (1982) are in substantial agreement with that of C. S. Johnson (1968a, 1968b), indicating critical bandwidths near 1 kHz at a center frequency of 10 kHz and approximately 10 kHz at a center frequency of 100 kHz. Figure 10.2 presents estimated critical bandwidths for both humans and bottlenose dolphins.

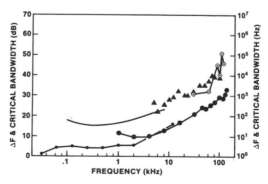

FIG. 10.2. Frequency sensitivity. The solid triangles are the critical ratios measured by Johnson (1968a), the circle points connected by a straight line are the critical ratios measured by Moore and Au (1982), and the large solid circles connected by a straight line are the differential discrimination data from Thompson and Herman (1975). The solid line depicts the critical ratios for humans by French and Steinberg (1947) and Hawkens and Stevens (1950), and the small solid dots connected by a straight line are the differential pitch sensitivity measurements made on human subjects by Shower and Biddulph (1931). Reprinted with permission from Johnson (1986).

For humans, relative frequency discrimination limens, or Weber fractions ($\Delta f/f$), are closely related to critical bandwidth—roughly 20 times smaller (Zwicker, Flottrop, & Stevens, 1957). This appears to be true as well for the bottlenose dolphin (C. S. Johnson, 1986). Jacobs (1972) and Herman and Arbeit (1972) independently collected frequency discrimination data from adult bottlenose dolphins, both with modified method of limits procedures combined with frequency-modulation detection tasks. Jacobs (1972) found that the range of greatest sensitivity was between 5 and 20 kHz, with Weber fractions between .002 and .004. Sensitivity dropped off by more than a factor of two for frequencies above 20 kHz and below 5 kHz. Jacobs concluded the region of greatest sensitivity to frequency differences lay below the region of peak absolute sensitivity. However, Jacobs' data were incomplete, as the subject died after only one-third of the planned experiment.

Herman and Arbeit (1972) and, later, Thompson and Herman (1975) collected frequency discrimination limens from a single adult bottlenose dolphin. In the first experiment of Herman and Arbeit (1972), discrimination thresholds were lower with practice, with FM stimuli of 2 Hz (versus 1 Hz) modulation, and with the highest tested center frequencies (27 and 36 kHz). The smallest Weber fractions were found between 6 and 36 kHz and were near .001 to .002.

In a second experiment, the same methodology was used with an extended set of higher frequencies. All FM stimuli were modulated at 2 Hz. Weber fractions of .002 to .004 were obtained for 36 and 50 kHz stimuli, and .011 for 70 kHz. The finding of relatively low thresholds at 50 kHz stands in contrast to the findings of Jacobs, and suggests that sensitivity to frequency differences may correspond more closely to absolute sensitivity. The lower thresholds for 2 Hz FM is consistent with human data (Shower & Biddulph, 1931). Since no FM frequencies greater than 2 Hz have been tested in this procedure with dolphins, it is entirely possible that dolphins are more sensitive to even higher rates (however, see Herman & Arbeit, 1973).

Thompson and Herman (1975) tested 14 center frequencies from 1 to 140 kHz in a modulation detection task. The results were consistent with Herman and Arbeit (1972) and Jacobs (1972) below 20 kHz, but were divergent from Jacobs' data at higher frequencies. Whereas Jacobs found a rapid decrease in sensitivity from 20 to 90 kHz (with associated mean Weber fractions of .004 and .011, respectively), Thompson and Herman reported a somewhat less precipitous drop over the same range (Weber fractions of approximately .003 and .006, respectively), and found a rapid roll-off only above 100 kHz. Their minimum Weber fractions were again near .002 and .004 over the most sensitive range of hearing. No responses were obtained for stimuli with 140 kHz center frequency. Figure 10.2 presents frequency discrimination limens for dolphins and human subjects.

Intensity perception.   Relatively few studies have directly examined the dolphin's sensitivity to above-threshold changes in sound level (Popper, 1980b), and much relevant data come from studies primarily concerned with other issues.

Not only would intensity discrimination be useful in echolocation, where presumably the loudness within narrow frequency bands might give clues to target distance, shape, size, and composition (Evans, 1973; Evans & Prescott, 1962; Norris, 1969; Thompson & Herman, 1975), but amplitude modulation may be meaningful in social signals as well (Gish, 1979; Lilly & Miller, 1961a, 1961b; Tyack, 1986).

At least two studies of amplitude discrimination have been conducted in Soviet laboratories. In one, a Black Sea dolphin was trained to judge whether amplitude modulation was present in a 30 s duration broadband noise. The obtained difference threshold was for 4–7% modulation (Burdin, Markov, Reznik, Skornyakov, & Chupakov, 1973). In a second study, two dolphins were trained to choose the louder of two trains of synthetic echolocation clicks. The observed difference limen decreased with increasing sensation level of the stimuli, and was near 1 dB for the highest tested sensation level, 45 dB (Vel'min & Dubrovskii, 1978).

Evans (1973) examined discrimination performance in an echolocation task by a bottlenose dolphin, and a boutu (*Inia geoffrensis*). The targets were 18-cm-long cork-neoprene cylinders, which varied in radius. The changes in radius effected 1 dB increments across stimuli. On each trial, a -19 dB (re: 1 μbar) standard was paired with a comparison stimulus. The bottlenose dolphin performed above chance on trials with the smallest difference, less than 1 dB.

C. S. Johnson (1971) derived estimates of amplitude sensitivity from two-tone masking data. In particular, Johnson used data for test signals close in frequency to the masker at 70 kHz, which presumably gave rise to beats. The estimated limens were near 1 dB for the 80 dB masker, and 2 dB for the 40 dB masker. The results are certainly preliminary, as they are based on a limited number of data, but are in general agreement with other data.

Temporal perception.   Estimates of duration may underlay passive and active sonar. Since dolphins emit an echo click only after the previous return has arrived, the interval between the leading edges of the outgoing pulse and the return may yield range information (Au, 1980; Murchison, 1980a, 1980b; Norris, 1969; Norris, Evans, & Turner, 1967). In addition, duration information may be a distinctive cue in the perception of whistle signals or other environmental sounds.

Yunker and Herman (1974) employed 9 or 25 kHz pure tone standards of 300, 600, or 1200 ms duration with an adult dolphin in a discrimination task. The estimated Weber fractions were not influenced by frequency for the dolphin and were between .06 and .08. The observed temporal resolutions would allow resolutions of target distances to an accuracy of 6–8%, for targets at moderate to large distances. However, the perception of range in echolocation may entail the estimation of "empty" intervals. Therefore, the data of Yunker and Herman may be more appropriately applied to the perception of "filled" intervals, such as whistle, burst-pulse, and other environmental sounds.

Time-separation putch (TSP) has also been proposed as an alternative cue for interval estimation, and hence, range estimation (Floyd, 1980; R. A. Johnson, 1980; Nordmark, 1960, 1970). For example, when two wide-band pulses are presented to humans in rapid succession, a tone is perceived whose pitch is inversely related to the interpulse interval. Similarly, some central mechanism may operate during echo-ranging, sensing the temporal distance between successive pulses, or the spectral distance between interference ripples, and may produce a corresponding TSP. Many experiments have employed trains of pulse pairs as models of natural outgoing clicks and returning echoes (Caine, 1976; R. A. Johnson, 1977, 1980). The obtained limens of Caine (1976) were much larger than those observed in actual echolocation tasks with comparable ranges. Murchison (1980a, 1980b) suggested that the performance of Caine's subject may have been degraded by the reverberant tank environment. In contrast, R. A. Johnson (1977, 1980) reported data from human subjects listening to trains of pulse pairs with intrapair delays from 1 to 10 ms. The results were similar in both form and magnitude to those from Murchison's dolphin subject.

However, a separate line of research initiated in Soviet laboratories calls into question the use of TSP cues in range determination. Vel'min and Dubrovskii (1975, 1976, 1978) conducted several experiments providing converging evidence suggesting a "critical interval" defining (a) the lower limit of interpulse separation yielding reliable temporal resolution for successive, *uncorrelated* signals, and (b) the upper limit of interpulse separation between successive, *correlated* signals yielding TSP percepts. Their estimates, along with other more recent data (Au & Moore, 1986; Moore, Hall, Friedl, & Nichtigall, 1984; Zanin & Zaslavskii, 1977) indicate that the critical interval is 250–300 μs.

Zanin and Zaslavskii (1977) tested human and dolphin subjects on an interpulse interval discrimination task, similar to other experiments by Vel'min and Dubrovskii (1976) and Caine (1976), but with an extended range of interpulse delays (ca. 50–30000 μs). In terms of difference limens, both human and dolphin subjects exhibited functions which appear as Weber functions with a pronounced, superimposed peak. For the dolphin subject, there were small values ($\Delta t/t = 0.1$) from the smallest delays to 200 μs, increases to a peak ($\Delta t/t = 0.4$) at 300 μs, a decline to about 500 μs ($\Delta t/t = 0.1$), and monotonically increasing values with further increases in pulse delays. The function for human subjects was similar in form over the tested range (1000–20000 μs), but the "superimposed" peak was near 6000 μs. Human subjects reported that they judged the stimuli on the basis of spectral color or pitch (TSP) for delays up to 5000 μs, above which the stimuli were perceived as discrete events and interval was judged in terms of temporal attributes. If we assume that there were analogous percepts in the dolphin, then we may conclude that the dolphin judged the delays on the basis of pitch up to about 300 μs, after which judgments were based on temporal percepts.

If dolphins perceive TSP for delays shorter than 300 μs, then it is doubtful that they play a role in range estimation. C. S. Johnson (1980) has noted that the shortest possible two-way path for a dolphin echolocation pulse would yield a travel time of approximately 500 μs, greater than the putative limit for TSP. Thus, it appears as though range perception may be dependent upon estimation of intervals in the time domain.

The critical interval concept has been corroborated by a recent masking study using masking signals uncorrelated with preceding signals (Moore et al., 1984). An echolocating bottlenose dolphin was first trained to judge whether or not an aluminum cylinder was present. Masking noise was then presented at various lagging delays relative to the dolphin's own echo returns. Using a modified method of constant stimuli, the interpolated detection threshold occurred with the masker lagging the echo by 265 μs. Moore et al. concluded that their results confirmed the critical interval as a limit of temporal resolution, and also that the unexpectedly high performance previously observed for short masking delays were probably due to perceived TSP components. They noted that the predicted TSPs corresponding to 11–125 μs delays (90–8 kHz) are well within the dolphin's hearing range. They concluded that TSP probably is not involved in range determination, but more likely underlies the perception of target attributes conveyed in secondary echoes, such as size, internal structure, and material composition.

Differences in the reported data of Zanin and Zaslavskii (1977) on one hand, and of Caine (1976), Murchison (1980a, 1980b), and R. A. Johnson (1977, 1980) on the other hand, are most perplexing. The difference limens obtained by Caine (1976) are generally much larger than those of other investigators. The close correspondence between dolphin (Murchison, 1980b) and human (R. A. Johnson, 1977) is also at variance with Zanin and Zaslavskii (1977). It is possible that, while Johnson's and Murchison's psychometric functions are similar in form, that the echolocating dolphin was judging temporal delays and that the human subjects were judging TSP cues. Future research should try to rectify these disparate results.

Binaural perception. An important piece of information about any sound source, be it a conspecific or an ensonified target, is its spatial location relative to the listening dolphin. In a series of experiments, Renaud and Popper (1975) trained a bottlenose dolphin to discriminate which of two closely spaced underwater speakers projected a sound. They determined the minimum audible angle (MAA), the smallest angle of separation for which there was reliably accurate performance, as a function of a number of experimental manipulations. The stimuli were trains of either pulsed tones or 35 μs clicks with peak energy near 63 kHz.

MAAs for pulsed tones varied only slightly as a function of center frequency. For 0° azimuth, MAAs were 2° to 3° for stimuli from 20 to 80 kHz, and somewhat higher for 6, 10, and 90 kHz pulses. MAAs were not significantly influenced by the various manipulations of the pulsed stimuli. However, MAAs were approximately 1.5° for azimuths of 15° and 345°, and near 5° for 30° and

330° azimuth. This trend is radically different from other terrestrial animals, including humans, whose MAAs are always smallest for 0° azimuth (Erulkar, 1972; Mills, 1958). That localization is best for slightly off-center sounds supports the "jaw-hearing" hypothesis (Norris, 1964, 1968, 1969, 1986). MAAs were .7°–.8° for trains of 35 μs clicks, indicating enhanced sensitivity to short-duration, rapid rise-time stimuli. This finding is consistent with those of electrophysiological experiments which have found the largest collicular evoked potentials pulsed stimuli with very rapid rise-times (Bullock et al., 1968; Bullock & Ridgway, 1972). Surprisingly, MAAs were nearly the same along the horizontal and vertical meridians, again in contrast to humans (Mills, 1958).

The shape of the receiving beam pattern (masking functions), and the derivative receiving directivity index (DI), are measures of how resistant the auditory system is to unwanted background noise, particularly noise arriving from directions away from the long axis of the echolocation beam (Urick, 1975). The shape of the receiving beam is a fundamental property of the auditory system which also influences spatial localization (Au & Moore, 1984). The receiving beam pattern is usually measured by presenting signal and masking stimuli at various angular separations, and examining the resulting masking functions (see Zaytseva, 1978).

Au and Moore (1984) mapped the horizontal and vertical receiving beam patterns with the subject of Renaud and Popper (1975). They collected thresholds for pure tones embedded in wideband masking noise as a function of spatial separation of the signal and masker. The results indicated maximum sensitivity for signals in front of the dolphin, 5° to 10° above the plane defined by the teeth. The beam patterns were tightly focused: the 3 dB vertical beamwidths were 30.4°, 22.7°, and 17.0°, respectively, for signal frequencies of 30, 60, and 120 kHz. Similarly, the 3 dB horizontal beamwidths were 59.1°, 32°, and 13.7°, respectively. The beamwidths were only slightly larger than those of outgoing echolocation clicks (Au et al., 1974; Au, Moore, & Pawloski, 1986). Although the horizontal beam patterns were symmetric about the longitudinal axis of the dolphin, the vertical beam pattern was asymmetric in that noise from below the head was a much more potent masker than noise from above the head. This asymmetry is again consistent with jaw hearing, which predicts shadowing of sounds from above the head.

Conclusion. Dolphin audiograms are similar in form and in minimum detectable sound level to human data, but with peak sensitivity nearly two orders of magnitude above that of humans and an upper hearing limit near 150 kHz. The sensitivity to a broad spectrum of sounds coincides with the broad-band production of sounds, from the low frequencies of the burst-pulse sounds, to the high frequencies present in echolocation pulses and whistle harmonics. Therefore, it appears that much of the acoustic energy vocally produced by dolphins may also be detected.

Masking and discrimination data indicate an impressive degree of frequency resolution and probably a large number of functional critical bands, or processing channels. The smallest Weber fractions for bottlenose dolphins are somewhat smaller than those for humans and probably arise from adaptations at the basilar membrane and acoustic nerve (Wever, McCormick, Palin, & Ridgway, 1971a, 1971b, 1971c).

Dolphins are very sensitive to small changes in intensity, and may operate over a large dynamic range. The difference thresholds reported by Evans (1973), C. S. Johnson (1971), and Vel'min and Dubrovskii (1978) were similar in magnitude (approximately 1 dB) to those for comparable frequency ranges for humans (Pollack, 1954).

Studies employing either tonal or click stimuli have found very fine temporal resolution. In addition, directional hearing studies reveal an acute localization sense and a resistance to masking noise even a few degrees from the main axis of the echolocation beam. The dolphin's keen temporal and spatial resolution may have evolved as a responses to ambient noise and reverberation (Grinnell, 1967; Moore et al., 1984).

Perception of Suprathreshold Sound Patterns

The psychophysical results reviewed above represent the limits of perception of simple sounds under favorable listening conditions. Empirically derived difference limens help to estimate the basic "digitization" units of an auditory code which may be submitted to further central processing. Models of dolphin auditory perception should incorporate these "front-end" processing abilities and constraints, such as peripheral filtering, as have recent models of dolphin echolocation (Altes, 1980), human vision (Marr, 1982), and human speech processing (Pisoni & Sawusch, 1975). However, the listening conditions that confront the active dolphin are most likely suboptimal, and the signals themselves may be composed of multiple dimensions.

There are many environmental and social sounds that wild dolphins may recognize, and which may convey important information to dolphins. These include sounds associated with aerial behaviors, such as leaps, and body slaps on the surface of the water, the low-frequency percussive sound associated with jaw-claps, the sounds associated with specific boats, and the sounds of prey (see Wood, 1973, and Norris, 1974 for anecdotes).

Studies employing relatively complex and/or natural stimuli have typically examined recognition of isolated discrete sounds or of serial patterns of sound (Batteau & Markey, 1968; Caldwell, Hall, & Caldwell, 1971a, 1971b; Herman & Arbeit, 1973; Thompson & Herman, 1977). The distinction between discrete and serial patterns is arbitrary, but is useful as an organizational principle. Discrete sounds in this context refers to those sounds that have largely static properties throughout their duration. Rather than exploring limits of discrimination, these experiments have emphasized recognition of patterns sampled from large sets of presumably distinctive signals. However, valuable information regarding dolphin audition may be derived from this work.

Perception of discrete sounds. In a series of investigations of discrimination learning and auditory short-term memory, Herman and his associates have employed a variety of discrete, complex sounds as experimental stimuli (Herman, 1975; Herman & Arbeit, 1973; Herman & Gordon, 1974; Herman & Thompson, 1982; Thompson, 1976; Thompson & Herman, 1977). The sounds were all derived from a basic set of components (CF, FM, AM), and each of the components could occur with any of a range of center frequencies and modulation rates. A sound was composed of one of the component sounds by itself, or of one of the components combined with a CF component. The center frequencies of all components ranged from 1 to 42 kHz, and the rate of both FM and AM modulation ranged from 1 to 40 Hz with equal duty cycles. The duration of each discrete sound varied according to the experiment, but was generally no more than 2.5 s.

An adult dolphin was successfully trained on auditory discriminations in both simple discrimination and matching tasks (Herman & Arbeit, 1973; Herman & Gordon, 1974) with the same types of stimuli. Rates of learning were rapid, and performance was generally high for most stimulus pairs. Some pairs were discriminated better than others, possibly due to perceptual factors. Herman and Arbeit (1973) found that pairs of stimuli with pulse rates (AM) from 1 to 7 Hz, and pairs with center frequency differences were associated with better performance. Performance was also better with greater numbers of differing acoustic dimensions between members of the stimulus pairs, implying the integration of cue information. The results suggest that with these novel stimuli, perceived pitch of the components may have been highly salient or heavily weighted in perceptual judgments.

Similar, distinctive stimuli were constructed for subsequent memory studies (Herman, 1975; Herman & Gordon, 1974; Thompson & Herman, 1977). In those experiments, the subject remembered individual sounds for at least 120 s, the longest delay tested (Herman & Gordon, 1974). Memory for individual sounds within a list of sounds was most highly influenced by position in the list. There was a strong recency effect, in that sounds at the end of the list were remembered almost perfectly, and earlier sounds remembered less well. Performance was still above chance (50% correct) for the second or third items of 6-item or 8-item lists (Herman, 1980, Fig. 8.8; Thompson & Herman, 1977). The data were similar in form and magnitude to that from human studies (Waugh & Norman, 1965), and indicate a long-lasting, high-fidelity acoustic memory.

There have been two receptive language experiments in which bottlenose dolphins were trained to recognize isolated sounds which denoted either chains of actions (Batteau & Markey, 1968), or individual objects, events, or qualifiers (Herman, 1980; Herman, Richards, & Wolz, 1984). Details of the sounds employed by Batteau and Markey are sketchy, but they appear to have been constant-amplitude sinusoids (transposed to the dolphins' range of best hearing) which tracked the center frequency of some component, such as the first formant, of trainers' spoken imperative commands. One subject reached a level of 85% correct responses in recognizing the contours of 12–13 isolated sounds and responding appropriately. Unfortunately, there is little description of the whistle patterns and no auditory analysis of performance (i.e., confusions) was conducted.

In a similar vein, Herman et al. (1984) designed a set of distinctive sound elements which served as acoustic "words" in an artificial language. An adult dolphin was trained to recognize sequences of these sounds as sentences in an imperative language. The sounds of the language were either unmodulated sine-wave, triangle-wave, or square-wave signals, or these same signals modulated by either sinewave, triangle-wave, or square-wave functions. Center frequencies ranged between 1 and 40 kHz and modulation rates varied from unmodulated to 50 Hz. Sounds were between .5 and 1.5 s in duration. Figure 10.3 displays schematic spectrograms of a subset of sound symbols. In formal tests with a blind observer, the averaged word-level performance for nouns and actions in a

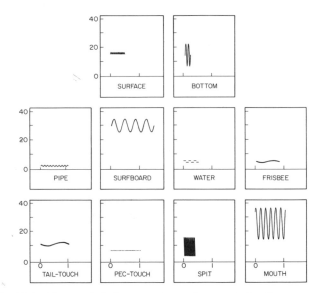

FIG. 10.3. The modulation waveform characteristics (frequency versus time plots) of selected sounds of an acoustic language. Frequency (0–40 kHz) is on the vertical axis and time in seconds on the horizontal axis. The sounds illustrated in the top row are the acoustic signals for the modifiers SURFACE and BOTTOM; the second row shows the sounds for the objects PIPE, SURFBOARD, WATER, and FRISBEE: the final row illustrates sounds for the actions TAIL-TOUCH, PEC-TOUCH, SPIT, and MOUTH. Reprinted with permission from Herman, Richards, and Wolz (1984).

variety of novel sentences was nearly 90% correct, far above that predicted by chance. Analyses of the data were in terms of semantic confusions, but there did not appear to be acoustic confusions.

Perception of the human voice.   The human voice is an acoustically rich and extensively studied signal, and its structure has been described elsewhere (Fant, 1960; Jakobson, Fant, & Halle, 1963; Peterson & Barney, 1952). Although the frequency band between approximately 1 kHz and 4 kHz carries most phonetic information, some distinctive information may occur above 4 kHz, particularly for some fricatives (French & Steinburg, 1947; Miller & Nicely, 1955).

Abundant anecdotal or circumstantial information exists suggesting recognition of human speech sounds by nonhumans. Accurate mimicry of a variety of speech sounds, such as that by the African grey parrot, *Psittacus erithacus* (Pepperberg, 1986), the beluga whale, *Delphinapterus leucas* (Ridgway, Carder, & Jeffries, 1985), and the bottlenose dolphin (Caldwell & Caldwell, 1972) implies a preceding discrimination (see section on vocal mimicry). However, only recently have any species been subjected to rigorous training and controlled testing. Nonhuman species that have demonstrated an ability to discriminate speech sounds include the domestic dog, *Canis familiaris* (Warden & Warner, 1928), the pigmy chimpanzee, *Pan paniscus* (Savage-Rumbaugh et al., 1986), the chinchilla, *Chinchilla laniger* (Kuhl & Miller, 1975, 1978), macaque monkeys, *Macaca fuscata* and *Macaca hemistrina* (Kuhl & Padden, 1983), and the Japanese quail, *Coturnix coturnix* (Kluender & Diehl, 1986). These studies have demonstrated that specialized, species-specific processes are not necessary for recognition of acoustic-phonetic segments (Kuhl, 1986; Kuhl & Miller, 1978).

In contrast to other species, relatively little formal research has been conducted on the dolphin's ability to recognize human speech sounds. However, there have been several informal attempts as part of language training programs. Lilly (1967, 1978) reported anecdotal accounts of dolphins recognizing spoken words in sentences, but never conducted controlled experiments. Informal training on speech recognition was conducted with an adult dolphin at KBMML (unpublished data) with stimuli projected through an underwater hydrophone and, at times, with stimuli spoken in-air by trainers. A number of word pairs were contrasted (i.e., "pec" versus "tail"), but none were successfully discriminated after many training sessions. The difficulty the subject encountered may have been related more to prior language training than to the subjective discriminability of the sounds.

Finally, the Dolphin Research Center at Grassy Key, Florida, housed an adult bottlenose dolphin that reportedly recognized 15 spoken English words and 27 spoken commands (Philip Morris Magazine, Winter, 1987). Previously, one of us (LH) observed the dolphin responding accurately to four different spoken commands, given by a trainer sitting on a dock next to the dolphin. Herman then conducted an informal test for social cues. The trainer was removed from dock-side, placed approximately 4.5 m away with his back to the dolphin. The trainer spoke into a microphone leading to an in-air speaker located at dockside. The dolphin responded to the four sounds correctly, indicating that he was under control of the human speech sounds.

Perception of conspecific vocalizations. Recognition of conspecific vocal signals is a prerequisite for their use in a native communication system. There are several anecdotes and data indicating potential vocal communication in the wild (Dreher & Evans, 1964; Evans & Dreher, 1962; Norris & Dohl, 1980a, 1980b; Watkins & Schevill, 1974; Wursig & Wursig, 1980). Although they provided no behavioral data, Norris and Dohl (1980a) noted that the whistles of resident Hawaiian spinner dolphins within a bay project outside the bay, and may function as a graded "no vacancy" sign to newcomers.

Several investigators have described listening behavior and "call and response," or antiphony in dolphins (Lilly & Miller, 1961b). In a study of five common dolphins (*Delphinus delphis*), Caldwell and Caldwell (1968) reported that if a pair of animals began whistling within about 300 ms of one another, one of the pair abruptly terminated its whistle until the other terminated. Dolphins apparently engage in signature whistle exchanges and burst-pulse exchanges, but not exchanges with mixed sound types (Caldwell & Caldwell, 1968; Gish, 1979; Lang & Smith, 1965; Lilly & Miller, 1961b; Watkins & Schevill, 1974). These behaviors suggest that dolphins at least recognize the two types of acoustic patterns. In addition, newly acquainted dolphins connected by an "acoustic-link" slowly decrease the amount of signature whistle exchanges after their original introduction. However, if one of the partners in a link is replaced, both members will again emit a large proportion of signature-type whistles (Gish, 1979; Lang & Smith, 1965). This habituation behavior implies recognition of, and habituation to, particular whistle patterns.

Fish and Lingle (1977) provide evidence for whistle recognition in a playback study in the field. In their study, they captured a large male spotted dolphin (*Stenella attenuata*) near Oahu, Hawaii, and recorded its nearly continuous vocalizations while aboard the capture vessel. The investigators later played the recorded sound back to members of the same herd and to another herd of spotted dolphins off the distant island of Hawaii. The dolphin herd off Oahu dispersed rapidly after each instance of playback, as if alarmed. The herd off Hawaii did not flee: instead animals approached the underwater speaker, even touching it. Herman and Tavolga (1980) have reviewed the data and hypothesized that "alarm may be conveyed by atypical variations . . . in the well-known call of familiar and possibly dominant individuals. These same variations in a stranger's call may have no impact because the normal 'baseline' characteristics are not known [and therefore variations are not recognized] (p. 173)."

Caldwell, Caldwell, and Hall presented data from a series of studies of "speaker identification" abilities of a single dolphin (Caldwell, Caldwell, & Hall, 1969, 1970, 1973; Caldwell, Hall, & Caldwell, 1971a, 1971b). Within a few sessions the subject learned to reliably sort the conspecific whistles by speaker (Caldwell et al., 1969, 1971a, 1971b). In further experiments, the dolphin was able to sort the whistles of up to eight conspecifics into two response categories (go/no-go), to sort whistles of other dolphin species by speaker, to remember the discrimination over delays up to seven months, and finally, to sort the stimuli accurately when only a single FM "loop" of a whistle was presented.

Unfortunately, detailed descriptions of both stimuli and methods were lacking in all these reports. It appears as though the dolphin may have been trained and tested with the same set of stimuli, without crucial transfer tests. If so, the dolphin may have learned the correspondence between individual stimuli and responses without actually applying sorting rules based on speaker identity.

Perception of serial patterns.   The recognition of serial acoustic patterns is a capacity which underlies several important human auditory functions, such as the perception of speech and music (Hulse, Cynx, & Humpal, 1984; Lashley, 1951; Mullennix and Pisoni, this volume; Roitblat, 1987). Studies exploring sensitivity to sequence have been conducted at this laboratory (Herman et al., 1984; Thompson, 1976; Thompson & Herman, 1974). As part of one experiment, a bottlenose dolphin was trained to sort 4 two-element sequences into two response categories (Thompson, 1976). After 7500 training trials, the subject learned to press one paddle after either the AC or BD sequences, and to press a second paddle after AD or BC sequences. Note that the problem could not be solved by using "local" strategies (cf. D'Amato & Salmon, 1982, 1984), such as responding to a stimulus in a particular temporal position.

Once the discrimination was learned, the duration of the silent interval between the sound elements was progressively increased in a modified staircase technique. Four experiments, each utilizing a slightly different methodology, all found nearly the same result: performance rapidly deteriorated with intersound intervals longer than about 2 sec. Error patterns did not indicate a simple failure to recall the first item of the sequences at longer delays. Thompson speculated that the dolphins may have perceived some "configural" auditory property of the sequences at short intervals, and that this property was destroyed at longer delays. This analysis is consistent with other research with humans suggesting that configural properties, or "emergent features," may be associated with sound elements which are spectro-temporally adjacent (Sawusch & Nochajski, 1982). Therefore, it is possible that the subject may not have heard the stimuli as sequences per se, but as four unique sounds that were perceived only at short durations (Thompson, 1976).

Herman et al. (1984) have recently reported powerful evidence for "fluent" recognition of sound sequences in a language learning experiment by two bottlenose dolphins. One dolphin was trained to recognize sequences of acoustic language symbols (see section on discrete sounds). Individual sounds were associated with objects, actions, or modifiers in the tutored language. The sentences were imperatives which directed the dolphin to carry out some sequence of actions, such as taking one acoustically named object to another acoustically named object. The subject was completely correct on 50% to 77% of the novel sentences presented in various syntactic forms, whereas chance responding would have yielded only 4% correct sequences. In addition, the dolphin correctly responded to semantically reversible sentences: different sequences of the same words that required different response chains. For example, FRISBEE FETCH SURFBOARD (glossed as "take the frisbee to the surfboard") required a different sequence of responses than SURFBOARD FETCH FRISBEE ("take the surfboard to the frisbee"). Because only the word order changed in complementary pairs of reversible sentences, we may conclude that the dolphin was sensitive to the sequence of the sounds.

Vocal mimicry. The results of mimicry experiments provide indirect evidence of auditory functioning. That an acoustic feature exists in a produced sound does not necessarily indicate perception of the attribute. However, mimicry responses are equivalent to other absolute perceptual judgments in that different points in a perceptual space are mapped onto distinctive, arbitrary responses. Mimicry data generally do not provide detailed psychophysical information, but do suggest important characteristics of complex auditory processing.

Dolphin mimicry data may be gleaned from a wide variety of playback studies (Dreher, 1966; Evans & Prescott, 1962; Lang & Smith, 1965; Richards, Bauer, Wolz, & Herman, 1981), acoustic-link studies (Gish, 1979; Lang & Smith, 1965; Lilly & Miller, 1961b), language experiments, and other experiments which specifically examined mimicry (Batteau & Markey, 1968; Caldwell & Caldwell, 1972; Lilly, 1962, 1965; Lilly, Miller, & Truby, 1968; Penner, 1966, as cited in Evans, 1973; Richards, Wolz, & Herman, 1984; Tyack, 1986). The common denominator of all these experiments has been the recording of vocal responses to auditory stimulation.

Several vocal mimicry studies which presented either human speech models (Lilly, 1965; Lilly et al., 1968), or whistle-like models (KBMML, unpublished data; Penner, 1966, as cited in Evans, 1973; Richards et al., 1984) have found a close correspondence between the durations of model sounds and mimics. These results are consistent with the fine duration discrimination reported in previous psychophysical studies (Yunker & Herman, 1974), and imply that duration of events may be a salient perceptual feature.

There are several reports of accurate matching of both absolute frequency and frequency modulation, or "FM contour," of synthetic or natural whistles (Caldwell & Caldwell, 1972; Gish, 1979; Penner, 1966, as cited in Evans, 1973; Richards et al., 1981; Richards et al., 1984; Tyack, 1986). Caldwell and Caldwell (1972) recorded a juvenile bottlenose dolphin which spontaneously mimicked the frequency and contour of a 10 kHz CF tone used as a test sound. Other studies have reported accurate mimicry of the modulation contour of synthetic whistles (Penner, 1966 as cited in Evans, 1973; Richards et al., 1981, 1984). Dolphins also apparently mimic natural conspecific whistles on occasion (Gish, 1979; Tyack, 1986). Mimicry of natural whistles may mediate the development of regional dialects within wild populations of dolphins (Graycar, 1976; Richards, 1986; Tyack, 1986).

Research at KBMML (Richards et al., 1981, 1984; Richards, 1986) has demonstrated mimicry of a number of acoustic parameters, such as duration, absolute frequency, FM contour, and AM contour. AM mimicry was surprising, as it was not explicitly reinforced during training. The subject mimicked amplitude changes in various stimuli, some of which were artifacts initially unknown to the investigators. The mimicry of an unreinforced dimension suggests that the dolphin had developed a generalized concept of mimicry.

Accurate mimicry of the human voice by odontocetes has been reported several times for bottlenose dolphins (Caldwell & Caldwell, 1972; Lilly, 1965, 1967) and for beluga whales (Ridgway et al., 1985). With the exception of Lilly et al. (1967), there has been little spectrographic analysis of dolphin mimics of the human voice, and phonetic quality has generally been judged by human ears. Although there is some degree of similarity between the harmonic structure of human voiced speech sounds and the odontocete burst-pulse sounds (Lilly et al., 1968; Ridgway et al., 1985; Watkins, 1967), odontocete sounds may lack a similar formant structure or noise segments. Humans are known to attach speech labels reliably to sounds which share only a few acoustic features with human speech sounds (Ralston, 1986; Ralston & Sawusch, 1985, 1986; Remez, Rubin, Pisoni, & Carrell, 1981), and human phonetic perception is subject to a variety of contextual effects (Warren, 1970). Therefore, descriptions of the acoustic-phonetic quality of dolphin mimics of human speech await spectrographic verification. However, the preliminary mimicry data are concordant with recognition studies, suggesting recognition of acoustic-phonetic features.

Two other serendipitous findings have emerged from mimicry research. The first is a shifting by an octave of the center frequency of a mimic whistle relative to models outside of the "preferred" whistling range of the dolphin (Penner, 1966, as cited in Evans, 1973; Richards et al., 1984). This phenomenon, which is common in humans, suggests that the dolphin perceives octave relationships. The second unexpected finding came from work on mimicry of human speech sounds (Lilly et al., 1968). In those studies, the duration of the interval between the end of the model sequence (a list of consonant-vowel and vowel-consonant syllables) and the beginning of the dolphin's mimic response was roughly equal to the duration of the silent intervals between model syllables. This effect was obtained even with tape-recorded versions of the model sequences, ruling out nonacoustic cuing. As the number of model syllables per trial was randomized within experimental blocks, the results imply that the dolphin may have been sensitive to correlated prosodic cues (pitch contour, duration, or loudness).

Conclusion.   Perceptual studies employing complex stimuli have generally agreed with, and have extended, knowledge gained from psychophysical experiments. These experiments have demonstrated that pitch, duration, frequency contour, and the presence of pulsing are salient dimensions. However, the preliminary research examining perception of FM and AM is somewhat contradictory. A few studies with complex stimuli have found maximum sensitivity at relatively low rates of modulation (circa 2–3 Hz). However, other experiments have reported recognition and mimicry of relatively high rates (circa 10 Hz) of FM, suggesting that the region of maximal FM sensitivity may be higher than previously believed. It is quite likely that dolphins may possess mechanisms specific for detecting and coding AM and FM, as suggested by the electrophysiological research of Bullock et al. (1968).

Preliminary data also indicate that the dolphin may be trained to recognize phonetic segments in human speech sounds. Even if the dolphin's peripheral auditory system approximates a 2–150 kHz band-pass filter, we would expect them to be able to discriminate a large percentage of acoustic-phonetic features, an ability useful in training contexts or in human/dolphin communication systems. Therefore, the limited success with human speech recognition by dolphins may be due primarily to a lack of adequate training and testing.

Dolphins appear to recognize several complex social signals generated by conspecifics, both vocal and nonvocal. Research on the perception of conspecific vocalizations needs to be replicated with greater experimental control and explicit transfer conditions. Further experiments combining similarity judgments, multidimensional scaling, and modern signal processing techniques may reveal the distinctive cues to which dolphins attend when listening to conspecific calls (Brown & Dooling, 1987; Sands, Lincoln, & Wright, 1982). A better understanding of the perception of natural social signals would enhance future attempts at establishing fluent, acoustically oriented artificial languages (Batteau & Markey, 1968; Dudok van Heel, Kamminga, & van der Toorn, 1982; Herman et al., 1984; Richards et al., 1984).

Results from mimicry studies have generally corroborated those of other listening experiments and suggest several acoustic parameters that may be salient or important in the perceptual world of the dolphin (i.e., duration, pitch, FM contour, and AM). There is also reason to believe that bottlenose dolphins may be sensitive to octave relationships, acoustic-phonetic information, and prosodic features of the human voice.

Dolphins are sensitive to temporal order, or sequence information. This has been demonstrated convincingly in one study of imposed language. This type of processing greatly expands the potential number of unique messages which may be communicated within that context. The occurrence and nature of syntactic patterns in native communication systems is unknown. Research is currently underway at KBMML exploring the perception of tonal sequences.

III. GENERAL CONCLUSIONS

In general, studies of sound production and perception of the bottlenose dolphin have confirmed and greatly extended early hypotheses. The sound production and perception systems of the dolphin consist of two distinct subsystems, one specialized for communicative and environmental sounds, and the other for echolocation. The "passive" auditory system operates primarily on energy below 20 kHz, and the echo system operates primarily on energy from 20 kHz to the upper range of hearing, near 130 kHz. The bandwidth of the combined systems of the bottlenose dolphin and other odontocetes may be the widest in the animal kingdom. Simultaneous production of echolocation clicks and whistles suggests that dolphins may perceptually process both types of information in parallel (Bel'kovich & Dubrovskiy, 1976; Bullock & Ridgway, 1972; Bullock et al., 1968; Ridgway et al., 1981; Zanin & Zaslavskii, 1977).

Although this chapter does not focus on echolocation, target dimensions which dolphins have successfully discriminated in controlled experiments may be briefly listed. Dolphin echolocation provides discrimination of auditory information that is correlated with a variety of target dimensions, including direction, range, size, shape, and material composition. Dolphins can detect metal spheres the size of a softball at ranges greater than the length of a football field (Au & Snyder, 1980; Murchison, 1980a, 1980b). Due to considerations of the emitted signal levels, transmission loss, and perceptual thresholds, the maximum functional detection range would probably not exceed one half kilometer (Evans & Dreher, 1962; Ayrapet'yants & Konstantinov, 1974). Dolphins may be able to detect other dolphins from their unreflected echolocation signals. If so, the maximum range of passive detection would probably be a little more than twice the active detection range. The range of ensonified targets is probably perceived in a temporal domain on the basis of the arrival time of the primary echo (C. S. Johnson, 1980; Moore et al., 1984; Vel'min & Dubrovskiy, 1975, 1976, 1978; Zanin & Zaslavskii, 1977). The error in range estimation is no greater than a few centimeters for standard ranges less than 10 m (Murchison, 1980a, 1980b).

Empirical data suggest that perception of spatial form is relatively coarse, as size differences less than 10 to 50% may not be reliably detected (Ayrapet'yants & Konstantinov, 1974; Barta, 1969; Nachtigall, 1980; Turner & Norris, 1966). Two- and three-dimensional forms may be discriminated, and the perception of form may be critically based on the processing of dynamic echo properties (Au, Schusterman, & Kersting, 1980; Barta, 1969; Nachtigall, Murchison, & Au, 1980). The material composition of targets may also be reliably discriminated

(Evans & Powell, 1967; Hammer & Au, 1980). TSP is probably the most salient in the perception of target qualities conveyed in secondary echoes, or in the perception of target echoes and temporally adjacent reverberation (Au & Hammer, 1980; Au & Turl, 1983; Hammer & Au, 1980; Moore et al., 1984).

The adaptive significance of echolocation is obvious in turbid coastal environments, in dark pelagic depths, and as part of nocturnal activity. Echolocation may provide a sort of "x-ray" vision, allowing detection of targets behind optically opaque and acoustically transparent objects, detection of targets in the (solar) shadows of larger objects, such as near rocks or reefs, and the discrimination of the internal composition and structure of objects. The echolocation system appears well-integrated with other sensory systems (Bagdonis, Bel'kovich, & Krushinskaya, 1970; Penner & Murchison, 1970). Presumably, the information from active sonar ultimately contributes to amodal representations of objects and events in the dolphin's three-dimensional environment (Herman & Forestell, 1985; Jerison, 1986).

The similarities between vocal patterns and auditory sensitivity suggest that the two systems have coevolved. Other investigators have proposed a similar process of coevolution of human speech production and hearing (Stevens, 1972). If there is a lock-and-key relationship between productive and receptive systems, then study of a perceptual system may profit from a preliminary examination of functionally important stimuli.

There remain a number of important questions and unresolved problems regarding dolphin "passive" audition. The literature suggests that there may be specialized mechanisms which mediate the perception of complex auditory characteristics, such as FM, AM, or spectrum shape. In addition, there may be lower-level grouping and segmentation processes similar to those in humans. As there is little relevant empirical data, future experiments should focus on their existence and function. One of the more interesting questions regards the perception of conspecific social vocalizations. Modified learning set experiments can test the dolphin's classification of vocalizations according to abstract properties such as speaker identity, cultural affiliation, emotional state, or any other arbitrary category. The salient perceptual dimensions of natural vocalizations may be revealed by multidimensional scaling studies in which the dolphin makes similarity judgments of pairs of whistles or other vocalizations. The inclusion of synthetic or signal-processed vocalizations in such experiments may help define the perceptual dimensions which underlie the various distinctions.

A better understanding of dolphin audition may be exploited in the design of maximally distinctive sound symbols for an artificial vocal language. Future work on artificial systems should pursue the development of a phoneme-like set of recombinable sound patterns which optimize perceptual distinctiveness and reproducibility (Batteau & Markey, 1968; Richards, 1986). Such a system would be desirable for its relative ease of use by the dolphin. Related communication research might also explore a system based on human speech sounds. Such a system would be desirable for its relative ease of use by humans.

The hearing capacities of dolphins observed in the wild and the laboratory suggest that dolphins could have actually been summoned by Arion's tune. And we can be confident that if Galatea has blessed the dolphin, as Arion requested, her gift was one of extraordinary hearing.

ACKNOWLEDGMENTS

Preparation of this paper was supported by Contract N00014-85-K-0210 from the Office of Naval Research, Grant BNS-8109653 from the National Science Foundation, and grants from the Center for Field Research, all to L. M. Herman. Thanks to Sherry Ralston for conversations and support during the writing of this chapter.

REFERENCES

Altes, R. A. (1980). Models for echolocation. In R. G. Busnel & J. F. Fish (Eds.), *Animal sonar systems* (pp. 625–671). New York: Plenum Press.

Anderson, S. (1971). Auditory sensitivity of the harbor porpoise *Phocoena phocoena*. In G. Pilerri (Ed.), *Investigations on Cetacea* (Vol. 3, pp. 255–259). Berne, Switzerland: Institute of Brain Anatomy, University of Berne.

Au, W. W. L. (1980). echolocation of the Atlantic Bottlenose Dolphin (Tursiops-truncatus) in open waters. In R.-G. Busnell & J. F. Fish (Eds.), *Animal sonar systems* (pp. 251–282). New York: Plenum Press.

Au, W. W. L., Floyd, R. W., & Haun, J. E. (1978). Propagation of Atlantic bottlenose dolphin echolocation signals. *Journal of the Acoustical Society of America, 64*, 411–422.

Au, W. W. L., Floyd, R. W., Penner, R. H., & Murchison, A. E. (1974). Measurement of echolocation signals of the Atlantic bottlenose dolphin, *Tursiops truncatus* Montagu, in open waters. *The Journal of the Acoustical Society of America, 56*, 1280–1290.

Au, W. W. L., & Hammer, C. E. (1980). Target recognition via echolocation by the bottlenose dolphin, *Tursiops truncatus*. In R.-G. Busnel & J. F. Fish (Eds.), *Animal sonar systems* (pp. 855–858). New York: Plenum Press.

Au, W. W. L., & Moore, P. W. B. (1983). Critical ratios and bandwidths of the Atlantic bottlenose dolphin (*Tursiops truncatus*). *Journal of the Acoustical Society of America*, Suppl. 1, *74*, S73.

Au, W. W. L., & Moore, P. W. B. (1984). Receiving beam patterns and directivity indices of the Atlantic bottlenose dolphin (*Tursiops truncatus*). *The Journal of the Acoustical Society of America, 75*, 255–262.

Au, W. W. L., & Moore, P. W. B. (1986). The perception of complex echoes by an echolocating dolphin. *Journal of the Acoustical Society of America, 80*, Suppl. 1, YY8.

Au, W. W. L., Moore, P. W. B., & Pawloski, D. (1986). Echolocation transmitting beam of the Atlantic bottlenose dolphin. *The Journal of the Acoustical Society of America, 80*, 688–691.

Au, W. W. L., Penner, R. H., & Kadane, J. (1982). Acoustic behavior of echolocating Atlantic bottlenose dolphins. *The Journal of the Acoustical Society of America, 71*, 1269–1275.

Au, W. W. L., Schusterman, R. J., & Kersting, D. A. (1980). Sphere-cylinder discrimination via echolocation of *Tursiops truncatus*. In R.-G. Busnell & J. F. Fish (Eds.), *Animal sonar systems* (pp. 859–862). New York: Plenum Press.

Au, W. W. L., & Snyder, K. J. (1980). Long-range detection in open waters by an echolocating Atlantic bottlenose dolphin (*Tursiops truncatus*). *Journal of the Acoustical Society of America, 68*, 1077–1084.

Au, W. W. L., & Turl, C. W. (1983). Target detection in reverberation by an echolocating Atlantic bottlenose dolphin (*Tursiops truncatus*). *The Journal of the Acoustical Society of America, 73*, 1676–1681.

Ayrapet'yants, E. Sn., & Konstantinov, A. I. (1974). *Echolocation in nature*. Nauka, Leningrad (JPRS 63328-2).

Bagdonis, A., Bel'kovich, V. M., & Krushinskaya, N. L. (1970). Interaction of analyzers in dolphins during discrimination of geometrical figures, *Journal of Higher Neural Activity, 20*, 1070–1075.

Barta, R. E. (1969). *Acoustical pattern discrimination by an Atlantic bottlenose dolphin*. Unpublished manuscript, Naval Undersea Center, San Diego, CA.

Batteau, D. W., & Markey, P. R. (1968). *Man/dolphin communication*. (Final Report, Contract N00123-67-1103. Dec. 1966–1967). China Lake, California, U.S. Naval Ordnance Test Station.

Bel'kovich, V. M., & Dubrovskii, N. A. (1976). *Sensory basis of cetacean orientation*. Izdatel'stov Nauka, Leningrad.

Brown, S. D., & Dooling, R. J. (1987). Perception of bird calls by budgerigars and humans: A multidimensional scaling analysis. *Journal of the Acoustical Society of America, 81*, Suppl. 1, 010.

Bulfinch, T. (1986). *Bulfinch's mythology*. New York: Random House.

Bullock, T. H., & Gurevich, V. (1979). Soviet literature on the nervous system and psychobiology of cetacea. *International Review of Neurobiology, 21*, 48–127.

Bullock, T. H., & Ridgway, S. H. (1972). Evoked potentials in the central auditory system of alert porpoises to their own and artificial sounds. *Journal of Neurobiology, 3*, 79–99.

Bullock, T. H., et al. (1968). Electrophysiological studies of the central auditory mechanisms in cetaceans. *Zeitschrift fur Vergleichende Physiologie, 59*, 117–156.

Burdin, V. I., Reznik, A. M., Skornyakov, V. M., & Chupakov, A. G. (1974). Study of communicative signals of Black Sea dolphins. *Akusticheskiy Zhurnal, 20*, 518–529.

Burdin, V. I., Markov, V. I., Reznik, A. M., Skornyakov, V. M., & Chupakov, A. G. (1973). Determination of the just noticeable difference for white noise in the Black Sea bottlenose dolphin (*Tursiops truncatus ponticus barabasch*). In H. Mills (Ed. and Trans.), *Morphology and ecology of marine mammals: Seals, dolphins, and porpoises*. New York: Wiley.

Busnel, R.-G. & Dziedzic, A. (1966). Acoustic signals of the pilot whale *Globicephala malaena*, and of the porpoises *Delphinus delphis* and *Phocoena phocoena*. In K. S. Norris (Ed.), *Whales, dolphins, and porpoises* (pp. 607–646). Berkeley: University of California Press.

Caine, N. G. (1976). *Time separation pitch and the dolphin's sonar discrimination of distance*. Unpublished master's thesis, San Diego State University, San Diego, CA.

Caldwell, D. K., & Caldwell, M. C. (1972). Vocal mimicry in the whistle mode by an Atlantic bottlenosed dolphin. *Cetology, 9*, 1–8.

Caldwell, M. C., & Caldwell, D. K. (1965). Individualized whistle contours in bottlenosed dolphins, *Tursiops truncatus*. *Nature, 207*, 434–435.

Caldwell, M. C., & Caldwell, D. K. (1967). Intraspecific transfer of information via the pulsed sound in captive odontocete cetaceans. In R.-G. Busnel (Ed.), *Animal sonar systems* (Vol. 2, pp. 879–936). Jouy-en-Josas, France: Laboratorie de Physiologie Acoustique.

Caldwell, M. C., & Caldwell, D. K. (1968). Vocalization of naive captive dolphins in small groups. *Science, 159*, 1121–1123.

Caldwell, M. C., & Caldwell, D. K. (1971). Statistical evidence for individual signature whistles in Pacific white-sided dolphins, *Lagenorhynchus obliquidens*. *Cetology, 3*, 1–9.

Caldwell, M. C., Caldwell, D. K., & Hall, N. R. (1969). *An experimental demonstration of the ability of an Atlantic bottlenose dolphin to discriminate between whistles of other individuals of the same species* (Tech. Rep. No. 6). Los Angeles, CA: Los Angeles Museum of Natural History Foundation.

Caldwell, M. C., Caldwell, D. K., & Hall, N. R. (1970). An experimental demonstration of the ability of an Atlantic bottlenose dolphin to discriminate between playbacks of recorded whistles of conspecifics. *Proceedings of the 7th Annual Conference on Biological Sonar and Diving Mammals* (pp. 141–158). Menlo Park, CA.

Caldwell, M. C., Caldwell, D. K., & Hall, N. R. (1973). Ability of an Atlantic bottlenosed dolphin (*Tursiops truncatus*) to discriminate between, and potentially identify to individual, the whistles of another species, the common dolphin (*Delphinus delphis*). *Cetology, 14,* 1–7.

Caldwell, M. C., Caldwell, D. K., & Miller, J. F. (1973). Statistical evidence for individual signature whistles in the spotted dolphin, *Stenella plagiodon. Cetology, 16,* 1–21.

Caldwell, M. C., Hall, N. R., & Caldwell, D. K. (1971a). Ability of an Atlantic bottlenosed dolphin to discriminate between, and potentially identify to individual, the whistles of another species, the spotted dolphin. *Cetology, 6,* 1–6.

Caldwell, M. C., Hall, N. R., & Caldwell, D. K. (1971b). Ability of an Atlantic bottlenose dolphin to discriminate between, and respond differentially to, whistles of eight conspecifics. *Proceedings of the 8th Annual Conference on Biological Sonar and Diving Mammals* (pp. 57–65). Menlo Park, CA: Stanford Research Institute.

Caldwell, M. C., Haugen, R., & Caldwell, D. K. (1962). High-energy sound associated with fright in the dolphin. *Science, 138,* 907–908.

D'Amato, M. R., & Salmon, D. P. (1982). Tune discrimination in monkeys (*Cebus apella*) and in rats. *Animal Learning and Behavior, 10,* 126–134.

D'Amato, M. R., & Salmon, D. P. (1984). Processing of complex auditory stimuli (tune) by rats and monkeys (*Cebus apella*). *Animal Learning and Behavior, 12,* 184–194.

Diercks, K. J. (1974). *A collection of foreign language papers on the subject of biological sonar systems* (Tech. Rep. 74–79). Applied Research Laboratory, University of Texas, Austin.

Diercks, K. J., Trochta, R. T., & Evans, W. E. (1973). Delphinid sonar: Measurement and analysis. *Journal of the Acoustical Society of America, 54,* 200–204.

Diercks, K. J., Trochta, R. T., Greenlaw, C. F., & Evans, W. E. (1971). Recording and analysis of dolphin echolocation signals. *Journal of the Acoustical Society of America, 49,* 1729–1732.

Dormer, K. J. (1979). Mechanisms of sound production and air recycling in delphinids: Cineradiographic evidence. *Journal of the Acoustical Society of America, 65,* 229–239.

Dreher, J. J. (1966). Cetacean communication: Small group experiment. In K. S. Norris (Ed.), *Whales, dolphins, porpoises* (pp. 529–543). Berkeley: University of California Press.

Dreher, J. J., & Evans, W. E. (1964). Cetacean communication. In W. N. Tavolga (Ed.), *Marine bio-acoustics* (pp. 373–399). Oxford, England: Pergamon Press.

Dudok van Heel, W. H., Kamminga, C., & van der Toorn, J. D. (1982). An experiment in two-way communication in *Orcinus orca* L. *Aquatic Mammals, 9,* 69–82.

Egan, J. P., & Hake, H. W. (1950). On the masking pattern of a simple auditory stimulus. *Journal of the Acoustical Society of America, 22,* 622–630.

Erulkar, S. D. (1972). Comparative aspects of spatial localization of sound. *Physiological Reviews, 52,* 237–260.

Evans, W. E. (1967). Vocalization among marine mammals. In W. N. Tavolga (Ed.), *Marine bio-acoustics* (Vol. 2, pp. 159–186). New York: Pergamon Press.

Evans, W. E. (1973). Echolocation by marine delphinids and one species of freshwater dolphin. *Journal of the Acoustical Society of America, 54,* 191–199.

Evans, W. E., & Dreher, J. J. (1962). Observations on scouting behavior and associated sound production by the Pacific bottlenosed porpoise (*Tursiops gilli* Dall). *Bulletin of the Southern California Academy of Sciences, 61,* 217–226.

Evans, W. E., & Maderson, P. F. A. (1973). Mechanisms of sound reproduction in delphinid cetaceans: A review and some anatomical considerations. *American Zoology, 13,* 1205–1213.

Evans, W. E., & Powell, B. A. (1967). Discrimination of different metallic plates by an echolocating delphinid. In R.-G. Busnel (Ed.), *Animal sonar systems: Biology and bionics* (Vol. 1, pp. 363–382). Jouy-en-Josas, France: Laboratorie de Physiologie Acoustique.

Evans, W. E., Prescott, J. H. (1962). Observations of the sound reproduction capabilities of the bottlenose porpoise: A study of whistles and clicks. *Zoologica, 47,* 212–128.

Fant, C. G. M. (1960). *Acoustic theory of speech production.* The Hague: Mouton.

Fish, J. F., & Lingle, G. E. (1977, December). Responses of the spotted porpoises, *Stenella attenuata,* to playbacks of distress (?) sounds of one of their own kind. *Proceedings of the 2nd Conference on the Biology of Marine Mammals,* San Diego, p. 34.

Fletcher, H. (1940). Auditory patterns. *Reviews of Modern Physiology, 12,* 47–65.

Floyd, R. W. (1980). Models of cetacean signal processing. In R.-G. Busnel & J. F. Fish (Eds.), *Animal sonar systems* (pp. 615–623). New York: Plenum Press.

Fraser, F. C. (1947). Sound emitted by dolphins. *Nature* (London), *160,* 759.

French, N. R., & Steinberg, J. C. (1947). Factors governing the intelligibility of speech sounds. *Journal of the Acoustical Society of America, 19,* 90–119.

Gannon, F. (1987, Winter). The days of the dolphins. *Philip Morris Magazine,* pp. 14–37.

Gish, S. L. (1979). *Quantitative analysis of two-way acoustic communication between captive Atlantic bottlenose dolphins* (*Tursiops truncatus* Montague). Unpublished doctoral dissertation. University of California, Santa Cruz.

Graycar, P. J. (1976). Whistle dialects of the Atlantic bottlenose dolphin, *Tursiops truncatus.* Doctoral thesis, University of Florida.

Green, D. M. (1976). *An introduction to hearing.* Hillsdale, NJ: Lawrence Erlbaum Associates.

Grinnel, A. D. (1967). Mechanisms for overcoming interference in echolocating animals. In R.-G. Busnel (Ed.), *Animal sonar systems: Biology and bionics* (Vol. 1, pp. 451–481). Joy-en-Josas, France: Laboratorie de Physiologie Acoustique.

Hall, J. D., & Johnson, C. S. (1972). Auditory thresholds of a killer whale *Orcinus orca* Linnaeus. *Journal of the Acoustical Society of America, 51,* 515–517.

Hamilton, P. M. (1957). Noise masked thresholds as a function of tonal duration and masking noise bandwidth. *Journal of the Acoustical Society of America, 29,* 506–511.

Hammer, C. E., & Au, W. W. L. (1980). Porpoise echo-recognition: an analysis of controlling target characteristics. *Journal of the Acoustical Society of America, 68,* 1285–1293.

Hawkins, J. E., & Stevens, S. S. (1950). The masking of pure tones and of speech by white noise. *Journal of the Acoustical Society of America, 22,* 6–13.

Herman, L. M. (1975). Interference and auditory short-term memory in the bottlenose dolphin. *Animal Learning and Behavior, 3,* 43–48.

Herman, L. M. (1980). Cognitive characteristics of dolphins. In L. M. Herman (Ed.), *Cetacean behavior: Mechanisms and functions* (pp. 149–209). New York: Wiley-Interscience.

Herman, L. M., & Arbeit, W. R. (1972). Frequency difference limens in the bottlenose dolphin: 1–70 KC/S. *Journal of Auditory Research, 2,* 109–120.

Herman, L. M., & Arbeit, W. R. (1973). Stimulus control and auditory discrimination learning sets in the bottlenose dolphin. *Journal of the Experimental Analysis of Behavior, 19,* 379–394.

Herman, L. M., & Forestell, P. H. (1985). Short-term memory in pigeons: Modality specific or code-specific effects? *Animal Learning and Behavior, 13,* 463–465.

Herman, L. M., & Gordon, J. A. (1974). Auditory delayed matching in the bottlenose dolphin. *Journal of the Experimental Analysis of Behavior, 21,* 19–26.

Herman, L. M., Richards, D. G., & Wolz, J. P. (1984). Comprehension of sentences by bottlenosed dolphins. *Cognition, 16,* 129–219.

Herman, L. M., & Tavolga, W. N. (1980). The communication systems of cetaceans. In L. H.

Herman (Ed.), *Cetacean behavior: Mechanisms and functions* (pp. 149–209). New York: Academic Press.

Herman, L. M., & Thompson, R. K. R. (1982). Symbolic, identity, and delayed matching of sounds by the bottlenosed dolphin. *Animal Learning and Behavior, 10,* 22–34.

Hulse, S. H., Cynx, J., & Humpal, J. (1984). Cognitive processing of pitch and rhythm structures by birds. In H. L. Roitblat, T. G. Bever, & H. S. Terrace (Eds.), *Animal cognition* (pp. 183–198). Hillsdale, NJ: Lawrence Erlbaum Associates.

Hult, R. (1982). Another function of echolocation for bottlenose dolphins *(Tursiops truncatus)*. *Cetology, 47,* 1–7.

Jacobs, D. W. (1972). Auditory frequency discrimination in the Atlantic bottlenose dolphin, *Tursiops truncatus* Montagu: A preliminary report. *Journal of the Acoustical Society of America, 52,* 696–698.

Jacobs, D. W., & Hall, J. D. (1972). Auditory thresholds of a freshwater dolphin, *Inia geoffrensis* Blainville. *Journal of the Accoustical Society of America, 51,* 530–533.

Jakobson, R., Fant, C. G. M., & Halle, M. (1963). *Preliminaries to speech analysis: The distinctive features and their correlates.* Cambridge, MA: MIT Press.

Jerison, H. J. (1986). The perceptual worlds of dolphins. In R. J. Schusterman, J. A. Thomas, & F. G. Wood (Eds.), *Dolphin cognition and behavior: A comparative approach* (pp. 347–359). Hillsdale, NJ: Lawrence Erlbaum Associates.

Johnson, C. S. (1967a). Sound detection thresholds in marine mammals. In W. N. Tavolga (Ed.), *Marine bio-acoustic* (Vol. 2, pp. 247–260). New York: Pergamon Press.

Johnson, C. S. (1968a). Relation between absolute threshold and duration-of-tone pulses in the bottlenosed porpoise. *Journal of the Acoustical Society of America, 43,* 757–763.

Johnson, C. S. (1968b). Masked tonal thresholds in the bottlenosed porpoise. *Journal of the Acoustical Society of America, 44,* 965–967.

Johnson, C. S. (1971). Auditory masking of one pure tone by another in the bottlenosed porpoise. *Journal of the Acoustical Society of America, 49,* 1317–1318.

Johnson, C. S. (1980). Important areas for future cetacean auditory study. In R.-G. Busnel & J. F. Fish (Eds.), *Animal sonar systems* (pp. 515–518). New York: Plenum Press.

Johnson, C. S. (1986). Dolphin audition and echolocation capabilities. In R. J. Schusterman, J. A. Thomas, & F. G. Wood (Eds.), *Dolphin cognition and behavior: A comparative approach* (pp. 347–359). Hillsdale, NJ: Lawrence Erlbaum Associates.

Johnson, R. A. (1977). Time difference pitch resolution in human and animal echolocation abilities. *Journal of the Acoustical Society of America, 62,* Suppl. 1, AA1.

Johnson, R. A. (1980). Energy spectrum analysis in echolocation. In R.-G. Busnel & J. F. Fish (Eds.), *Animal sonar systems* (pp. 673–693). New York: Plenum Press.

Johnson, R. A., & Titlebaum, E. L. (1976). Energy spectrum analysis: A model of echolocation processing. *Journal of the Acoustical Society of America, 60,* 484–491.

Kellogg, W. N. (1953). Ultrasonic hearing in the porpoise, *Tursiops truncatus. Journal of Comparative and Physiological Psychology, 46,* 446–450.

Kellogg, W. N., & Kohler, R. (1952). Reactions of the porpoise to ultrasonic frequencies. *Science, 116,* 250–252.

Kluender, K. R., & Diehl, R. L. (1986). Japanese quail categorize [d] across allophonic and talker variation. *Journal of the Acoustical Society of America, 80,* Suppl. 1, ZZ11.

Kuhl, P. K. (1986). Reflections on infants' perception and representation of speech. In J. S. Perkell & D. H. Klatt (Eds.), *Invariance and variability in speech processes* (pp. 19–30). Hillsdale, NJ: Lawrence Erlbaum Associates.

Kuhl, P. K., & Miller, J. D. (1975). Speech perception by the chinchilla: Voiced-voiceless distinction in alveolar-plosive consonants. *Science, 190,* 69–72.

Kuhl, P. K., & Miller, J. D. (1978). Speech perception by the chinchilla: Identification functions for synthetic VOT stimuli. *Journal of the Acoustical Society of America, 63,* 905–917.

Kuhl, P. K., & Padden, D. M. (1983). Enhanced discriminability at the phonetic boundaries for the place feature in macaques. *Journal of the Acoustical Society of America, 73*, 1003–1010.

Lawrence, B., & Schevill, W. E. (1956). The functional anatomy of the delphinid nose. *Bulletin of the Museum of Comparative Zoology, 114*, 103–197.

Lilly, J. C. (1962). Vocal behavior of the bottlenose dolphin. *Proceedings of the American Philosophical Society, 106*, 520–529.

Lilly, J. C. (1963). Distress call of the bottlenose dolphin: Stimuli and evoked behavioral responses. *Science, 139*, 116–118.

Lilly, J. C. (1965). Vocal mimicry in *Tursiops:* Ability to match numbers and durations of human vocal bursts. *Science, 147*, 300–301.

Lilly, J. C. (1967). *The mind of a dolphin.* New York: Doubleday.

Lilly, J. C. (1978). *Communication between man and dolphin.* New York: Crown Publishers.

Lilly, J. C., & Miller, A. M. (1961a). Sounds emitted by the bottlenose dolphin. *Science, 133*, 1689–1693.

Lilly, J. C., & Miller, A. M. (1961b). Vocal exchanges between dolphins. *Science, 134*, 1873–1876.

Lilly, J. C., Miller, A. M., & Truby, H. M. (1968). Reprogramming of the sonic output of the dolphin: Sonic

Lang, T. G., & Smith, H. A. P. (1965). Communication between dolphins in separate tanks by way of an electronic acoustic link. *Science, 150*, 1839–1844.

Lashley, K. S. (1951). The problem of serial order in behavior. burst count matching. *Journal of the Acoustical Society of America, 43*, 1412–1424.

Mackay, R. S. (1980). Dolphin air sac motion measurements during vocalization by two noninvasive ultrasonic techniques. In R.-G. Busnel & J. F. Fish (Eds.), *Animal sonar systems* (pp. 933–935). New York: Plenum Press.

Madsen, C. J., & Herman, L. M. (1980). Social and ecological correlates of cetacean vision and visual appearance. In L. M. Herman (Ed.), *Cetacean behavior: Mechanisms and functions.* New York: Wiley-Interscience.

Marr, D. (1982). *Vision.* San Francisco, CA: Freeman.

McBride, A. F., & Hebb, D. O. (1948). Behavior of the captive bottlenose dolphin (*Tursiops truncatus*). *Journal of Comparative Physiology and Psychology, 41*, 111–123.

Miller, G. A., & Nicely, P. E. (1955). An analysis of perceptual confusions among some English consonants. *Journal of the Acoustical Society of America, 27*, 338–352.

Mills, A. W. (1958). On the minimum audible angle. *Journal of the Acoustical Society of America, 30*, 237–246.

Moore, P. W. B., & Au, W. W. L. (1982). Masked pure-tone thresholds of the bottlenosed dolphin (*Tursiops truncatus*). *Journal of the Acoustical Society of America, 72*, S42.

Moore, P. W. B., Hall, J. D., Friedl, J., & Nachtigall, P. E. (1984). The critical interval in dolphin echolocation: What is it? *Journal of the Acoustical Society of America, 76*, 314–317.

Morris, R. J. (1986). The acoustic facility of dolphins. In M. M. Bryden & R. Harrison (Eds.), *Research on dolphins* (pp. 369–399). Oxford, England: Clarendon Press.

Murchison, A. E. (1980a). Detection range and range resolution of echolocating bottlenose porpoise (*Tursiops truncatus*). In R.-G. Busnel & J. F. Fish (Eds.), *Animal sonar systems* (pp. 43–70). New York: Plenum Press.

Murchison, A. E. (1980b). Maximum detection range and range resolution in echolocating bottlenose porpoises, *Tursiops truncatus* (Montague). Doctoral dissertation, University of California, Santa Cruz.

Nachtigall, P. E. (1980). Odontocete echolocation performance on object size, shape and material. In R.-G. Fish & J. F. Fish (Eds.), *Animal sonar systems* (pp. 71–96). New York: Plenum Press. In L. A. Jeffress (Ed.), *Cerebral mechanisms in behavior* (pp. 112–136). New York: Wiley.

Nachtigall, P. E., Murchison, A. E., & Au, W. W. L. (1980). Cylinder and cube shape discrimination by an echolocating blindfolded bottlenosed dolphin. In R.-G. Busnel & J. F. Fish (Eds.), *Animal sonar systems* (pp. 945–947). New York: Plenum Press.

Nordmark, J. (1960). Perception of distance in animal echolocation. *Nature* (London), *188*, 1009–1010.

Nordmark, J. (1970). Time and frequency analysis. In J. V. Tobias (Ed.), *Foundations of modern auditory theory* (Vol. 1, pp. 57–83). New York: Academic Press.

Norris, K. S. (1964). Some problems of echolocating cetaceans. In W. N. Tavolga (Ed.), *Marine bio-acoustics* (Vol. 1, pp. 317–336). Oxford, England: Pergamon Press.

Norris, K. S. (1968). The evolution of acoustic mechanisms in odontocetes. In E. T. Drake (Ed.), *Evolution and environment.* New Haven, CT: Yale University Press.

Norris, K. S. (1969). The echolocation of marine mammals. In H. T. Andersen (Ed.), *The biology of marine mammals* (pp. 391–421). New York: Academic Press.

Norris, K. S. (1974). *The porpoise watcher.* New York: Norton.

Norris, K. S. (1980). Peripheral sound processing in odontocetes. In R.-G. Busnel & J. F. Fish (Eds.), *Animal sonar systems* (pp. 495–509). New York: Plenum Press.

Norris, K. S. (1986). Sound production in dolphins. *Marine Mammal Science, 2,* 233–235.

Norris, K. S., & Dohl, T. P. (1980a). Behavior of the Hawaiian spinner dolphin, *Stenella longirostris. Fishery Bulletin, 77,* 821–849.

Norris, K. S., & Dohl, T. P. (1980b). The structure and function of cetacean schools. In L. M. Herman (Ed.), *Cetacean behavior: Structure and function* (pp. 211–261). New York: Wiley-Interscience.

Norris, K. S., Evans, W. E., & Turner, R. N. (1967). Echolocation in an Atlantic bottlenose porpoise during discrimination. In R.-G. Busnel (Ed.), *Animal sonar systems: Biology and bionics* (Vol. 1, pp. 409–443). Jouy-en-Jouy, France: Laboratorie de Physiologie Acoustique.

Norris, K. S., & Mohl, B. (1983). Can odontocetes debilitate prey with sound? *American Naturalist, 122,* 85–104.

Penner, R. H., & Murchison, A. E. (1970). Experimentally demonstrated echolocation in the Amazon River porpoise, *Inia geoffrensis* (Blainville). *Naval Undersea Center Technical Publication, 187,* 1–25.

Pepperberg, I. M. (1986). Acquisition of anomalous communicatory systems: Implications for studies on interspecies communication. In R. J. Schusterman, J. A. Thomas, & F. G. Wood (Eds.), *Dolphin cognition and behavior: A comparative approach* (pp. 289–302). Hillsdale, NJ: Lawrence Erlbaum Associates.

Peterson, G. E., & Barney, H. L. (1952). Control methods used in the study of vowels. *Journal of the Acoustical Society of America, 24,* 175–184.

Pisoni, D. B., & Sawusch, J. R. (1975). Some stages of processing in speech perception. In A. Cohen & S. G. Nooteboom (Eds.), *Structure and process in speech perception.* New York: Springer-Verlag.

Plomp, R., & Bouman, M. A. (1959). Relation between hearing threshold and duration of tone pulses. *Journal of the Acoustical Society of America, 31,* 749–758.

Pollack, I. (1954). Intensity discrimination thresholds under several psychophysical procedures. *Journal of the Acoustical Society of America, 26,* 1056–1059.

Popper, A. N. (1980a). Behavioral measures of odontocete hearing. In R.-G. Busnel & J. F. Fish (Eds.), *Animal sonar systems* (pp. 469–481). New York: Plenum Press.

Popper, A. N. (1980b). Sound emission and detection by delphinids. In L. M. Herman (Ed.), *Cetacean behavior: Mechanisms and functions* (pp. 1–52). New York: Wiley-Interscience.

Ralston, J. V. (1986). *Auditory and phonetic perception of stop consonant place of articulation information.* Unpublished doctoral dissertation, State University of New York at Buffalo.

Ralston, J. V., & Sawusch, J. R. (1985). Perception of sinewave analogs of stop consonant place information II. *Journal of the Acoustical Society of America, 77,* Suppl. 1., HH8.

Ralston, J. V., & Sawusch, J. R. (1986, November). *Auditory and phonetic codes in stop-consonant perception.* Paper presented at the 27th meeting of the Psychonomic Society, New Orleans.

Remez, R. E., Rubin, P. E., Pisoni, D. B., & Carrell, T. D. (1981). Speech perception without traditional speech cues. *Science, 212,* 947–950.

Renaud, D. L., & Popper, A. N. (1975). Sound localization by the bottlenose porpoise (*Tursiops truncatus*). *Journal of Experimental Biology, 63,* 569–585.

Reyesenback de Haan, F. W. (1957). Hearing in whales. *Acta Otolaryngolica, 134* (Suppl.), 1–114.

Richards, D. G. (1986). Dolphin vocal mimicry and vocal object labeling. In R. J. Schusterman, J. A. Thomas, & F. G. Wood (Eds.), *Dolphin cognition and behavior: A comparative approach* (pp. 273–288). Hillsdale, NJ: Lawrence Erlbaum Associates.

Richards, D. G., Bauer, G. B., Wolz, J. P., & Herman, L. M. (1981, December). *Reponses of dolphins, Tursiops truncatus, to playbacks of natural and computer-generated sounds.* Paper presented at the Biennial Conference on the Biology of Marine Mammals, San Francisco.

Richards, D. G., Wolz, J. P., & Herman, L. M. (1984). Vocal mimicry of computer-generated sounds and vocal labeling of objects by a bottlenosed dolphin, *Tursiops truncatus. Journal of Comparative Psychology, 98,* 10–28.

Ridgway, S. H., Bullock, S. H., Carder, D. A., Seeley, R. L., Woods, D., & Galambos, R. (1981). Auditory brainstem response in dolphins. *Proceedings of the National Academy of Sciences of the United States of America, 78,* 943–1947.

Ridgway, S. H., Carder, D. A., & Jeffries, M. M. (1985). Another "talking" male white whale [Abstract]. *Proceedings of the 6th Biennial Conference on the Biology of Marine Mammals.*

Roitblat, H. L. (1987). *Introduction to comparative cognition.* San Francisco, CA: Freeman.

Sands, S. F., Lincoln, C. E., & Wright, A. A. (1982). Pictorial similarity judgments and the organization of visual memory in the rhesus monkey. *Journal of Experimental Psychology: General, 111,* 369–389.

Savage-Rumbaugh, S., McDonald, K., Sevcik, R. A., Hopkins, W. D., & Rubert, E. (1986). Spontaneous symbol acquisition and communicative use by pigmy chimpanzees (*Pan paniscus*). *Journal of Experimental Psychology: General, 115,* 211–235.

Sawusch, J. R., & Nochajski, T. H. (1982). Stimulus integrality in the auditory coding of speech. Paper presented at the 23rd meeting of the Psychonomic Society, Minneapolis.

Scharf, B. (1970). Critical bands. In J. V. Tobias (Ed.), *Foundations of modern auditory theory* (Vol. 1, pp. 157–202). New York: Academic Press.

Schevill, W. E., & Lawrence, B. (1953a). Auditory response of a bottlenose porpoise, *Tursiops truncatus,* to frequencies above 100 kc. *Journal of Experimental Zoology, 124,* 147–165.

Schevill, W. E., & Lawrence, B. (1953b). High-frequency auditory responses of a bottlenosed porpoise, *Tursiops truncatus* (Montagu). *Journal of the Acoustical Society of America, 25,* 1016–1017.

Schevill, W. E., & Lawrence, B. (1956). Food-finding by a captive porpoise (*Tursiops truncatus*). *Brevoria, 53,* 1–16.

Seaton, W. H., & Trahiotis, C. (1975). Comparison of critical ratios and critical bands in the monaural chinchilla. *Journal of the Acoustical Society of America, 57,* 193–199.

Shower, E. G., & Biddulph, R. (1931). Differential pitch sensitivity of the ear. *Journal of the Acoustical Society of America, 3,* 275–287.

Stevens, K. N. (1972). The quantal nature of speech: Evidence from articulatory-acoustic data. In P. B. Denes & E. E. David, Jr. (Eds.), *Human communication: A unified view.* New York: McGraw-Hill.

Thompson, R. K. R. (1976). *Performance of the bottlenose dolphin (Tursiops truncatus) on delayed auditory sequences and delayed auditory successive discriminations.* Unpublished doctoral dissertation, University of Hawaii.

Thompson, R. K. R., & Herman, L. M. (1974, April). *Auditory sequence discrimination and delayed discriminations in the Atlantic bottlenose dolphin.* Paper presented at the meeting of the Western Psychological Association, Los Angeles.

Thompson, R. K. R., & Herman, L. M. (1975). Underwater frequency discrimination in the bottlenose dolphin (1–140 kHz) and the human (1–8 kHz). *Journal of the Acoustical Society of America, 57,* 943–948.

Thompson, R. K. R., & Herman, L. M. (1977). Memory for lists of sounds for the bottle-nosed dolphin: Convergence of memory processes with humans? *Science, 195,* 501–503.

Turner, R. N., & Norris, K. S. (1966). Discriminative echolocation in a porpoise. *Journal of the Experimental Analysis of Behavior, 9,* 535–544.

Tyack, P. L. (1986). Whistle repertoires of two bottlenose dolphins, *Tursiops truncatus:* Mimicry of signature whistles? *Behavioral Ecology and Sociobiology, 18,* 251–257.

Urick, R. J. (1975). *Principles of underwater sound.* New York: McGraw-Hill.

Vel'min, V. A., & Dubrovskii, N. A. (1975). On the analysis of pulsed sounds by dolphins. *DAN SSSR, 225,* 229–232, as cited in Bel'kovich, V. M., & Dubrovskii, N. A. (1976). *Sensory basis of cetacean orientation* (Izdatel'stov Nauka, Leningrad).

Vel'min, V. A., & Dubrovskii, N. A. (1976). The critical interval of active hearing in dolphins. *Soviet Physical Acoustics, 22,* 351–352.

Vel'min, V. A., & Dubrovskii, N. A. (1978). Auditory perception by bottlenose dolphins of pulsed sounds. In V. Ye. Sokolov (Ed.), *Marine mammals: Results and methods of study* (pp. 90–98). Moscow: Nauka Publications.

Warden, C. J., & Warner, L. H. (1928). Sensory capacities and intelligence of dogs. *Quarterly Review of Biology, 3,* 1–28.

Warren, R. M. (1970). Perceptual restoration of missing speech sounds. *Science, 167,* 392–393.

Watkins, W. A. (1967). The harmonic interval: Fact or artifact in spectral analysis of pulse trains. In W. N. Tavolga (Ed.), *Marine bio-acoustics* (Vol. 2, pp. 15–43). Oxford, England: Pergamon Press.

Watkins, W. A., & Schevill, W. E. (1974). Listening to Hawaiian spinner dolphins, *Stenella longirostris,* with a three-dimensional hydrophone array. *Journal of Mammalogy, 55,* 319–328.

Waugh, N. C., & Norman, D. A. (1965). Primary memory. *Psychological Review, 72,* 89–104.

Wegel, R. L., & Lane, C. E. (1924). The auditory masking of one pure tone by another and its probable relation to the dynamics of the inner ear. *Physiological Reviews, 23,* 266–285.

Wever, E. G., McCormick, J. G., Palin, J., & Ridgway, S. H. (1971a). The cochlea of the dolphin, *Tursiops truncatus:* General morphology. *Proceedings of the National Academy of Science, 68,* 2381–2385.

Wever, E. G., McCormick, J. G., Palin, J., & Ridgway, S. H. (1971b). The cochlea of the dolphin, *Tursiops truncatus:* The basilar membrane. *Proceedings of the National Academy of Science, 68,* 2708–2711.

Wever, E. G., McCormick, J. G., Palin, J., & Ridgway, S. H. (1971c). The cochlea of the dolphin, *Tursiops truncatus:* Hair cells and ganglion cells. *Proceedings of the National Academy of Science, 68,* 2908–2912.

White, M. J., Norris, J., Ljungblad, D., Baron, K., & di Sciara, G. (1978). *Auditory thresholds of two beluga whales.* (Hubbs Sea World, Technical Report 78–109). San Diego.

Wood, F. G. (1953). Underwater sound production and concurrent behavior of captured porpoises, *Tursiops truncatus* and *Stenella plagiodon. Bulletin of Marine Science of the Gulf and Caribbean, 3,* 120–133.

Wood, F. G. (1973). *Marine mammals and man.* Washington, DC: Luce.

Woods, D. L., Ridgway, S. H., Carder, D. A., & Bullock, T. H. (1986). Middle- and long-latency auditory event-related potentials in dolphins. In R. J. Schusterman, J. A. Thomas, & F. G. Wood (Eds.), *Dolphin cognition and behavior: A comparative approach* (pp. 347–359). Hillsdale, NJ: Lawrence Erlbaum Associates.

Wursig, B. (1986). Delphinid foraging strategies. In R. J. Schusterman, J. A. Thomas, & F. G. Wood (Eds.), *Dolphin cognition and behavior: A comparative approach* (pp. 347–359). Hillsdale, NJ: Lawrence Erlbaum Associates.

Wursig, B., & Wursig, M. (1979). Behavior and ecology of bottlenose porpoises, *Tursiops truncatus*, in the south Atlantic. *Fishery Bulletin, 77,* 399–442.

Wursig, B., & Wursig, M. (1980). Behavior and ecology of the dusky porpoises, *Lagenorhyncus obscurus*, in the south Atlantic. *Fishery Bulletin, 77,* 871–890.

Yunker, M. P., & Herman, L. M. (1974). Discrimination of auditory temporal differences by the bottlenose dolphin and by the human. *Journal of the Acoustical Society of America, 56,* 1870–1875.

Zanin, A. V., & Zaslavskii, G. L. (1977). Temporal resolving power of the auditory analyzer of the dolphin Tursiops truncatus. *Zhurnal Evolyutsionnoi Biokhimii i Fiziologii, 13,* 491–493.

Zaytseva, K. A. (1978). Role of directivity of dolphin auditory analyzer in isolating signal from noise. In V. Ye. Sokolov (Ed.), *Marine mammals: Results and methods of study* (pp. 99–105). Moscow: Nauka Publications.

Zwicker, E. (1961). Subdivision of the audible frequency range into critical bands (Frequenzyruppen). *Journal of the Acoustical Society of America, 33,* 248.

Zwicker, E., Flottorp, G., & Stevens, S. S. (1957). Critical bandwidth in loudness summation. *Journal of the Acoustical Society of America, 29,* 548–557.

Editorial Comments on Hulse

This article describes research on the perception of complex arbitrary sound patterns by European starlings. The author draws his theoretical ideas from the realm of human music perception, specifically, in this case, the fact that humans are excellent perceivers of relative pitch. That is, they learn melodies by attending to the higher or lower pitch relationships that exist in a melody from one note to the next (see chapter by Carterette and Kendall). They do not remember the absolute pitch of sounds very well at all. Because of the propensity for relational perception, humans recognize a familiar melody regardless of the key in which it is played—or whether it is played in a high or low range at the top or bottom of the piano keyboard.

Research is based on a comparative approach which emphasizes that the proper null hypothesis in comparative psychology is the assumption that all species are equal in their capacity to process acoustic information. This hypothesis has the property that it is easily rejected in an area of research where one is often led subtly to presume that species are in fact different. The presumption of equal species capacity can lead to questions which might not otherwise be asked.

These theoretical strategies are applied to research on relative pitch perception in arbitrary sound patterns by songbirds. In a surprising twist, the data suggest that unlike humans songbirds are not very adept at processing relative pitch. Given patterns which to humans would be easily solved on the basis of "higher than" or "lower than" pitch relations, birds preferred to distinguish the patterns by attending to isolated pitch features in their structure. That is, they used absolute pitch strategies to code the stimuli—although other experiments showed that they could use relative pitch perception when pressed to do so. The role of absolute pitch perception in natural avian communication remains to be explored, but these results are certainly reminiscent of those described by Moody and Stebbins for monkeys (Chapter 12). It is possible that birdsong is coded significantly by the absolute frequency information contained in the syllables and phrases that comprise it. Perhaps the same is true for the communicative utterances of other species. In any case, the research shows once again that much of profit can be learned by applying principles of human cognition to a comparative analysis of animal behavior.

11 Comparative Psychology and Pitch Pattern Perception in Songbirds

Stewart H. Hulse
Johns Hopkins University

INTRODUCTION

This article describes some comparative research with songbirds that rests uniquely upon fact and theory drawn from human cognitive psychology. The consequences of that research are twofold. First, new light has been shed upon some sound dimensions to which songbirds are especially sensitive in acoustic perception, dimensions which they may use in acoustic communication. Second, certain principles of acoustic perception have been highlighted that, by contrast, may be unique to humans.

I first discuss a general theoretical orientation to comparative psychology that has helped guide the resarch program. Next, I describe the domain in human cognitive psychology that has provided the major theoretical impetus for the research. I then outline the results of some experiments on pitch perception in songbirds that was stimulated by theory. Finally, I discuss some implications of the research for natural acoustic communication in songbirds.

I. HYPOTHESES IN COMPARATIVE PSYCHOLOGY

A comparative psychologist faces an unusual and subtle problem when developing ideas for research. The problem is fundamental yet it, and especially its implications, may be overlooked. If not overlooked, the problem may nevertheless be addressed without explicit consideration. And it becomes exquisitely acute in comparative research on complex cognitive processes. That topic enjoys a great deal of recent attention in psychology and encompasses the research described in this chapter. The problem is this: What should one choose for the proper null hypothesis in comparative research?

The problem, though fundamental, is indeed subtle. That is so because the very idea of a comparative analysis of behavior starts, virtually by definition, with a stress upon *differences* in behavior across species. It is the concept of species variation that evokes the interest of the comparative psychologist. Faced with a world of differences, the comparative psychologist may be led to formulate research problems in terms of differences, and therein lies a trap. If a problem is expressed for study in terms of differences, it may lead to a null hypothesis also expressed in differences. And such a null hypothesis is incapable of disproof on purely logical, to say nothing of practical grounds. Put quite simply, how do you *disprove* the hypothesis that two behaviors are *different?*

Things work much better on a null hypothesis of species *identity.* One can disprove on both logical grounds and by practical means the null hypothesis that some aspect of the behavior of two or more species is identical. All that is required is some appropriately controlled situation in which the behavior in question differs such that the null hypothesis can be rejected with an appropriate confidence level. A null hypothesis of species identity, then, is the proper one for comparative psychology—and the general solution to the problem posed at the outset.

Once expressed, the problem—and its solution—seem trivial, perhaps to the point of absurdity. But there are implications of the solution and the thinking that lies behind it that are deep and potentially profound. For example, here is C. Lloyd Morgan's famous canon expressed in his *Comparative Psychology* (1894):

> In no case may we interpret an action as the outcome of the exercise of a higher psychical activity, if it can be interpreted as the outcome of an exercise of one which stands lower in the psychological scale. (p. 53)

Morgan's statement was a plea for parsimony stimulated by the then-current use of the anecdotal method in comparative psychology and the free and uncritical attribution of human capacities to nonhuman animals (Romanes, 1882). But note that it is a plea based on a concept of implicit functional *differences*, namely, *higher* versus *lower* psychical activity. And it provides no *a priori* grounds for establishing a higher versus lower metric. The canon invites, subtly but inexorably, analytic predispositions based on presumed differences in behavior.

Morgan's expression of his plea in terms of differences, especially differences in "psychic activity," may have encouraged American radical behaviorism to embrace the canon as a justification for rejecting the comparative study of cognitive function—in the name of parsimony. And this, in turn, may have contributed to the dearth of comparative research on cognitive function in America for three quarters of a century. A full discussion of this and similar issues is far beyond the scope of this chapter and is under development elsewhere, but certain points are especially relevant for the effort at hand and may be mentioned briefly.

If one adopts truly a comparative strategy based on a null hypothesis of species identity, one is encouraged, even compelled, to ask questions that might not otherwise seem worth entertaining. For example, consider the issue of language in nonhuman primates. An a priori assumption of species differences may well have discouraged comparative research on a possible nonhuman capacity for language for a long time. It wasn't until the middle of the 20th Century—50 years or more since Morgan's statement—that serious research was undertaken for the first time, for example, the Hayes' work with the chimpanzee, Viki (Hayes & Hayes, 1951). That research began with an impeccable null hypothesis of identity—Viki was going to vocalize and talk just like humans—and it wasn't long before that null hypothesis was rejected convincingly. Viki never learned to utter more than a few words, like "cup," for example. Of course, the Gardners (Gardner & Gardner, 1969) soon came along with an insight into the reason for the Hayes' failure (chimpanzees do not possess the necessary articulatory apparatus to vocalize like humans)—and obtained evidence with sign language suggesting the null hypothesis of species identity for language capacity could be rejected only with much greater difficulty. Furthermore, the conditions that lead to rejection are still under intensive study, with important comparative data still emerging rapidly (e.g., Savage-Rumbaugh, McDonald, Sevcik, Hopkins, & Rubert, 1986). Interestingly enough, too, the contribution of those working on chimpanzee language is probably just as important for the research it has stimulated on *human* language development and the knowledge and further perspective we have so acquired. Chomsky (e.g., 1968) may be right when he adopts an hypothesis of difference and presumes that language is uniquely and biologically human, but it is ironic that we have learned so much about human language because we have seriously entertained the idea that Chomsky's viewpoint on this issue is wrong.

Note that the adoption of an hypothesis of identity does not substitute for insightful techniques and analytic methods. The Gardners succeeded where the Hayes failed because the Gardners were able to find a more productive method for asking the same question. That is in no way to denigrate the Hayes' effort; they began with the strongest form of an identity hypothesis, and that is the place to start.

Nor does an identity hypothesis excuse the comparative psychologist from rigorous application of the rules of science—especially when studying cognitive function. Morgan was right in rejecting the anecdotal method. Hypotheses must be entertained only with full appreciation of tight and concise operational definitions and with impeccable empirical rigor.

II. THEORETICAL ROOTS FOR A COMPARATIVE STUDY OF COMPLEX ACOUSTIC PERCEPTION

The research described in later sections of this chapter was stimulated by a direct application of a null hypothesis of species identity. Quite specifically, it was presumed that songbirds would behave like people (a) in their ability to process acoustic information that was presented in serial order, and (b) in their perception of pitch and rhythmic structures fashioned after principles of human music perception. There was no special faith that these hypotheses would prove to be true; indeed, intuition and many other considerations suggested it would not be hard to disprove them. But if salient and clever expressions of the hypothesis of identity could be selected, then in the process of disproof, we might learn something useful about *both* human and avian acoustic perception. From a comparative viewpoint, much, perhaps more, can be learned about function in a species from instances where function fails to generalize than instances where it does.

Of course, the interesting possibility remained that we would fail to reject the identity hypothesis and, in some important respects, human and avian acoustic processing would prove to be identical—unless proved otherwise by still further experimentation based on identity hypotheses. Given the nature of acoustic signals constructed with music in mind, that would have interesting implications about many perceptual processes, such as relational constancies (which have been difficult to demonstrate in nonhuman animals), as we shall see.

Let us consider the relevant background from which the specific identity hypotheses emerged.

Cognition and Serial Pattern Perception

There is a ubiquitous property of perception and performance that underlies many things that people do. That is the ability to perceive, organize, and utilize information that occurs in serial order. Our facility with problems of serial organization leads to many things. We learn to speak and read a language. We come to appreciate and enjoy the flow of music and to perform the highly complex motor tasks that must be mastered to play musical instruments. We learn to read maps and to find our way from place to place in the environment.

Theoretical ideas about serial order in behavior stem from Aristotelian principles of association. They found a formal home in the 19th and early 20th centuries with the physiological model of the reflex and the reflex arc, a model that was formalized in more general terms by Hull (1931) and Skinner (1934). Their model was essentially that of an associatively based, linear, reflex chain, a model that, until the late 1940s, dominated not only theories of animal psychology but also theories of human motor and verbal learning. Then Lashley (1951), in a truly seminal article, drew fresh attention to the problem of serial order in behavior—in particular, to the inadequacies of the associative model in handling many forms of human perception and motor performance. He found common examples in human language where meaning depended crucially upon the location of a word in a structure (the sentence) that had a *hierarchical* as opposed to a linear form. He noted that pianists could play arpeggios much faster than any model allowed that depended upon peripheral feedback to organize the flow of behavior. The serial organization of behavior begged for a top down, pre-programmed process.

Lashley's thinking was an impetus for many new developments. It was a statement found compatible by those, such as Chomsky and G. A. Miller, who began to develop the field of psycholinguistics in the later 1950s. It encouraged a model of human thought and memory based on the computer metaphor that began to take shape at about the same time (Miller, Galanter, & Pribram, 1960). Most important for the topic at hand, Lashley's thoughts stimulated theory and research on the problem of serial order in behavior most generally conceived, an effort that began in the early 1960s.

Fifteen years later, general theories of human serial pattern learning had become reasonably well formed (Jones, 1974, 1978; Restle, 1970, 1972; Simon, 1972; Simon & Kotovsky, 1963). Although the theories differed in detail, they shared many common properties.

Symbols and Alphabets. All theories start with an assumption that serial patterns are constructed from sets of *symbols* that form *alphabets* (Hulse & O'Leary, 1982; Jones, 1978; Simon & Kotovsky, 1963). A symbol is any stimulus event that is discriminably different from other stimulus events. That is, any set of stimulus events possesses the properties of a nominal scale (Stevens, 1951). Sets of such symbols form alphabets when the symbols are *ordered*. That is, the symbols must be arranged so the set also possesses the properties of an ordinal scale. Alphabets may, of course, also possess equal-interval and ratio properties (Hulse & Cynx, 1986; Stevens, 1951).

Alphabets, Rules, and Patterns. The application of *rules* to alphabets generates *serial patterns*. Given an initialization point in an alphabet, that is, the first symbol of the pattern, a rule or set of rules describe the process necessary to generate the next symbol(s) in the pattern. Most theories of serial pattern learning include REPEAT, NEXT, REVERSE, and INVERSE rules, although others may be added as well. Rules are often applied to alphabets to generate formally complex, hierarchically organized serial patterns as contrasted with formally simple, linear serial patterns.

Learning Serial Patterns. A great deal of research has been done with a great many alphabets (ranging from letters to numbers to tones from musical scales) to study how people learn serial patterns, and to discover the mechanisms they use in the process (e.g., Boltz, Marshburn, Jones, & Johnson, 1985; Deutsch & Feroe, 1981; Garner & Gottwald, 1968; Greeno & Simon, 1974; Hulse & Dorsky, 1979; Jones, 1974, 1978; Jones & Zamostny, 1975; Restle, 1970, 1972; Royer & Garner, 1966; Simon & Kotovsky, 1963). A number of generalizations have come from that research. For example, people parse patterns into groups of symbols that are bounded by rule changes. That is they tend to *chunk* a pattern into subgroups. People tend to extrapolate patterns. When asked to extend a pattern, they add a symbol based on a simple extension of the rule structure they have learned—although there is nothing in the formal structure of a pattern that demands this process. People find patterns with complex as compared with simple formal structure more difficult to learn. A valid general definition of pattern complexity is hard to come by, but complexity is often correlated, for example, with the number of different rules contained by the pattern.

Music as a Serial Pattern

Musical melodies possess all the formal requirements of serial patterns. All musical scales are, in fact, based on a log scale of frequency that meets all the requirements of an equal-ratio scale. Therefore, all musical scales are alphabets. All musical scales are also based on the interval of an *octave* between two tones, an interval in which the frequency of one tone is double that of the other. Musical scales differ in the size of the intervals that separate neighboring tones within an octave. For example, the chromatic scale divides the octave into 12 equal intervals (semitones) on the log scale of frequency, while the whole-tone scale divides the octave into 6 equal intervals (whole tones). The diatonic scale so characteristic of classical Western music is a mixture of whole tones and semitones.

Melodies are generated by applying rules to the alphabet of the musical scale. For example,

CDEDEFEFG

describes a melody, a *melodic contour,* based on a diatonic scale in the key of C major. The melody is initialized on middle C, the tonic of the scale (with a fundamental frequency of 256 Hz near the center of the piano keyboard), and subsequent notes are based on NEXT rules overarched hierarchically by another NEXT rule. The melody is not unlike something Bach might have used to begin a prelude or fugue. Of course, Bach would never have left matters there (he would have added other simultaneous melodic contours to form vertical *harmonic structure,* for example), and rule structures in the hands of any composer rapidly become complex. In fact, the composer usually tries to break rules ingeniously in the service of musical interest and compositional elegance and mood.

Many of the perceptual principles that hold for serial patterns in general hold for music in particular. For example, the perception of melodic contours generalizes easily to other musical alphabets—other keys, for example. A familiar melody written in the key of C major will be readily identified if it is transposed 5 semitones higher to the key of F major (a shift in overall *tone height*). Given time between a rendition of the melody in C major and its repetition in F major, many people may not even notice the shift. Melodies transpose equally well with shifts in tone height from one octave to another, a phenomenon known as *octave generalization*. In fact, one early model for musical perception (Deutsch, 1969; Shepard, 1965) represents the scales from which melodies are built as a helix coiling upwards about a vertical frequency axis marked in octave intervals. Given scale locations across octaves are represented at the same circular coordinate on the helix, implying that they are perceptually similar. Later models build on these earlier ideas to elaborate the early model substantially (Deutsch & Feroe, 1981; Shepard, 1982).

The foregoing indicates that people generally have excellent memory for the pitch *relations* between the successive notes that comprise a melody. If the pitch relations are constant (that is, the ratios of the frequencies of neighboring tones are constant), perceptual constancy is maintained even though the actual frequencies involved may change substantially. As a matter of fact, people generally have *poor* memory for *absolute* frequencies in music. Not many have perfect pitch—an ability, loosely speaking, to name a given musical note upon hearing it, or to identify accurately the key in which a given melody is played.

III. COMPARATIVE RESEARCH ON PITCH PATTERN PERCEPTION

The theoretical principles of human serial pattern perception and music perception I have just discussed suggested some comparative research on acoustic perception in nonhuman animals. At the time the research was undertaken, much was known about the fundamental psychophysical attributes of hearing in many species (e.g., Dooling, 1982; Stebbins, 1970). And a good deal was understood about the functional significance of acoustic communication, such as that associated with birdsong (e.g., Greenewalt, 1968; Marler, 1960; Kroodsma & Miller, 1982; Thorpe, 1961). However, virtually nothing was known directly about any general principles governing more *complex* acoustic perception in animals—especially the perception of arbitrary acoustic patterns. There had been no attempt to look at birdsong, for example, as an event possibly representative of—or based on—more general perceptual processes.

To that end, I and my colleagues began research on acoustic perception in songbirds based on some things we knew about serial pattern perception and music perception in humans. The strong hypothesis was an identity hypothesis—we presumed that songbirds would perceive pitch patterns just like people, an hypothesis that immediately yielded some ideas for experiments. The hypothesis had another useful property, as we have seen: if wrong, it would be easy to disprove.

In selecting species for study, any might have sufficed in principle, but European starlings (*Sturnus vulgaris*) were chosen because they were easy to obtain and, as matters developed, easy to maintain and train in the laboratory.

Furthermore, and most important, they are excellent mimics (Kroodsma, 1982)—good a priori evidence that they could learn acoustic patterns and were not locked perceptually to some species-specific song. This was important because the research was to start with sound patterns that did not occur in nature.

Experimental procedures were straightforward (Hienz, Sinnott, & Sachs, 1977; Hulse, Cynx, & Humpal, 1984). Birds were first taught with operant techniques to peck at one lighted disk on the wall of a sound attenuating chamber for a food reward. Then, in a baseline discrimination task, the birds learned that pecks on that disk started one of two sound patterns, Pattern A or Pattern B. Shortly, after a 4-s listening period, a second disk lit up. If Pattern A played, a peck on the second disk ended the sound pattern and produced food. If Pattern B played, a peck on the second disk ended the sound pattern and produced an immediate time out—the key and chamber lights darkened for 10 s. If the bird withheld a peck in the presence of Pattern B for 4 s, the pattern and the trial ended. In all cases, the next trial began 5 s later. Daily sessions were typically 0.5 to 1 hr long; in some experiments, they were 3 hr long.

Successful discrimination appeared when the birds responded rapidly with short latencies on the second disk to Pattern A and with long latencies (approaching or equal to 4 s) to Pattern B. Given initial acquisition of this GO/NO-GO discrimination, the experiments then explored the factors controlling the baseline discrimination. Typically, transfer tests were used which studied changes in discrimination behavior with altered baseline stimuli. If a stimulus change produced a change in discrimination, that change was presumed to identify a functionally significant aspect of the acoustic stimulus. However, if a stimulus change failed to disrupt discrimination behavior, the change was presumed to be functionally irrelevant. In this way, we could uncover, step by step, those perceptual processes the birds could use to process complex acoustic patterns.

Relative and Absolute Pitch Pattern Perception and the Frequency Range Constraint

The first experiments were designed to study songbirds' perception of relative pitch in complex pitch patterns. Those experiments quickly turned into a study of absolute pitch perception as well because the birds behaved very much as if they were attending to certain absolute aspects of the acoustic stimuli.

Rising and Falling Pitch Patterns.   The first experiment (Hulse et al. 1984) asked two simple questions, as a matter of fact the simplest we could think of based on considerations of serial pattern learning and pitch perception: Could songbirds learn to discriminate patterns that rose in pitch from patterns that fell in pitch? That is, could the birds learn to make a *relational* discrimination? Based on human acoustic perception, that discrimination should be learned with ease (Deutsch, 1978). Second, given that the birds learned the discrimination, what features of the stimuli controlled perceptual processing?

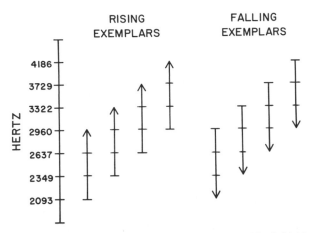

FIG. 11.1.   Rising and falling four-tone exemplars used for initial baseline training. The frequencies (in Hertz) for the tones are arranged at
equal intervals on a log scale, the whole-tone musical scale.

To these ends, starlings learned to discriminate between the classes of four-
tone rising and falling patterns displayed in Fig. 11.1 (Hulse et al. 1984). The
patterns all contained tones with frequencies located within one octave. The
tones divided the octave into 6 equal intervals; hence the patterns were based on a
whole-tone, log scale of frequency. Across the set of rising or falling patterns,
there was substantial overlap in tone frequencies. All patterns were generated by
the computer with a temporal structure such that each tone was 100 msec long
with a 100-msec intertone interval. Sequences of four tones were separated by an
intersequence interval of 800 msec. Thus, during a 4-sec listening period initiated by a starting peck, the birds heard a repeating pattern that configured a
sequence into 4-tone groups. Four starlings learned the rising/falling discrimination within 2 to 4 weeks. At that time, latencies were on the order of 0.6 s for
patterns associated with the GO contingency. Latencies approached 4 s for
patterns associated with the NO-GO contingency. Apparently, songbirds learned
a relational discrimination with ease.

The next step was to ascertain how much and what type of information the
birds required from each pattern to decide whether it fell in the class of rising or
falling patterns. In some test sessions, patterns were shortened to 3 or 2 tones to
see how much relative information the birds required to solve the discrimination.

Other transfers tested for the possibility the birds were not using a relative
pitch strategy at all. Instead, they might have been using an absolute pitch
strategy in which they coded a pattern as rising or falling based on the absolute
frequency of the pattern's first or last tone. Although the patterns were designed
with substantial overlap in tone frequencies, most patterns began or ended with a
unique frequency. To test for the possibility the birds were utilizing absolute
pitch information, we introduced occasional probe stimuli against background

trials of the baseline rising/falling discrimination. The probe trials incorporated a single tone of a given frequency, with frequency varying from trial to trial. If the birds were coding on the basis of absolute frequency, they ought to give latencies characteristic of rising exemplars when tested with low frequencies, because all rising exemplars began on low frequencies in the range. Similarly, the birds should produce latencies characteristic of falling exemplars when tested with high frequencies, because all falling exemplars began on high frequencies in the range.

Other probe stimuli pitted a possible absolute strategy against a relative strategy directly. Here, probe patterns began on a given frequency, but "went the wrong way." For example, in baseline training the 4-tone pattern beginning on 3322 Hz always fell to 2349 Hz. In the transfer, the pattern became a 3-tone pattern that rose in pitch to 4186 Hz. If the birds were responding on absolute pitch alone, they ought to classify the pattern as a falling pattern because it began on a high frequency in the range. If, however, they were capable of using relative pitch, they ought to classify the pattern as rising because it did, in fact, ascend in pitch.

The results of the transfer tests based on pattern length showed that the starlings required only two tones to discriminate rising from falling patterns. However, their performance improved the more information they received, i.e., the longer the pattern. As Fig. 11.2 shows, the latency differences between rising and falling patterns became smaller as stimuli moved from repeated 4-tone baseline stimuli to 4-, 3-, and 2-tone probe stimuli. Of course, there were no latency differences for single tones (arbitrarily designated by the computer as "rising" or "falling").

The simple conclusion that songbirds require only a minimum of relative pitch information to process rising and falling patterns is colored substantially, however, by the results of the other transfer tests. These provided clear evidence that the birds used both relative and *absolute* frequency to solve the discrimination. Thus, as Fig. 11.2 shows, there was a gradual overall shift in response latencies for *both* rising and falling patterns as frequencies moved from low to high in the one-octave test range. The latency differences associated with rising as compared with falling patterns maintained themselves, but were biased by the effect associated with the change in absolute frequency. The effect of absolute frequency alone appeared in its purest form when relative pitch information was removed by using single tones on probe trials. Latencies decreased by more than half as probe stimuli moved from low to high frequencies.

The course of latency changes displayed in Fig. 11.2 follows sensibly from reinforcement conditions for stimuli associated with GO and NO-GO stimuli. Thus, rising sequences—associated with nonreinforcement for which a long-latency NO-GO reaction was appropriate—began on low frequencies. Falling sequences—associated with reinforcement for which a short-latency GO response was appropriate—began on high frequencies. The birds simply generalized this inherent bias as frequencies moved about in the range.

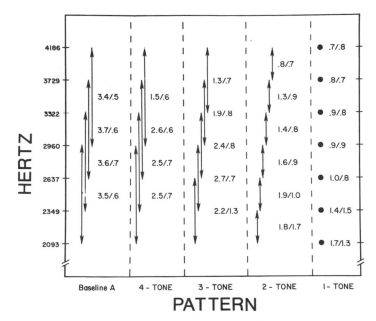

FIG. 11.2.   Mean response latencies for each exemplar under initial Baseline conditions in which exemplars repeated through a listening period, and for exemplars of varying length heard just once on a trial. The latencies to the left of the slash are reaction times on NO-GO trials for rising exemplars; those on the right are reaction times on GO trials for falling exemplars. The data for single tones were arbitrarily classified by the computer as rising or falling.

It is tempting to conclude that the birds were processing all patterns on the basis of absolute frequency alone. Figure 11.1 shows this could have happened because within each rising and falling exemplar there is a frequency unique to that exemplar—in spite of great overlap in frequencies across exemplars. In designing the stimuli, we exhibited the human predilection for processing on the basis of relative pitch and failed to control completely for the possible use of absolute pitch cues. For example the initial frequencies of each rising exemplar (except that beginning on 2960 Hz, the middlemost frequency in the range) are unique to each pattern. So are the terminal frequencies.

To test for the possible exclusive use of absolute pitch, we introduced some probe stimuli that pitted an absolute against a relative pitch strategy. These probe stimuli started, say, on a high frequency normally associated with a falling pattern and "went the wrong way," rising instead of falling. Consider, for example, a 3-tone probe exemplar beginning on 3322 Hz and rising to 3729 Hz and 4186 Hz. In baseline training, all exemplars beginning on 3322 Hz fell in frequency and produced short latencies. Here, however, the pattern rose in frequency. If the birds responded on the probe pattern on the basis of absolute pitch, they should give short latencies characteristic of rapid GO responding to high frequencies. If, however, they responded on the basis of relative pitch, they should give long latencies characteristic of NO-GO responding to rising patterns. As Fig. 11.2 shows, the birds responded to the probe stimuli in a relative way, producing, in this case, long latencies characteristic of rising patterns.

To sum up, these initial results suggest that songbirds process complex acoustic patterns using *both* relative and absolute pitch. They appear to respond to the formal relations that define whether a pattern rises or falls in pitch. However, they also respond differentially to the absolute frequency of the tones from which patterns are built.

Octave Generalization and the Frequency Range Constraint.   We obtained further evidence that songbirds are sensitive to absolute pitch when we tested starlings, cowbirds (*Molothrus ater*), and one male mockingbird (*Mimus polyglottus*) for octave generalization (Hulse & Cynx, 1985). Recall that humans typically maintain perceptual constancy for melodies that are shifted up or down an octave in pitch. That is, human melody perception works on a relational basis, with perceptual constancy appearing for successive pitch relations maintaining constant frequency ratios. On the basis of our strong hypothesis that songbirds perceive pitch patterns like humans, we expected all three bird species to show octave generalization, too, The use of cowbirds and mockingbirds would add another comparative dimension to the research; mockingbirds are among the best mimics among songbirds, while cowbirds show no particular mimicking ability (Kroodsma & Miller, 1982). However, cowbirds are nest parasites, suggesting that like mimicking species, they do attend to the song of other species and show some a priori flexibility in acoustic perception.

To test for octave generalization, after training the birds on the 4-tone rising/falling stimuli, the frequencies of the baseline stimuli were halved or doubled (to lower or raise the frequencies an octave, respectively) in separate transfer tests.

When this was done, the results were striking and unexpected (on the strong hypothesis of species identity). With the first shift, which was down an octave in frequency, all birds regardless of species lost the rising/falling discrimination instantly. Performance is shown in Fig. 11.3. The figure indicates stable discrimination for the three days prior to the transfer, and a sudden loss of the discrimination in the first transfer session. Although the figure does not show it, the discrimination was lost from the outset of the session. Three of the four starlings, H1, H3, and H4, relearned the discrimination in the new frequency range in 8, 20, and 29 sessions—as compared with 15, 25, and 34 sessions in original baseline training. Thus there was some evidence of savings, but probably only marginal evidence because initial training was no doubt extended by factors irrelevant to the discrimination, such as initial accommodation to the test apparatus and procedures. In an absolute sense, relearning in the new range took

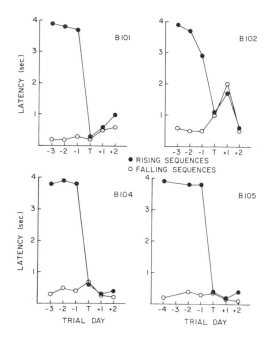

FIG. 11.3. The frequency range constraint. Response latencies on NO-GO trials for rising sequences and GO trials for falling sequences for four starlings. Days −3, −2, and −1 occurred just prior to an octave shift downward in frequency, Day T was the day of the shift, and Days +1 and +2 were the days just after the shift. The discrimination was immediately and completely lost with the shift on Day T.

many sessions under conditions where we would expect rapid recovery of the discrimination if positive transfer had prevailed. The fourth bird (H2), in fact, failed to relearn after 48 sessions in the novel range.

The discrimination returned immediately with full vigor for all four birds when stimuli were shifted back to the baseline range, indicating the downward transfer had not had some catastrophic effect on memory. However, the discrimination disappeared immediately once again when stimuli were suddenly shifted an octave above the baseline range. The data virtually duplicate those appearing in Fig. 11.3. Once again, there was only small evidence of savings in the novel frequency range (Birds H1, H3, and H4 relearned in 17, 24, and 9 sessions, respectively). In this case, bird H2 did relearn the discrimination in 31 sessions.

The behavior of the two cowbirds and the mockingbird was qualitatively identical to that of the starlings. All learned the baseline discrimination, and all lost it immediately with the octave shift to the lower range. For the cowbirds, only one recovered reliable discrimination in the novel range (after 26 sessions), and it never reached a criterion of a 2-s difference between GO and NO-GO stimuli achieved during initial discrimination. The mockingbird showed little sign of relearning after 32 sessions in the novel range. Once again, however, both cowbirds and the mockingbird recovered the discrimination rapidly when returned to baseline stimuli.

Another test with new birds trained the rising/falling discrimination initially in *two* ranges, leaving a gap of unused frequencies in between. After learning the discrimination in both ranges (the birds lost the discrimination and had to relearn it, of course, when shifted from the first to the second range), they were shifted to rising and falling patterns in the novel frequency gap. This was a very strong test for positive transfer of the rising/falling discrimination because generalization of the discrimination should summate from both the high and low range into the gap. However, once again, the birds immediately lost the rising/falling discrimination.

At this point, a natural question occurred. Perhaps the birds were incapable of transferring the discrimination to *any* novel stimuli. Perhaps they were truly locked to the absolute frequencies of the individual tones incorporated in the initial discrimination. As a test for this possibility, birds were given a session of familiar baseline rising and falling patterns. Within the session, they heard occasional rising and falling *probe* patterns with novel frequencies chosen from the familiar range in which they had learned the discrimination initially. The frequencies in the novel patterns were a semitone away from baseline frequencies, an interval easily discriminable by the birds. Here, there was immediate transfer to the novel probe patterns: the starlings performed just as well as they did for standard baseline patterns. Apparently, the earlier losses of discrimination were confined to novel frequencies *outside a range made familiar by extensive training*. For this reason, Jeffrey Cynx, in part of his dissertation (Cynx, Hulse, & Polyzois 1986), named the phenomenon the *frequency range constraint*.

Further work has shown that starlings are exquisitely sensitive to the frequency boundaries of the training range; the frequency range constraint appears with minimal frequency shifts outside the range. Cynx trained birds with the usual 4-tone rising and falling sequences (Cynx et al. 1986). Then occasional unreinforced probe patterns were introduced that incorporated frequencies such that the initial one, two, or three tones were outside the familiar training range. The starlings lost the discrimination when just two initial tones of the probe patterns were outside the range. In a second experiment, Cynx eliminated all relative pitch information by using 4-tone probe sequences of a single repeating frequency. Frequencies were chosen to span both the familiar training range and novel ranges an octave above and below the training range. Sequence frequencies were separated by a semitone on a log scale of frequency. Results of this experiment showed latency changes associated with sequences covering frequencies outside the training range that were virtually identical to those obtained in the earlier experiment for 4-tone patterns that rose or fell in pitch. As frequencies changed within the training range, latencies for sequences of a single frequency did not differ as much as latencies for 4-tone rising or falling patterns that began with the same frequencies, but there was still a substantial and reliable shift. Most important, shifts in response latency characteristic of the range constraint appeared for high- and low-range sequences with frequencies that were just one semitone removed from the baseline range. This suggests that the sharpness of the constraint boundary may approach the difference limen for frequency.

Further experiments addressed primarily at other issues have provided additional evidence supporting both the existence and the generality of the frequency range constraint. In their study of the perception of frequency contours, for example, Hulse and Cynx (1986) found that starlings trained with the usual 4-tone baseline rising and falling patterns responded to the ordinal, as opposed to the equal-interval or ratio, properties of the patterns. Overlying this, however, was the familiar predominant tendency to respond to the absolute frequency location of the test stimuli within the baseline range.

Relative Pitch Perception Without Absolute Pitch Cues

The range constraint and the salience of absolute pitch perception were discovered, as we have seen, because of a partial confound between relational and absolute pitch cues in baseline discriminative stimuli (cf. Fig. 11.1). What would happen to discrimination if the confound were removed, and starlings were presented with a set of rising and falling pitch stimuli in which absolute pitch was removed as a potential differentiating cue? Would the birds learn under these conditions, or would they fail to do so—reflecting once again a dependence on absolute frequency perception?

Suzanne Page addressed these questions directly (Page, Hulse, & Cynx, in press). She prepared a set of 64 stimulus patterns, half of which rose or fell in pitch, respectively. Patterns could be 2, 3, or 4 tones long, and they were based on semitone intervals. The set of stimuli included frequencies spanning the range 988 to 2217 Hz (i.e., an octave plus two whole tones). The patterns were constructed such that a tone with a given frequency provided no consistent information about whether subsequent tones would rise or fall in pitch, or how many of them there would be.

The stimulus set embodied the strategy that the relational concept of rising versus falling pitch could be taught by using many exemplars for which the only common feature was the rising/falling pitch relation in question. The strategy was patterned after that used in teaching natural concepts to animals (e.g., Herrnstein, Loveland, & Cable, 1976), although to our knowledge, this was the first attempt to do so with acoustic stimuli.

The results of the experiment were straightforward: after as many as 30,000 trials, four starlings showed no evidence whatsoever of learning the rising/falling pitch discrimination. A second stage of Page's research showed that four new birds could learn to distinguish rising from falling patterns if the set was reduced to eight exemplars and patterned after those of Fig. 11.1, i.e., if absolute pitch was reintroduced as a potential cue. So the initial failure to learn was not due to some incapacity to process pitch information unique to Page's conditions as compared with those prevailing in earlier research. A third stage of the research was especially interesting, however. Here, the birds trained on the 8-exemplar set were tested with exemplars from the initial 64-exemplar set. Under these conditions, the birds could now classify some of the initial stimuli on the basis of their pitch relations. Perhaps the initial 32-exemplar set contained just too much information (e.g., the patterns varied not only in pitch structure but also in length) for the birds to manage at one time. In any case, some preliminary training on a simpler and smaller 8-exemplar set appeared to have set the stage for more successful processing of rising/falling pitch relationships. These are complicated data currently undergoing further analysis—especially with respect to the role of absolute and relative pitch perception in the third stage of the experiment.

All the foregoing leads to an obvious question: if songbirds are so good at adopting absolute pitch strategies in situations designed to induce relative pitch perception, how would they do if asked directly to manage absolute pitch? We are addressing that question now.

IV. CONCLUSIONS AND SPECULATIONS

What are we to make of these results? To summarize, first, it appears that at least three species of songbirds depend extensively on the absolute pitch properties of complex acoustic patterns to perceive and code them for discrimination. This propensity reveals itself in three ways, two direct and one indirect. First, the predilection to use absolute pitch appears through the loss of discrimination between two relationally defined pitch patterns when the patterns are shifted outside a familiar frequency range—the frequency range constraint. Second, the constraint appears as a response bias even within a familiar baseline range; if possible, birds are heavily predisposed to discriminate patterns on the basis of whether they are high or low in the familiar range. Third, when absolute pitch cues are removed from a relational pitch discrimination, evidence to date shows they cannot learn to make the relational discrimination.

It is too soon, however, to follow these data to the strong conclusion that songbirds process arbitrary acoustic patterns solely on the basis of absolute frequency. That is, it is too soon to conclude that they are incapable of learning pitch relationships—such as rising or falling relationships—among neighboring tones. For example, data from the Hulse et al. (1984) experiment in which patterns "went the wrong way" and rose or fell from high or low frequencies in contradiction to baseline conditions suggest that songbirds can process relative pitch information. Data from Page's experiment, which are still under analysis, also suggest relative pitch discrimination at work. Most important, there is a strong suggestion in the literature that at least one species of songbird, the black-capped chickadee (*Parus atricapillus*), makes relational transpositions in its own song (Hulse & Cynx, 1986; Ratcliffe & Weisman, 1985). All of our work to date has been with arbitrary, nonnatural stimuli; the fact that relative perception may be at work in nature is provocative and obviously worth further exploration. In fact, given the complex pitch changes that are the hallmark of the syllables and phrases of birdsong, it is difficult to imagine that such pitch information is without functional significance.

Null Hypotheses

Rejection of the null hypothesis of species identity with regard to relational pitch pattern perception has been accomplished with ease. There is some evidence that songbirds process relative pitch, but they fail to do so under conditions where humans would certainly succeed with facility. But what have we learned in this case as a consequence of the rejection of the identity hypothesis?

First, we have learned something new about the methods songbirds do use, in fact, to process pitch. The most striking observation from all the work to date is the potent role of absolute frequency in songbirds's perception of complex arbitrary sound patterns. The full scope of that form of perception remains to be explored in songbirds—especially in their own natural communication—but enough has been done to show that absolute frequency perception is a major factor under the conditions explored thus far.

Second, we have gained fresh perspective on *human* pitch perception. Humans are disposed to use relative as contrasted with absolute pitch, and that was well known, of course, before the research began. But now we are poised to ask, for example, why humans are so poor at absolute pitch perception when at least three avian species are so good at it. What conditions predispose humans to use relative over absolute pitch? Why is it that some people do nevertheless possess absolute or perfect pitch, and what are the factors and conditions leading to and controlling the process?

Finally, we are led to ask about the distribution of relative and absolute perception across all species. Is the predisposition for relational perception unique to humans? Is that for absolute perception unique to avian species? How about nonhuman primates or other mammals, for example? One can never do an exhaustive search, but it should be practical to get at least some sense of the extent to which humans and other animals do or do not share relational and absolute perception. That is important not only practically, but also theoretically; there has been at least one claim that cognitive relational capacities are reserved solely for humans—or "language-trained" chimpanzees (Premack, 1983). But above all, the failure of the hypothesis of identity has led to some interesting and meaningful new questions to ask—to be phrased for future research, of course, in the form of further identity hypotheses.

ACKNOWLEDGMENTS

Suzanne Page and Richard Braaten joined me in many discussions about this material and provided good critical reviews of the article. They have my thanks for their many suggestions and comments. I have also benefitted in many ways from the contributions of Jeffrey Cynx, and he has my appreciation, too. Thanks also to the Johns Hopkins undergraduates, too many to name, who have helped to conduct the work. The research and the preparation of this chapter were supported by National Science Foundation Research Grants BNS 8310246 and BNS 8606307.

REFERENCES

Boltz, M., Marshburn, E., Jones, M. R., & Johnson, W. R. (1985). Serial-pattern structure and temporal-order recognition. *Perception and Psychophysics, 37,* 209–217.

Chomsky, N. (1968). *Language and mind.* New York: Harcourt, Brace, & World.

Cynx, J., Hulse, S. H., & Polyzois, S. (1986). A psychophysical measure of pitch discrimination loss resulting from a frequency range constraint in European Starlings (*Sturnus vulgaris*). *Journal of Experimental Psychology: Animal Behavior Processes, 12,* 394–402.

Deutsch, D. (1969). Music recognition. *Psychological Review, 76,* 300–307.

Deutsch, D. (1978). The psychology of music. in E. C. Carterette & M. P. Friedman (Eds.), *Handbook of perception* (Vol. 10, pp. 191–224). New York: Academic Press.

Deutsch, D., & Feroe, J. (1981). The internal representation of sequences in tonal music. *Psychological Review, 88,* 503–522.

Dooling, R. J. (1982). Auditory perception in birds. In D. E. Kroodsma & E. H. Miller (Eds.), *Acoustic communication in birds* (Vol. 1, pp. 95–130). New York: Academic Press.

Gardner, R. A., & Gardner, B. T. (1969). Teaching sign language to a chimpanzee. *Science, 165,* 664–672.

Garner, W. R., & Gottwald, R. L. (1968). The perception and learning of temporal patterns. *The Quarterly Journal of Experimental Psychology, 20,* 97–109.

Greenewalt, C. H. (1968). *Bird song: Acoustics and physiology.* Washington, D.C.: Smithsonian Institution Press.

Greeno, J., & Simon, H. A. (1974). Processes for sequence production. *Psychological Review, 81,* 187–198.

Hayes, K. J., & Hayes, C. (1951). The intellectual development of a home-raised chimpanzee. *Proceedings of the American Philosophical Society, 95,* 105–109.

Herrnstein, R. J., Loveland, D. H., & Cable, C. (1976). Natural concepts in pigeons. *Journal of Experimental Psychology: Animal Behavior Processes, 2,* 285–302.

Hienz, R. D., Sinnott, J. M., & Sachs, M. B. (1977). Auditory sensitivity of the redwing blackbird and the brownheaded cowbird. *Journal of Comparative and Physiological Psychology, 91,* 1365–1376.

Hull, C. L. (1931). Goal attraction and directing ideas conceived as habit phenomena. *Psychological Review, 38,* 487–506.

Hulse, S. H., & Cynx, J. (1985). Relative pitch perception is constrained by absolute pitch in songbirds (*Mimus, Molothrus, Sturnus*). *Journal of Comparative Psychology, 99,* 176–196.

Hulse, S. H., & Cynx, J. (1986). Interval and contour in serial pitch perception by a Passerine bird, the European Starling (*Sturnus vulgaris*). *Journal of Comparative Psychology, 100,* 215–228.

Hulse, S. H., Cynx, J., & Humpal, J. (1984). Absolute and relative pitch discrimination in serial pitch perception by songbirds. *Journal of Experimental Psychology: General, 113,* 38–54.

Hulse, S. H., & Dorsky, N. (1979). Serial pattern learning by rats: Transfer of a formally defined stimulus relationship and the significance of nonreinforcement. *Animal Learning and Behavior, 7,* 211–220.

Hulse, S. H., & O'Leary, D. K. (1982). Serial pattern learning: Teaching an alphabet to rats. *Journal of Experimental Psychology: Animal Behavior Processes, 8,* 260–273.

Jones, M. R. (1974). Cognitive representations of serial patterns. In B. Kantowitz (Ed.), *Human information processing: Tutorials in performance and cognition.* Hillsdale, NJ: Lawrence Erlbaum Associates.

Jones, M. R. (1978). Auditory patterns: Studies in the perception of structure. In E. C. Carterette & M. P. Friedman (Eds.), *Handbook of perception* (Vol. 8, pp. 255–288). New York: Academic Press.

Jones, M. R., & Zamnosty, (1975). Memory and rule structure in the prediction of serial patterns. *Journal of Experimental Psychology: Human Learning and Memory, 104,* 295–306.

Kroodsma, D. E., & Miller, E. H. (Eds.). (1982). *Acoustic communication in birds* (Vols. I and II). New York: Academic Press.

Lashley, K. S. (1951). The problem of serial order in behavior. In L. H. Jeffress (Ed.), *Cerebral mechanisms in behavior.* New York: Wiley.

Marler, P. (1960). Bird songs and mate selection. In W. E. Lanyon & W. N. Tavolga (Eds.), *Animal sounds and communication* (pp. 348–367). Washington, D.C.: American Institute of Biological Sciences.

Miller, G. A., Galanter, E., & Pribram, K. H. (1960). *Plans and the structure of behavior.* New York: Holt.

Morgan, C. L. (1894). *An introduction to comparative psychology.* New York: Scribner's Sons.

Page, S. C., Hulse, S. H., & Cynx, J. (in press). Relative pitch perception in the European starling (*Sturnus vulgaris*): Further evidence for an elusive phenomenon. *Journal of Experimental Psychology: Animal Learning and Behavior.*

Premack, D. (1983). The codes of man and beast. *The Behavioral and Brain Sciences, 6,* 125–167.

Ratcliffe, L., & Weisman, R. G. (1985). Frequency shift in the *fee bee* song of the black-capped chickadee. *Condor, 87,* 555–556.

Restle, F. A. (1970). Theory of serial pattern learning: Structural trees. *Psychological Review, 77,* 481–495.

Restle, F. A. (1972). Serial patterns: The role of phrasing. *Journal of Experimental Psychology, 92,* 385–390.

Romanes, G. J. (1882). *Animal intelligence.* London: Kegan, Paul, Trench.

Royer, F. L., & Garner, W. R. (1966). Response uncertainty and perceptual difficulty of auditory temporal patterns. *Perception and Psychophysics, 1,* 41–47.

Savage-Rumbaugh, S., McDonald, K., Sevcik, R. A., Hopkins, W. D., & Rubert, E. (1986). Spontaneous symbol acquisition and communicative use by Pygmy Chimpanzees (*Pan paniscus*). *Journal of Experimental Psychology: General, 115,* 211–235.

Shepard, R. (1965). Approximation to uniform gradients of generalization by monotone transformations of scale. In D. I. Mostofsky (Ed.), *Stimulus generalization.* California: Stanford University Press.

Shepard, R. (1982). Structural representations of musical pitch. In D. Deutsch (Ed.). *The psychology of music* (pp. 343–390). New York: Academic Press.

Simon, H. A. (1972). Complexity and the representation of patterned sequences of symbols. *Psychological Review, 79,* 369–382.

Simon, H. A., & Kotovsky, K. (1963). Human acquisition of concepts for sequential patterns. *Psychological Review, 70,* 534–546.

Skinner, B. F. (1934). The extinction of chained reflexes. *Proceedings of the National Academy of Sciences, 20,* 234–237.

Stebbins, W. C. (Ed.). (1970). *Animal psychophysics.* New York: Appleton-Century-Crofts.

Stevens, S. S. (1951). Mathematics, measurement, and psychophysics. In S. S. Stevens (Ed.), *Handbook of experimental psychology* (pp. 1–49). New York: Wiley.

Thorpe, W. (1961). *Birdsong.* Cambridge, England: Cambridge University Press.

Editorial Comments on Moody and Stebbins

Frequency modulation seems to be a common feature of sounds that are used in communication by most species. That is true for human language, for the coo contact calls uttered by Japanese macaques, and for the signals of rodents. In a series of experiments they describe in this chapter, Moody and Stebbins have set out to study the characteristics of frequency modulated stimuli when they must be discriminated from unmodulated stimuli near threshold. The experiments are designed to determine not just what monkeys *do* perceive about frequency modulated calls, but what they *can* perceive about such calls—especially when the calls are modified systematically. Only by analytic procedures of this type can we determine in a more general sense the factors that govern acoustic perception.

The results of the experiments show to an extraordinary degree that monkeys are prone to make discriminations near threshold on the basis of absolute frequency characteristics of modulated and unmodulated stimuli. That is, for example, they prefer to make comparisons between the frequency of a standard stimulus and the initial frequency of a comparison stimulus instead of noting that the standard maintains a steady frequency while the comparison rises. Only by designing stimulus sets that eliminated the possibility of absolute frequency perception was it possible to show that monkeys could, in fact, use frequency modulation as a relevant cue for successful discrimination. Although species and experimental situations differ in substantial detail, these results are certainly reminiscent of Hulse's experiments with birds (Chapter 11) which show substantial dependence on absolute frequency cues for successful acoustic pattern discrimination.

Of course, as Moody and Stebbins are quick to point out, Japanese macaques have been shown to depend extensively on frequency modulation in their natural communication. So all these results are not to say that monkeys are incapable, indeed sometimes depend greatly upon, frequency modulation and relational pitch perception. The point is that for many animals, monkeys included, the use of relational pitch perception may be a secondary strategy which is used when discrimination based on absolute pitch perception fails.

12

Salience of Frequency Modulation in Primate Communication

David B. Moody
William C. Stebbins
Kresge Hearing Research Institute and University of Michigan

INTRODUCTION

Acoustic communication signals can be well described by specifying the changes that occur in the spectral content of the signals over time; that is, by specifying the amplitude of each frequency component in the signal at each instant. Standard devices used for the analysis of acoustic signals, such as the Sonograph, are in fact designed to provide graphic representations of exactly those parameters by producing a plot of frequency as a function of time, with amplitude indicated by the darkness of the tracing.

One of the most striking commonalities among communication signals that is revealed by frequency-time analysis is that when the frequency of a continuous vocalization changes, it does so gradually, not in discrete steps. It does not matter whether one is examining the mating call of a frog, the song of a bird, the call of a monkey, or the speech of a human. In each case, frequency changes are characterized by sweeps (sometimes called glides) from a high frequency to a low one, or vice versa. In this chapter, we use the more generic term "frequency modulation" (FM) to refer to change in frequency over time. In some cases, such as the songs of birds, such frequency changes may occur very rapidly, and may not be discriminable, to our ears, as gradual changes at all; rather, they sound like chirps. In other cases, such as the calls of some monkeys, the frequency modulation is much more gradual, and is plainly discernible.

It is the ubiquity of these frequency sweeps in such a wide variety of communication signals that makes them intriguing to study in their own right. It should be noted, however, that the mere presence of such signal components does not confer upon them any unique importance in the communication systems of the organisms that produce them. It is quite possible, and perhaps even likely, that the presence of frequency sweeps reflects a lack of efficiency of the acoustic

353

production apparatus in generating step-like frequency changes during continuous acoustic output, as opposed to reflecting some perceptual specialization that has led to preferential selection of frequency sweeps for inclusion in the communicative repertoire. As reported in the next section, however, it has been demonstrated in a variety of contexts that such sweeps are information-bearing components of communication signals, and that there are elements in the auditory system that respond preferentially to the occurrence of stimuli that change in frequency over time.

As auditory physiologists began to abandon the simple clicks and pure tones that had been the mainstays of much of the early work in the field and began working with more complex, biologically relevant stimuli, it became clear that stimuli that changed in frequency over time had effects that could not be predicted by observations with simpler stimuli. One of the earliest studies to use such frequency modulated stimuli was one by Whitfield and Evans (1965), who examined the responses of auditory cortical neurons to such stimuli in the unanesthetized cat. Most of their work was with stimuli that were sinusoidally frequency modulated; that is, stimuli for which a graph of frequency over time would resemble a sine wave, and which therefore have a frequency periodicity equal to the modulation frequency.

With such modulated stimuli, Whitfield and Evans demonstrated that responses of the majority of units they studied could not be predicted from responses to steady tones. For example, they found many units with considerably wider response areas for FM tones than for steady tones. Approximately 10% of the units they studied could not be made to respond at all to steady tones, but rather responded only when the tones were modulated. They also found many units that responded periodically to modulated stimuli; some units responding when the frequency was rising, and some when it was falling. When these units were tested with unidirectional frequency sweeps, they were shown to respond as predicted from the sinusoidal modulation data; that is, units that responded to the increasing portions of sinusoidally modulated stimuli also responded only to rising frequency sweeps, and vice-versa. In addition, preferential responding to sweep direction could be demonstrated for much higher rates of frequency change with linear frequency sweeps than could be shown with sinusoidally modulated stimuli. With these data, it then became obvious that FM stimuli are potentially very important and unique stimuli to the auditory nervous system and that the physiological mechanisms are in place for their detection and discrimination.

Research carried out with human speech sounds has also amply demonstrated the importance of FM in the perception of the speech code. It has been shown, for example, that differences in the slopes of the frequency sweeps (called formant transitions) in the initial 40–50 msec of the second and third formants of the speech sounds such as /ba/ and /da/ are responsible for the perceived differences between those sounds. When those transitions are increasing in frequency, the sound is heard as a /ba/; while decreases in frequency are heard as /da/. Liberman, Cooper, and Shankweiler (1967) have suggested that ". . . the second formant transition is a major cue for all consonants . . . , and is probably the single most important carrier of linguistic information in the speech signal" (p. 434).

When these frequency transitions are isolated from other components of the speech sounds and used as stimuli in psychoacoustic experiments with humans, they also appear to have some unique properties. For example, there seem to be two different modes of processing depending on the duration of the sweep. Thresholds for detecting sweeps less than about 300 ms in duration depend on the total frequency excursion of the sweep; while for sweeps longer than that duration, thresholds depend on the rate at which the frequency changes (Arlinger, Jerlvall, Ahren, & Holmgren, 1977; Nabelek & Hirsh, 1969; Pollack, 1968). A second example of the unique properties of frequency transitions comes from selective adaptation studies using unidirectional sweeps as adapting and test stimuli. These studies have suggested the presence of channels in the auditory system that are specifically sensitive to such stimuli (Gardner & Wilson, 1979; Tansley & Regan, 1979), although a more recent experiment has suggested caution in interpreting the results of such studies (Moody, Cole, Davidson, & Stebbins, 1984). A final example of the special properties of frequency sweeps is provided in an experiment by Schwartz and Tallal (1980) that used synthesized stop consonants in which the formant transitions were either 40 or 80 msec in duration. They found that the right ear advantage (REA) that characterizes the perception of certain speech sounds was much greater for the normal 40-msec transitions than for the 80-msec transitions. They concluded that the hemispheric specialization indicated by a REA depends, at least in part, on the rate of change of formant transitions in speech sounds.

Many nonhuman primate species have been shown to produce vocalizations that are characterized by tonal frequency transitions (e.g., Green, 1975; Grimm, 1967; Lillehei & Snowdon, 1978; Marler, 1970, 1972; Marler & Hobbett, 1975; Rowell & Hinde, 1962; Waser, 1977). Only a relatively limited subset of these vocalizations has been subjected to extensive analysis, and only the Green (1975) study on the Japanese macaque (*M. Fuscata*) provides data on correlations between the call structure and the context in which the call occurs. One class of vocalizations that Green studied were contact-soliciting "coo" calls. He described seven subdivisions of these coo calls based on their acoustic structure, and showed how the occurrence of each subdivision was correlated with a particular social situation.

Among other features, these calls differed in certain characteristics of frequency modulation. For example, calls in which there is a frequency inflection (i.e., a transition from rising to fall frequency) early in the call, smooth-early-highs (SEH), tend to be emitted by juvenile monkeys sitting calmly alone and looking around. A very similar vocalization with the frequency inflection late in the call, a smooth-late-high (SLH), is emitted by an estrous female during the earliest stages of sexual solicitation. Although the calls are acoustically similar enough to be considered to lie on a continuum of temporal position of frequency inflection, there was essentially no overlap observed in the social situations in which the calls were emitted.

In part because of the acoustic similarity but functional dissimilarity of these calls, they have been used in a number of laboratory studies of primate communication that have illustrated the importance of the frequency transitions in determining the functional significance of the calls. In one of the first of these studies, both Japanese monkeys and control species were trained to release a response lever to presentations of one class of call, and to continue to hold the lever when examples of the other class were presented. The training stimuli included a variety of examples of each type of call that differed in several dimensions including duration and average pitch. The animals were trained first with one member of each class; for example, to release to a particular SEH and hold through a particular SLH. As the monkeys learned that discrimination, additional stimuli were added to the experiment so that the animals had to learn to ignore irrelevant differences such as pitch or duration and to respond on the basis of temporal position of the frequency inflection.

At this stage of the experiment, it became apparent that there was a difference in rate of acquisition of the discrimination between the Japanese monkeys, for whom the temporal cue was thought to be relevant in their communication system, and the control species. Although both groups acquired the initial discrimination between one smooth-early high and one smooth-late high at about the same rate, the Japanese monkeys learned much more rapidly when additional examples of the two types of call were added to the stimulus set (Zoloth et al., 1979). Such an outcome could indicate either that the position of the frequency inflection was an important aspect of the call, or that the Japanese monkeys were in general more adept at making auditory discriminations.

To test the hypothesis that the frequency inflection was the important determinant of these results, the smooth-early and smooth-late stimuli were lumped together and then rearranged into two new sets according to their initial pitch. This new stimulus set consisted of one set of stimuli with starting pitches below 600 Hz and another set of stimuli with starting pitches greater than that frequency. Both smooth-early and smooth-late stimuli were included in each of the new stimulus sets, and thus temporal position of the frequency inflection was no longer a relevant cue. This new set of stimuli was referred to as the "pitch-relevant" set, while the original set was referred to as "peak-relevant." When another group of animals was trained on this new discrimination, a difference in rate of acquisition was also observed, but the difference was the opposite of that observed in the peak-relevant discrimination: the control species acquired this pitch-relevant discrimination more rapidly than did the Japanese macaques (Zoloth et al., 1979). This finding provides a strong indication that modulation, or at least change in direction of modulation, is a highly salient feature of acoustic communication signals for Japanese monkeys.

This conclusion was also supported by observations on these same animals of a differential ear advantage in making the discrimination. When making the peak-relevant discrimination, the Japanese monkeys were more accurate, in terms of percent correct responses, when the stimuli were presented to the right ear, suggesting processing primarily by the left hemisphere. With the pitch-relevant discrimination, the Japanese monkeys showed either a left-ear advantage or no ear advantage. In all cases but one, the control species showed no ear advantage for either feature of the vocalizations (Petersen, Beecher, Zoloth, Moody, & Stebbins, 1978). These right-ear, left-hemisphere advantages suggest that Japanese macaques lateralize the processing of communication sounds much as humans lateralize the processing of speech (see, for example, Springer, 1971; Studdert-Kennedy & Shankweiler, 1970). The specificity of the effect to the peak-relevant dimension would support the notion that the temporal position of a frequency inflection is a communicatively relevant dimension for the Japanese monkeys.

The importance of hemispheric specialization in the peak-relevant discrimination was demonstrated in a study by Heffner and Heffner (1984, 1986) in which they used the same stimuli as those used by Zoloth et al. (1979) and Petersen et al. (1978), and trained their subjects to make the peak-relevant discrimination. They then ablated portions of the auditory cortex and showed that the animal's ability to make the peak-relevant discrimination was impaired when the left auditory cortex was lesioned, but not when the lesion was on the right side. If the lesion was a left-auditory-cortex-only lesion, the animals were able to relearn the peak discrimination in 5–15 sessions. If the lesion was bilateral, the ability to learn the peak-relevant discrimination was lost, although the animals were able to make other auditory discriminations. Thus, although the left hemisphere seemed to be involved in making the original discrimination for all subjects, they could apparently compensate for loss of the left hemisphere if the right hemisphere was available.

Our technique for demonstrating that a particular dimension of a complex stimulus is relevant in determining discrimination performance is to present a set of stimuli that are varied along that dimension in an orderly way, and to note changes in performance as a function of that dimension (e.g., Terrace, 1966). In the case of the "peak-relevant" continuum, the dimension of interest is the temporal position of the frequency inflection. In order to vary only that dimension of the Japanese monkey communication sounds, it was necessary to generate artificial examples of smooth-early-high and smooth-late-high stimuli using computer synthesis techniques. Once a pair of stimuli had been generated that differed only in the temporal position of the frequency peak and that was differentially responded to in an appropriate manner by subjects trained to discriminate the two natural classes, it was then possible to present the entire continuum of

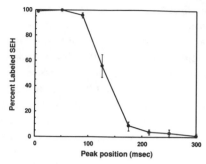

FIG. 12.1. Percentage of presentations of synthetic "coo" stimuli from a continuum of temporal position that were labeled as smooth early highs. Data are the means from 5 animals, and the error bars indicate ±1 SEM. Three of the subjects were trained to release to stimuli with the inflection early in the call, and two were trained to release when the peak was late in the call. Thus for three of the subjects, a SEH label consisted of making the behavioral response and for the remaining subjects, it consisted of withholding the response. Data from May, Moody, & Stebbins (1986).

peak positions to the subjects without differential reinforcement for either response or nonresponse and thus to determine the extent to which that dimension controlled their discrimination performance. The results of that operation, shown in Fig. 12.1 (May, Moody, & Stebbins, 1986) clearly demonstrate that the temporal position of the frequency inflection was a key determinant of the discrimination between different classes of communication sounds. The abruptness of the transition between response and nonresponse suggests that this dimension may demonstrate another characteristic found in human speech perception; namely, categorical perception. Data bearing on this possibility are not directly relevant to the topic of this chapter, but are discussed in Moody, Stebbins, and May (in press) and May (1987).

These studies in which frequency-modulated stimuli have been shown to have particular relevance to the auditory system, or to acoustic communication, demonstrate that such stimuli fall into a class that sets them apart from simpler stimuli such as pure tones, clicks, and noise bands. In order better to understand the specializations that exist for dealing with frequency modulation, we would argue that it is necessary to begin to study that feature in analytical isolation; that is, to study responses to stimuli that, as much as possible, vary only along the single dimension of modulation. The questions that are asked and the answers that are obtained in such studies are fundamentally different than in many of the studies that have been mentioned. No longer is the question one of what a subject *does* when presented with a stimulus containing frequency modulation; rather, the question becomes one of what a subject *can do* when required to discriminate between stimuli that differ along some dimension of frequency modulation. Both the *does* and the *can do* questions are important, but without a full understanding of the answers provided by the *can do* experiments, we would argue that it is not possible to appreciate fully the results of the *does* studies. Conversely, as we have already seen, experiments of the *does* class provide important input in guiding the direction of the *can do* studies.

In the remainder of this chapter, we describe a set of experiments that have been carried out using as stimuli linearly frequency modulated sinusoids; that is, stimuli that start at a particular frequency and increase or decrease at a fixed rate to some other frequency. The question being asked by these studies is straightforward: Under various stimulus configurations, what is the minimum amount of modulation necessary to discriminate a modulated stimulus from one that is unmodulated?

I. METHODS FOR STUDYING FM DISCRIMINATION

These experiments were carried out on both pigtail (*M. nemestrina*) and bonnet (*M. radiata*) monkeys. Although previous work (Beecher, Petersen, Zoloth, Moody, & Stebbins, 1979; Petersen et al., 1978; Zoloth et al., 1979) had demonstrated specializations for dealing with modulation in the Japanese macaque, that species was not used in the present series of studies because we were interested in more general specializations rather than those that might be unique to one species.

For testing, the animals were placed in standard primate restraint chairs and secured inside a double-walled, soundproof room. They were then fitted with earphones mounted on universal joints to allow some head movement. Small food pellets could be delivered to a trough mounted near the animal's mouth. A metal cylinder, which was part of a contact-sensitive switching circuit, was mounted within easy reach of the monkey and served as the response device. In the center of the cylinder was a small cue light that served to indicate the experimental contingencies and that provided feedback to the animal.

The procedure employed in these studies was a variant of one that had been successfully used to measure frequency and intensity discrimination thresholds and which is described in some detail in Moody, Beecher, and Stebbins (1976). Each of the studies discussed below required variations in the basic procedure, particularly with regard to the trial configuration. These variations are discussed as the particular experiments are described.

In the basic procedure, the subject was required to make contact with the response cylinder when the cue light began to flash. At that time, and for as long as contact was maintained, the cue light remained on without flashing, and an acoustic stimulus was repetitively presented to the right ear of the animal. Following a variable period that averaged 4 sec and during which a standard, unmodulated stimulus was presented, a test trial occurred. The test trial was a 2-

sec interval during which the stimulus was changed from the standard to one of eight comparison stimuli which were linear upsweeps. If the subject responded by releasing contact with the cylinder during the 2-sec trial, a banana-flavored food pellet was delivered, the cue light was turned off for 5 sec, and a correct detection of modulation was recorded.

On approximately 20% of the trials, the stimulus was not switched from standard to comparison, rather the standard stimulus continued to be presented. These trials, called "catch trials," were included in the procedure to assess the likelihood that some of the responses that occurred on regular trials were, in fact, false reports (guesses) that were not related to the change from standard to comparison stimuli. If a response occurred on one of these catch trials, no food pellet was delivered, and the cue light was turned off for 5 sec. This "time out" contingency, which was actually in effect for any releases of the key, except those that occurred during a trial, served as a mild punisher and effectively reduced the number of such responses. If responses occurred on more than 20% of the catch trials in a given session, the data from that session were discarded.

Throughout these studies, the method of constant stimuli was used to measure thresholds. Comparison stimuli were selected at random from a set of eight, and percent correct detections of each comparison was determined. Threshold was calculated by linear interpolation if necessary, as the stimulus value that produced 50% correct detections. As described below, this procedure was slightly modified for a later study to deal with an unusual pattern of responses to catch trials.

The stimuli used in these studies were all digitally synthesized and presented by a computer with a 12-bit digital-to-analog converter clocked at a rate at least 4 times the highest frequency in the sweep. All stimuli were synthesized with 5-msec cumulative-Gaussian (ogival) rise and fall times. The parameters studied in the experiments described below include frequency of the sweeps, duration of the sweeps, mode of presenting test trials, and effects of stimulus context.

Because the stimuli were linear sweeps, there were three dimensions of the stimuli that were interdependent; that is, that could not be varied independently. Those dimensions were duration, frequency excursion, and rate of frequency change. For example, if two stimuli of the same duration differed in amount of frequency change, then, of necessity, the rate of change also differed. Similarly, if the stimuli had a constant rate of change, but differed in excursion, then they must also differ in duration. The following results are in terms of excursion, but it is important to understand that the dimension determining discrimination performance may be rate of change or some interaction of rate and excursion.

II. RESULTS OF MODULATION THRESHOLD STUDIES

The purpose of the first experiment was to determine modulation detection thresholds at a number of different frequencies. Frequencies tested were 0.25,

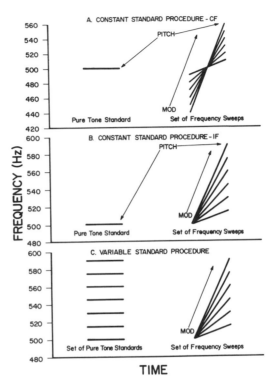

FIG. 12.2. Schematic diagrams of the stimulus sets used in the linear modulation detection experiments. In the CF procedure shown in Panel A, the frequency sweeps were centered at 500 Hz, the frequency of the standard tone. In the IF procedure (Panel B), the sweeps started at the 500-Hz frequency of the standard tone, and in the Variable Standard procedure (Panel C), the sweeps also started at 500 Hz, but a number of different pure tone standards were employed. From Moody, May, Cole, & Stebbins (1986).

0.5, 1.0, 2.0, and 4.0 kHz. The lowest three frequencies were from the range normally encountered in tonal primate vocalizations such as their "coo" calls. The 2.0 kHz stimulus is on the upper limit of that range, and the 4.0 kHz stimulus is above the normal range of this class of vocalizations.

The stimulus set, shown schematically for 500-Hz stimuli in Fig. 12.2A, consisted of a fixed standard stimulus at one of the test frequencies, and a set of increasing frequency sweeps centered at the same test frequency. Stimuli were specified in terms of total excursion; for example, a sweep from the 500-Hz set with a 60-Hz excursion would start at 470 Hz and increase at a constant rate to 530 Hz. A typical trial configuration from this first experiment is shown in Fig. 12.3A. The tone segments were 200 msec in duration, and were separated by 200-msec silent intervals. A test trial consisted of five successive presentations of a given modulated stimulus.

Modulation thresholds from the three subjects tested in this experiment are shown in Fig. 12.4. For each of the subjects, the greatest sensitivity to modulation occurs at 500 Hz, although thresholds at 250 Hz and 1 kHz are similar to those measured at the minimum. In other words, sensitivity to modulation is most acute for those frequencies that occur in tonal communication signals. Only one subject, M145, produced thresholds at 4 kHz, and the remaining two subjects produced stable thresholds at 2 kHz only after extended testing (67 sessions

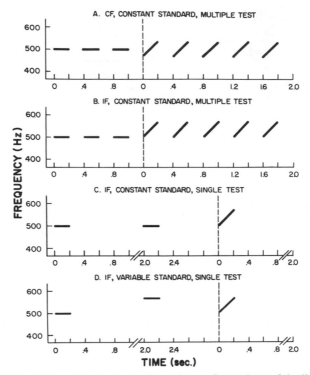

FIG. 12.3. Schematic diagrams of the trial configurations of the linear modulation detection experiments. In the procedure illustrated in Panel A, a single frequency standard stimulus was repeatedly presented, followed after a variable period of time by repeatedly presented comparisons centered at the frequency of the standard. The procedure illustrated in Panel B was the same as that in Panel A except that the sweeps all started at the frequency of the standard. In the procedure shown in Panel C, a single standard stimulus was presented only once every 2 s, and a trial consisted of a 2-s interval starting with a single presentation of a sweep that starts at the frequency of the standard. The procedure illustrated in Panel D was the same as that in Panel C except that the frequency of the standard was different from one presentation to the next. From Moody et al. (1986).

for M131 and 72 sessions for M146). The lower thresholds shown in this figure for M145 were characteristic of this animal throughout most phases of the study, although the magnitude of the difference was less for the stimulus configuration used in subsequent experiments.

In Fig. 12.5, the data from M145 are compared to thresholds from humans for detection of linear modulation (Arlinger et al., 1977) and with monkey (Stebbins, 1975) and human (Nordmark, 1968) frequency difference thresholds. Al-

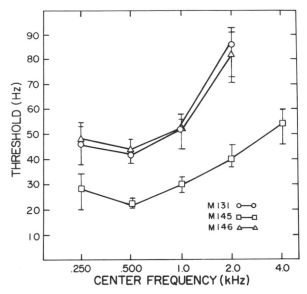

FIG. 12.4.   Thresholds for detection of linear frequency modulation for three monkeys. The CF procedure was used and the stimulus duration was 200 msec.

though, in all cases, the monkey thresholds are greater than comparable thresholds from humans, the general shape of the corresponding functions is remarkably similar as is the relationship between the two different types of function. For both species the modulation detection functions are essentially flat from 0.25 to 1 kHz, whereas difference thresholds continue to increase throughout the frequency range.

In the next experiment, the center frequency of the stimuli was held constant at 500 Hz as in Fig. 12.2A and thresholds were determined at stimulus durations of 100, 200, 400, 800, and 1600 msec. The interstimulus interval was held constant at 200 msec, but the number of stimulus presentations during a test trial was varied to maintain a trial duration between 1.8 and 2.0 sec. The number of presentations was 6 for the 100-msec stimuli (1.8-sec trial), 5 for the 200-msec stimuli (2.0-sec trial), 3 for the 400-msec stimuli (1.8-sec trial), 2 for the 800-msec stimuli (2.0-sec trial), and 1 for the 1600-msec stimuli (1.8 sec trial). Because more of the shorter stimuli are presented in each trial, giving greater opportunity for detection of modulation, it might be expected that those stimuli would yield lower thresholds.

The results of this experiment are shown by the open-circle functions in Fig. 12.6. Each of the animals shows lowest thresholds for the 800-msec duration and, with the exception of M131, highest thresholds to the shorter durations. For M131, the thresholds are about the same for the 100- and 1600-msec stimuli.

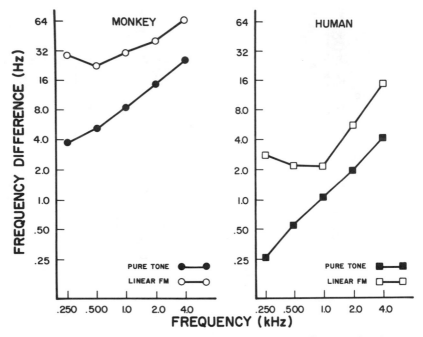

FIG. 12.5. Frequency modulation and frequency difference thresholds at various standard frequencies for macaque monkeys and humans. The values shown for frequency modulation (Linear FM) thresholds represent the differences between the starting and ending frequencies of the just-detectable FM sweeps. For frequency difference (pure tone) thresholds, the values shown are the frequency differences between the standard and just detectable comparison stimuli. The monkey linear FM data are those of M-145 from Fig. 12.4; the monkey frequency difference thresholds are from Stebbins, (1975); the human linear FM data are from Arlinger et al., (1977), and the human frequency difference thresholds are from Nordmark (1968). From Moody et al. (1986).

Thus the prediction of a lower threshold as the result of the greater number of presentations of the short stimuli is not supported by these data. These results are similar to those obtained by Sergeant and Harris (1962) from human observers using a slightly different procedure and sweeps that started at 1500 Hz. Those results showed a minimum at a slightly longer duration (2.0 sec), but for durations between 100 and 1600 msec, the slope of the function relating threshold excursion to duration was remarkably similar to that from the present data.

One explanation for the increase in threshold at longer durations that was noted for all subjects is that they may have responded before the end of the longer stimuli, and thus may not have heard the entire frequency excursion. If, for example, the subject initiated a response after only 400 msec of a stimulus that was 1600 msec in duration and had an excursion of 20 Hz, then that response was based on only the first quarter of the sweep; in other words, on only a 5-Hz excursion. Because the results reported here are based on the entire sweep excursion, then there would be a tendency to overestimate threshold for the longer durations. In the present study, response latencies were measured from the onset of the first sweep in a test trial to the occurrence of the release response. Frequency distributions of these latencies reveal that responses often occurred well before the longer stimuli had terminated, thus supporting this explanation of the increased thresholds at 1600 msec.

   Because of the procedure used to present these FM sweeps, a potential cue existed for detecting the onset of a trial that was not related to modulation per se. That cue, which is illustrated in Fig. 12.2A, is the frequency difference that occurs between the end of a standard, unmodulated stimulus and the end of the first comparison (modulated) stimulus on a trial. This difference, which we will refer to as a pitch or discrete-frequency cue, varied with the excursion of the modulated stimuli, and could have been used as a basis for discriminating the

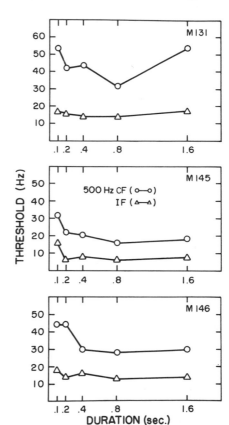

FIG. 12.6. Thresholds for detection of linear modulation for three subjects at various stimulus durations as measured in the CF and IF conditions. Values are total excursions of the just detectable sweep at each duration. From Moody et al. (1986).

transition between unmodulated and modulated stimuli that marked the onset of a trial. Although the parallels between the monkey data and comparable data from humans suggested that both were reflecting similar fundamental auditory abilities, a simple test of the pitch cue seemed necessary.

This test consisted of modifying the stimulus set such that the comparison stimuli, instead of being centered at 500 Hz, now all started at 500 Hz. All other aspects of this experiment, which we refer to as the "initial frequency" (IF) condition were the same as in the previous "center frequency" (CF) condition. However, if the animals were using the pitch difference between the end of a standard stimulus to the end of the first comparison stimulus, then thresholds with this new stimulus set should be half those obtained with the CF set. In other words, if a subject was able to report a 15-Hz difference between a standard and the final frequency in a CF stimulus, that stimulus would have a total excursion of 30 Hz from 485 Hz to 515 Hz. If the subject used the same strategy with an IF stimulus, that stimulus would have an excursion from 500 Hz to 515 Hz, half that of the CF stimulus. Although the same cue is used in both cases, the threshold would be lower because the subject was attending only to the difference between the end of a standard and the end of a comparison and therefore was ignoring the half of the CF sweep that was below the frequency of the standard.

The results from this experiment are shown as the lower functions in each panel of Fig. 12.6. In every case, the modulation thresholds from the IF condition are lower, by at least half, than those of the CF condition. In addition, there is almost no evidence in these data of duration effects of the magnitude of those seen in the CF condition. Given the apparent significance of modulated signals in the acoustic communication signals of animals, these findings are rather surprising. The implication of the reduced thresholds is that the subjects were using discrete frequency cues rather than cues inherent in the modulation itself; that is, the discriminations were made by comparison of frequencies sampled at particular temporal points in successive tone pulses rather than by detecting the presence of change within a modulated sweep.

This finding is especially significant because of the difficulty normally encountered in training animals to report frequency differences between successively presented tone pulses. In our experience, and in the anecdotally reported experience of other workers in the field, frequency discrimination is one of the most difficult auditory discriminations to train subjects to perform and from which to obtain replicable results across subjects. A rather extensive literature on selective attention to components of complex stimuli (e.g., Mackintosh, 1977; Mostofsky, 1970) suggests that, given a choice of two or more redundant cues on which to base a discrimination (such as, in this case, frequency difference and frequency modulation), subjects will choose that cue that is most salient to them. That literature also suggests that subjects can be made to attend to "nonpreferred" cues by making "preferred" cues unreliable. Given our subjects' apparent reliance on the discrete frequency cues available to them, the question became one of determining the conditions under which the modulation cue would be used as a basis for making the discrimination.

It was first necessary to determine the effect, if any, of one additional cue that was present during a trial, and that also could be used as the basis for making the required discrimination without attending to modulation. That cue, which can be seen in Fig. 12.3B, was the discrete frequency difference that existed between the end of one comparison stimulus in a trial, and the beginning of the next comparison stimulus. By attending to and reporting that difference, subjects could successfully perform the required task in all except the 1600-msec condition where only a single sweep was presented. To eliminate that cue within a trial, the procedure illustrated in Fig. 12.3C was employed. In that procedure, a stimulus, either standard or comparison, was presented once every 2 sec. The subject had the 2-sec interval following onset of a comparison stimulus in which to respond and thus to report the presence of modulation. Because the comparison stimuli were not repeated during the trial, the frequency difference between the end of one comparison and the start of the next was eliminated as a cue, although the subjects could still respond on the basis of differences between the end of a standard and the end of a subsequent comparison. This variation of the procedure will be referred to as the IF-single procedure as opposed to the previous IF-multiple procedure.

The results from the IF-single procedure are illustrated by the closed triangles of Fig. 12.7. Also contained in that figure are the results previously shown from the IF-multiple procedure. The principal difference between the two sets of functions occurs at the shortest stimulus durations where the IF-single thresholds are longer than those from the IF-multiple presentation procedure. At longer durations, thresholds are about the same, or in some cases even lower than IF-multiple thresholds. The higher thresholds at shorter durations might be attributed to the greater load placed on memory in this IF-single procedure. In the IF-multiple procedure, a constant interstimulus interval (ISI) of 200 msec separated each stimulus presentation, and the hypothesis was that comparisons were being made across that interval. In the present IF-single procedure, stimuli were presented once every 2 sec, so that a 100-msec stimulus was separated from the next stimulus by 1.9 sec rather than 200 msec. At least in humans, however, we have gathered preliminary data that suggests that, over a fairly wide range of interstimulus values, there was no effect of ISI on frequency discrimination thresholds. It should also be noted that, even for the 1600-msec duration, there was an increase in ISI from 200 to 400 msec, but no change, or perhaps a reduction, in thresholds.

A second explanation for the longer thresholds at shorter durations is that the IF-single procedure was designed to reduce the number of opportunities for making comparisons between the end of one comparison and the beginning of the next. As there were more opportunities to make such comparisons for short duration stimuli, then if that cue was in fact being used as the basis for the

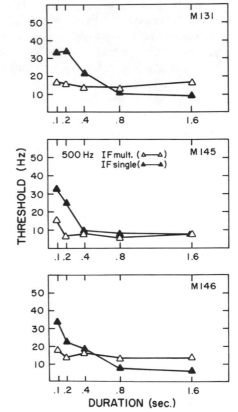

FIG. 12.7. Thresholds for detection of linear modulation for three subjects at various stimulus durations as measured in the IF-multiple standard and IF-single standard conditions. Values are total excursions of the just detectable sweep at each duration. From Moody et al. (1986).

discrimination, the effect of the procedural change would be expected to be greater on the shorter stimuli than on the longer ones. Once again, the data suggest that animals were using some sort of frequency comparisons between discrete frequency points within successively presented stimuli rather than using cues contained within the modulated comparisons, at least for short duration stimuli at threshold.

The next variation of the testing procedure was designed to make comparisons between discrete frequency points in successive stimuli a completely unreliable cue on which to base the discrimination. This variation was based on the IF-single procedure, but instead of presenting a fixed-frequency standard stimulus, standards were randomly selected from a set of eight different fixed frequencies that encompassed the range of frequencies contained within the comparison stimuli. Catch trials occurred presented on 50% of all trial presentations and consisted of presentation of one of the standard stimuli. Catch-trial responses were recorded separately for each standard stimulus. The stimulus set from this procedure is illustrated schematically in Fig. 12.2C and the trial configuration is

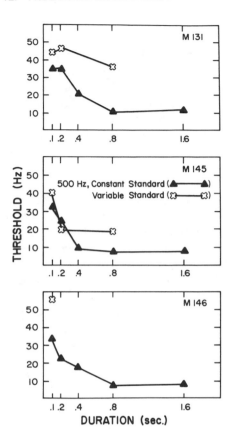

FIG. 12.8. Thresholds for detection of linear modulation for three subjects at various stimulus durations as measured in the constant standard (i.e., IF-single standard) and variable standard conditions. Values are total excursions of the just detectable sweep at each duration. Because of equipment limitations, thresholds could not be obtained under the variable standard condition for 1.6-s stimuli. From Moody et al. (1986).

illustrated in Fig. 12.3D. Because successively presented standard stimuli were of different frequencies in this "variable-standard" procedure, responses based on frequency differences between successively presented stimuli would, in most cases, be punished by the occurrence of a time out; only the modulation contained within a single comparison stimulus would be a reliable cue on which to base the discrimination.

Thresholds from the variable-standard procedure are shown as the open symbols in Fig. 12.8 along with thresholds from the fixed-standard procedure (i.e., the IF-single procedure). Equipment limitations prevented determination of thresholds from the 1600-msec duration. When subjects were first placed on this task, behavior was greatly disrupted as would be expected if the hypothesis about use of discrete frequency differences was correct. Many unreinforced responses were initially made to successively presented standards, and catch-trial response rates increased dramatically. Similar changes were seen in the data from human subjects who were also running on this procedure. After further training with comparison stimuli having considerably increased modulation excursions, behavior began to come under control of modulation per se and to stabilize at criterion accuracy. One exception was M-146 for whom, even after extended training, thresholds could only be obtained for the 100-msec duration.

In all cases except one (M-145, 200 msec), thresholds are considerably above those from the fixed-standard condition, and as can be seen by comparison with Fig. 12.6 and 12.7, are higher than most of those contained at comparable durations under any of the other testing conditions. Because this procedure requires attention to changes contained within a stimulus; that is, to modulation, we believe that the thresholds represented here are the best estimates of sensitivity to modulation.

Data obtained from responses to catch trials, however, revealed that at least some responses may have been based on cues other than modulation. The assumption normally made with catch-trial responses is that they represent random releases that are unrelated to the stimulus presented. Under such an assumption, it would be predicted that such responses would be equally distributed across all catch trials regardless of the frequency of the standard stimulus presented. Under the variable-standard procedure, especially early in training, it was clear that catch trial responses were concentrated on trials where particular standards were presented; in particular, on those trials where the frequency of the standard was near the terminal frequency of the comparison stimulus nearest threshold. For frequency differences that were above threshold, however, it was also clear that the subjects were responding appropriately; that is, releasing to modulated stimuli, and holding through unmodulated stimuli. One of the most obvious examples of this finding is illustrated in Fig. 12.9. For the 515-Hz stimuli; that is for a 515-Hz pure tone standard, and a 500-515 Hz modulated comparison, responding is actually somewhat more frequent to the standard stimulus than to the comparison, even though responses to the standard were never reinforced, and were, in fact, punished. Although the magnitude of the effect in this example is perhaps more extreme than was typical, it was by no means unique. Similar results were obtained for all subjects tested on this procedure, including humans, and for the monkeys they persisted to a lesser extent throughout testing. The implication of these data, we believe, is that for stimuli near threshold the auditory system confuses modulated stimuli with pure tones that are different from some reference stimulus; or in other words, that linear sweeps may be encoded by the auditory system as discrete frequency shifts. One of the difficulties with this interpretation is that it requires an internal reference stimulus that is derived either from the starting frequency of the sweeps or the lowest frequency standard stimulus; in other words, that the subjects utilize some sort of pitch memory.

This interpretation is, however, compatible with the findings of Nabelek, Nabelek, and Hirsh (1970) from an experiment in which human subjects were required to match the pitch of an FM sweep with a pure tone. For stimuli in which the product of frequency excursion and duration was less than some critical value, they found subjects could easily make the match. For stimuli

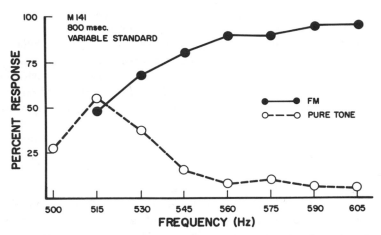

FIG. 12.9. Percent of presentations of both standard (pure tone) and comparison (modulated) stimuli on which subject M-141 responded during the 2-s trial. The data for the comparison stimuli are plotted as a function of the terminal frequency of the sweep, all of which started at 500 Hz. From Moody et al. (1986).

greater than the critical value, judgments were more variable, and subjects reported great difficulty in making the matches. The suggestion of these findings, then, is that the stimuli that were easily matched sounded more like the pure tones. Other support is obtained from studies in which modulated segments of biologically relevant stimuli are replaced with pure tones. One such study by Blumstein and Stevens (1980), replaced the formant transitions in formants 2, 3, and 4 of stop consonants with pure tones and showed that subjects could still discriminate the consonants even when the duration of the trailing vowel sound was significantly reduced. Similarly, Gerhardt (1986) mentions that replacing the FM components of the stereotyped mating calls of tree frogs with pure tones does not reduce the attractiveness of the calls to female frogs. In Japanese monkey calls, however, May (personal communication) has shown that calls in which frequency transitions are replaced by frequency steps; that is, modulation is replaced by tone segments, are not acceptable substitutes to trained Japanese monkeys for the modulated calls. May et al., (1986), have also shown that most other acoustic manipulations of those calls also result in stimuli that are unacceptable to the monkeys.

Perhaps the most noteworthy difference between the stimuli that were employed in the studies that have been described and many naturally occurring stimuli is that the latter contain frequency inflections; that is, transitions from rising to falling frequency, or vice versa, or from changing to steady frequency. The experimental stimuli used in the above studies, however, were all linear sweeps that started at one frequency and ended at a different frequency, with no change in direction of the sweep. In an effort to begin to make better approximations of more biologically relevant stimuli using sinusoidal components and to investigate the role of inflections in determining sensitivity to modulation, we began a series of experiments with stimuli containing such inflections.

These stimuli were produced by combining segments that were linearly modulated, or that were of constant frequency. They were synthesized so that the frequency of the start of one component was the same as the frequency of the end of the previous component and so that there was a continuous phase transition from one component to the next; that is, so that there was no abrupt discontinuity in the waveform at the transitions between components. An additional feature of these combined stimuli was that they were configured so that they all started and ended at 500 Hz. Thus, the subjects should have been unable to make discriminations based on discrete frequencies represented at the endpoints of the sweeps. As in the previous experiment, standard stimuli of different frequencies were employed, the comparison stimulus set consisted of a range of modulation excursions, and the subject's task was to report the presence of modulation.

The stimulus configurations tested in this experiment are illustrated in the left portion of Fig. 12.10. Stimulus configurations 1–3 are linear sweeps such as those used in previous studies, configurations 4–12 all contain frequency inflections, and in configurations 13–15, the inflections have been replaced by either a noise burst (13 and 14) or silence (15). The right portion of the figure presents relative modulation thresholds. These data, which represent medians of several determinations, have been normalized such that the largest threshold for each animal is represented as 100%, and other thresholds are represented as a percentage of that threshold. This normalization of the data was necessary because the absolute values of thresholds varied by a factor of 2 across subjects. In all cases, highest thresholds were found for linear sweeps; for two of the subjects these occurred with 200-msec downsweeps (configuration 2), and were 62.5 Hz for M-131 and 28 Hz for M-146. For the third subject, M-141, the highest threshold was 39 Hz for an 800-msec upsweep (configuration 3). With the exception of configuration 4 which was a 100-msec upsweep followed by a 100-msec downsweep, most of the inflection-containing stimuli had thresholds that were on the order of 50% of the maximum thresholds obtained at configurations 1, 2, and 3. The higher thresholds for configuration 4 may represent the inherently higher thresholds for short sweeps noted above.

These lower thresholds for stimulus configurations that contain inflections suggest that the presence of such inflections is an important feature of frequency-modulated stimuli in terms of making them easier to detect. When such inflections are replaced with noise bands, as in configurations 13 and 14, detectability was reduced for M-141 and M-146 when compared to configuration 12, which was identical except that it contained a frequency inflection at its halfway point. Replacing the noise band in configuration 14 with silence (configuration 15) produces somewhat less impairment for M-146, but somewhat more for M-141.

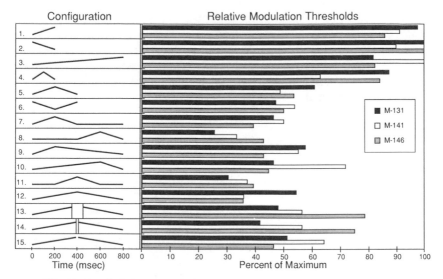

FIG. 12.10. Relative modulation detection thresholds obtained from three subjects for different stimulus configurations. On the left, the configurations are schematically illustrated, and on the right, thresholds are plotted as a percent of the maximum threshold produced at any of the configurations for each subject. The enclosed bars in the middle of configurations 13 and 14 represent the presence of low-pass noise.

The thresholds of M-131, which were the highest in terms of frequency excursion, seem unaffected by changes at the inflection point of the stimulus.

Although the set of inflection-containing stimuli all start and end at 500 Hz, and therefore should eliminate the discrete frequency cue between the endpoints of the modulated stimuli and the unmodulated standard stimuli, there was still increased responding observed on particular catch trials, notably those on which pure tones were presented that were at and below the maximum excursions of the near-threshold comparison stimuli. This increase, which we have attributed to confusion between modulated and unmodulated tones near threshold, suggests that the inflection point in these stimuli may serve as a temporal marker that is used by the animal to indicate a point in the stimulus at which instantaneous frequency should be sampled. Such sampling, since it would occur at frequency inflection points, would provide optimum information about maxima and minima in the spectrum of a communication signal. Stevens (1980) has attributed a similar function to certain acoustic events in human speech, most notably rapid spectral change.

In discussing the data from the various testing conditions with linear sweeps, we suggested that the animals seemed to be coding the sweeps according to the terminal frequency. However, the fact that thresholds for inflection-containing stimuli are lower than those for linear sweeps implies that the sweeps may be recoded as frequencies contained within the sweeps, but not those of the endpoints, since there should be no difference in thresholds if terminal frequency was the cue being used in the case of sweeps. In other words, the auditory system may perform some frequency-averaging operation on the sweeps that it does not perform on the inflected stimuli.

III. CONCLUDING COMMENTS

In this chapter, we have described a series of experiments that have examined the ability of nonhuman primates to detect the presence of an acoustic component that is commonly found in their communication signals; namely, frequency modulation. Evidence from a number of sources suggested that FM is a distinctive feature that conveys communicative significance and that is selectively responded to by the auditory system. The results of the experiments described in this chapter all support the notion that FM is *special* to the auditory system, but not in the sense that modulation is easier to detect than, for example, discrete frequency differences. Rather, it would appear that processing occurs in the system that, at least near the threshold for modulation detection, results in the recoding of modulation into a discrete frequency percept. Discriminations are then made based on those percepts.

It has also become apparent from these experiments that the strategies used to detect modulation vary depending on the mode of stimulus presentation and on the extent to which the test stimuli resemble the structure of natural calls. On the basis of these observations, we believe that there is much to be learned about the perception of frequency change by further modeling of natural call structure; both by increasing the complexity of stimuli such as were used in these experiments, and by artificially manipulating the structure of naturally occurring calls.

One would expect, and indeed it has been shown in many species, that a congruence should exist between the sounds that are used for communication and the specializations of the auditory system for perceiving those sounds. Such a congruence can develop through selective incorporation into the communication system of those sounds for which perceptual specializations exist and/or by selecting those specializations that are most suited for dealing with the sounds the species can readily produce. The primary difference between these two alternatives is whether the primary selection is for sounds because of available perceptual abilities or for perceptual ability because of available sound repertoire. Since the results that have been discussed suggest a perceptual translation of one stimulus feature (modulation) into a different one (discrete frequency), it would seem unlikely that modulation was differentially selected as a feature of communication sounds. Rather, it seems more likely that modulation is a feature that is prevalent in acoustic production, and that specific perceptual abilities may have been developed to deal with that feature.

ACKNOWLEDGMENTS

The research reported in this chapter was supported by NSF grant BNS 81-18027 and by NIH Program Project grant NS-05785.

The authors wish to express their appreciation to the many students who helped to gather these data, and especially to thank Mary A. Norat, Brad May, and Dorothy M. Cole, without whose help these experiments could have not been done.

REFERENCES

Arlinger, S. D., Jerlvall, L. B., Ahren, T., & Holmgren, E. C. (1977). Thresholds for linear frequency ramps of a continuous pure tone. *Acta Otolaryngologica, 83*, 317–327.

Beecher, M. D., Petersen, M. R., Zoloth, S. R., Moody, D. B., & Stebbins, W. C. (1979). Perception of conspecific vocalizations by Japanese macaques. *Brain, Behavior, and Evolution, 1*, 443–460.

Blumstein, S. E., & Stevens, K. N. (1980). Perceptual invariance and onset spectra for stop consonants in different vowel environments. *Journal of the Acoustical Society of America, 67*, 648–662.

Gardner, R. B., & Wilson, J. P. (1979). Evidence for direction-specific channels in the processing of frequency modulation. *Journal of the Acoustical Society of America, 66*, 704–709.

Gerhardt, H. C. (1986). Recognition of spectral patterns in the green treefrog: neurobiology and evolution. *Experimental Biology, 45*, 167–178.

Green, S. (1975). Communication by a graded vocal system in Japanese monkeys. In L. A. Rosenblum (Ed.), *Primate Behavior* (Vol. 4, pp. 1–102). New York: Academic Press.

Grimm, R. V. (1967). Catalog of sounds of the pig-tailed macaque (*Macaca nemestrina*). *Journal of Zoology,* (London), *152*, 361–373.

Heffner, H. E., & Heffner, R. S. (1984). Temporal lobe lesions and the perception of species-specific vocalizations by macaques. *Science, 226*, 75–76.

Heffner, H. E., & Heffner, R. S. (1986). Effect of unilateral and bilateral auditory cortex lesions on the discrimination of vocalizations by Japanese macaques. *Journal of Neurophysiology, 56*, 683–701.

Liberman, A. M., Cooper, F., & Shankweiler, D. (1967). Perception of the speech code, *Psychological Review, 74*, 431–461.

Lillehei, R., & Snowdon, C. T. (1978). Individual and situational difference in the vocalizations of young stumptail macaques (*M. arctoides*), *Behaviour, 65*, 270–271.

Mackintosh, N. J. (1977). Stimulus control: Attentional factors. In W. K. Honig & J. E. R. Staddon (Eds.), *Handbook of Operant Behavior* (pp. 481–513). Englewood Cliffs, NJ: Prentice Hall.

Marler, P. R. (1970). Vocalizations of East African monkeys. I. Red colobus. *Folia Primatologica, 13*, 81–91.

Marler, P. R. (1972). Vocalizations of East African monkeys. II. Black & white colobus. *Behaviour, 42*, 175–197.

Marler, P. R., & Hobbett, L. (1975). Individuality in long-range vocalizations by wild chimpanzees. *Zeitschrift Fur Tierpsychologie, 38*, 97–109.

May, B. (1987). Significant features and perceptual categories in the vocal signals of Japanese macaques. Doctoral dissertation, University of Michigan.

May, B., Moody, D. B., & Stebbins, W. C. (1986). *Significant features in Japanese monkey "coo" calls.* Abstracts of the ninth midwinter research meeting, Association for Research in Otolaryngology, pp. 108–109.

Moody, D. B., Beecher, M. D., & Stebbins, W. C. (1976). Behavioral Methods in Auditory Research. In C. A. Smith & J. A. Vernon (Eds.), *Handbook of auditory and vestibular research methods* (pp. 439–497) Springfield, IL: C. C. Thomas.

Moody, D. B., Cole, D., Davidson, L. M., & Stebbins, W. C. (1984). Evidence for a reappraisal of the psychophysical selective adaptation paradigm. *Journal of the Acoustical Society of America, 76,* 1076–1079.

Moody, D. B., May, B., Cole, D. M., & Stebbins, W. C. (1986). The role of frequency modulation in the perception of complex stimuli by primates. *Experimental Biology, 45,* 219–232.

Moody, D. B., Stebbins, W. C., & May, B. (in press). Auditory perception of communication signals by Japanese monkeys. In W. C. Stebbins & M. A. Berkley (Eds.), *Comparative perception—Volume II: Complex signals.* New York: Wiley.

Mostofsky, D. I. (1970). *Attention: Contemporary theory and analysis.* New York: Appleton-Century-Crofts.

Nàbelek, I. V., & Hirsh, I. J. (1969). On the discrimination of frequency transitions. *Journal of the Acoustical Society of America, 45,* 1510–1519.

Nàbelek, I. V., Nàbelek, A. K., & Hirsh, I. J. (1970). Pitch of tone bursts of changing frequency. *Journal of the Acoustical Society of America, 48,* 536–553.

Nordmark, J. (1968). Mechanisms of frequency discrimination. *Journal of Acoustical Society of America, 44,* 1533–1540.

Petersen, M. R., Beecher, M. D., Zoloth, S. R., Moody, D. B., & Stebbins, W. C. (1978). Neural lateralization of species-specific vocalizations by Japanese macaques (*Macaca fuscata*). *Science, 202,* 324–327.

Pollack, I. (1968). Detection of the rate of change of auditory frequency. *Journal of Experimental Psychology, 77,* 535–541.

Rowell, T. E., & Hinde, R. A. (1962). Vocal Communication by the rhesus monkey (*Macaca mulatta*). *Proceedings of the Zoological Society of London, 138,* 279–294.

Schwartz, J., & Tallal, P. (1980). Rate of acoustic change may underlie hemispheric specialization for speech perception. *Science, 207,* 1380–1381.

Sergeant, R. L., & Harris, J. D. (1962). Sensitivity to unidirectional frequency modulation. *Journal of the Acoustical Society of America, 34,* 1625–1628.

Springer, S. (1971). Ear asymmetry in a dichotic detection task. *Perception and Psychophysics, 10,* 239–241.

Stebbins, W. C. (1975). Hearing of the anthropoid primates: a behavioral analysis. In E. L. Eagles (Ed.), *The nervous system: Human communication and its disorders* (Vol. 3, pp. 113–124), New York: Raven Press.

Stevens, K. N. (1980). Acoustic correlates of some phonetic categories. *Journal of the Acoustical Society of America, 68,* 836–842.

Studdert-Kennedy, M., & Shankweiler, D. (1970). Hemispheric specialization for speech perception. *Journal of the Acoustical Society of America, 48,* 579–594.

Tansley, B. W., & Regan, D. (1979). Separate auditory channels for unidirectional frequency modulation and unidirectional amplitude modulation. *Sensory Processes, 3,* 132–140.

Terrace, H. S. (1966). Stimulus Control. In W. K. Honig (Ed.), *Operant behavior: Areas of research and application* (pp. 271–344). New York: Appleton-Century-Crofts.

Waser, P. (1977). Individual recognition, intragroup cohesion, and spacing: Evidence from sound playback to forest monkeys. *Behaviour, 60,* 28–74.

Whitfield, I. C., & Evans, E. F. (1965). Responses of auditory cortical neurons to stimuli of changing frequency. *Journal of Neurophysiology, 28,* 655–672.

Zoloth, S. R., Petersen, M. R., Beecher, M. D., Green, S., Marler, P., Moody, D. B., & Stebbins, W. C. (1979). Species-specific perceptual processing of vocal sounds by monkeys. *Science, 204,* 870–873.

Editor's Comments on Kuhl

One of the most challenging issues in speech perception is distinguishing between effects that can be attributed to the operation of general auditory system processes and those that require a more *specialized* phonetic mechanism. The study of speech perception by animals and human infants provides a critical contribution to the "special mechanisms debate." Animals clearly exhibit auditory-level processing but presumably do not have access to the kind of phonetic-level processing mechanism that has been postulated for humans. Prelinguistic human infants might be expected to fall somewhere in between at least on some tasks—exhibiting the rudiments of complex speech perception behavior characteristic of adult humans.

In this chapter, Kuhl provides an elegant review of the most recent work on speech perception by animals and human infants. Kuhl describes experiments demonstrating that animals whose hearing is similar to that of humans perceive a number of speech sound contrasts categorically, as do humans. These results indicate that at least in some instances, auditory-level processing may be sufficient for categorical perception. Human infants also show a surprising degree of sophistication in perceiving speech sounds revealing evidence of auditory and auditory-visual equivalence classes for certain speech sounds.

13

On Babies, Birds, Modules, and Mechanisms: A Comparative Approach to the Acquisition of Vocal Communication

Patricia K. Kuhl
University of Washington

INTRODUCTION

The vocal repertoires of animals constitute one of the most noticeable differences among them. The song of a bird, the croak of a frog, the sonar signals of a bat, the sounds that crickets make, and the calls of whales are strikingly different. Hearing any one of these signals allows us to name the animal that produced it. Birds do not croak like frogs, bats do not call like whales, and crickets do not chirp like birds. Vocalizations are a species' signature; they identify animals as members of one group rather than another.

Like birds, bats, and frogs, babies will produce a species-specific signal at a very young age—one that identifies them as members of the human species. The signal is "canonical babbling," repetitive consonant-vowel syllables such as /mamamama/ or /dadadada/. My 8-month-old baby has just begun this type of babbling, and in doing so she has produced the first observable sign that she will acquire language. Although I had heard infant babbling many times in the course of my research, I was awestruck at the regularity in its form and the precision of its timing when it occurred in my own child, and was somewhat surprised by its failure to occur early in response to my ever-constant modeling. I was reminded that this milestone of human speech occurs at the appointed time regardless of the language in which the infant is being reared, the educational background and socioeconomic status of the infant's parents, the infant's general motor and intellectual capabilities (within normal limits), and (apparently) parent prompting.

Acquisition of conspecific signals does not appear to be left to chance. All male swamp sparrows sing, all male humpbacks call, and all normal babies babble. Such obligatory behavior must be well protected from the nuances of individual development. Nature seems to have put a premium on ensuring that all appropriate members of the species produce the right signal at the right time.

What ensures this? How does nature guarantee that infants of a species will learn to produce one set of sounds as opposed to another? Are we protected from incorrect learning by restrictions on what we can hear? or on what our vocal tracts can produce? Certainly production constraints narrow the options some- what: birds cannot croak, given their vocal apparatus, and whales cannot produce birdsong, given theirs. Simple sensory limitations account for others: Crickets probably cannot hear speech, and frogs probably cannot hear the sonar signals produced by bats. In some instances, then, the selection of signals for reproduc- tion by the young is limited by fairly peripheral constraints, either motor or sensory.

But what of the remaining cases? Swamp sparrows produce signals that are quite different from their not-so-distant relatives, the song sparrow (see Marler, 1973, for review). The humpback whale's vocal signals differ greatly from those produced by other whales. Vocal tract constraints cannot explain these dif- ferences; nor can peripheral auditory constraints. And what of human infants? Why do they mimic speech rather than other reproducible signals? Peripheral constraints alone cannot explain the vocal repertoires of babies and birds. Experi- ence has been shown to play a critical role. Birds who are socially isolated or deafened will not produce conspecific song (Marler, 1973), and babies who are born deaf will not produce canonical babbling (Oller, 1986) nor learn to talk normally. But even here there is a further complication. The required auditory experience must be of the right kind. Hearing just any species' vocalizations is not sufficient to promote learning. Song sparrows will not produce their own song when they hear only the swamp sparrow song; nor will song sparrows learn to produce the swamp sparrow's song. Similarly, their is evidence suggesting that young infants do not mimic nonspeech auditory events (Kuhl & Meltzoff, 1988).

What accounts for selective vocal learning and selective imitation? How do infants of a species know which signals are the right kind?

Here, ethologists interested in birds and speech scientists interested in babies find themselves in the same box. We both have to explain what it is that allows the infant of the species to learn selectively. Ethologists have approached the problem by manipulating what the bird hears and observing what the bird eventually produces. But because speech scientists cannot experimentally manip- ulate what babies hear, our approach in studying human infants has been to conduct experiments involving auditory perception. We examine what babies can perceive, and use these data to test theories concerning the nature of the mechanisms underlying speech perception in infants.

These experiments reveal that human infants exhibit a remarkable sensitivity to human speech (see Kuhl, 1987a, for recent review). They appear to have an innate ability to perceive the universal set of phonetic[1] distinctions that are

---

[1]The term *phonetic* is used to signify any difference in any language that is sufficient to dis- tinguish two words. The term *phonemic* is used to specify distinctions that are used in a particular language.

appropriate for speech in any language. Moreover, the work discussed in this chapter shows that infants recognize complex equivalences between phonetically equal events—between two phonetically equal but discriminably different auditory events (Kuhl, 1979a, 1983, 1985a), between phonetically equal events delivered to two different modalities, as when an auditorily presented speech sound is related to the sight of a person producing that sound (Kuhl & Meltzoff, 1982, 1984a), and when an auditory event, produced by someone else, is related to the motor movements necessary to reproduce it oneself (Kuhl & Meltzoff, 1982, 1988). How are these complex equivalences detected? Is it simply infants' general sensory and cognitive processes that account for these remarkable abilities—or is there something more?

The production side poses similar questions. Normal speech will not occur unless the infant can hear, but given this, and given exposure to a specific language, influences of the mother tongue will appear quite early. By the end of the first year, young children already sound like infants being reared in a particular language environment; they have an *accent*. The American infant will sound distinctly different from a Russian, French, African, or Chinese infant (e.g., de Boysson-Bardies, Sagart, & Durand, 1984). Thus, vocal learning is affected by the infant's linguistic environment. But this learning is somehow restricted to sounds that are speech. How does the mechanism specify the signal to be learned, so as to restrict vocal learning to speech as opposed to other sounds in the environment? As in birds, the constraints on learning are not peripheral ones; neither motor limitations nor perceptual limitations account for infants' selectivity in learning. Their vocal learning must be guided by something more.

The *something more* that we subscribe to in explaining both innate perceptual abilities and selective vocal learning is the notion that for each species in which vocal communication plays a critical role, specialized perceptual mechanisms exist. These special mechanisms are as unique to the species as the sounds that are produced by that species. Thus, we say it is the bird's *auditory template* and the baby's *speech module* that explain why birds sing and babies babble, and why both display early perceptual recognition of their conspecific signals.

Accepting that infants demonstrate both innate perceptual abilities and early restrictions on vocal learning, the challenge to theory is to describe the mechanisms that underlie these abilities. What kinds of mechanisms are they? What information do they specify? Are the mechanisms dedicated to the processing of conspecific signals? Do they involve perceptual systems, production systems, or both?

The purpose of this chapter is to review the current status of our answers to these questions regarding the human infant's acquisition of speech. Important phenomena regarding infants' perception and production of speech are reviewed and two theories that have been advanced to explain these abilities are described. The comparative approach is shown to have made two important contributions to the study of special mechanisms in human infants. Experiments on animals' perception of speech have provided critical data on the question of specialized mechanisms. More generally, theory building has benefited from the interchange between developmental ethologists and developmental speech scientists who have examined each other's methods, data, and arguments.

I. MODULES AND MECHANISMS

There are two very different characterizations of infants' "initial state" regarding speech (Kuhl, 1986a, 1987a). One account argues that, from the start, the perceptual mechanisms underlying speech in infants include a phonetic-level representation of speech. On this view infants are born with an "innate phonetics"—linguistic-unit representations, either segments or features, preexist in the child in some form. It is this representation, one necessarily involving mechanisms that evolved especially for speech, that explains infants' abilities to detect complex equivalences.

The second account is quite different. On this view, there is no preexisting phonetic-level representation of speech; no formal description of phonetic units exists innately. By this account phonetic-level representations are formed later, perhaps as infants begin to map various acoustic forms onto objects and events in the world. According to this model, infants' initial speech perception abilities are attributable to their more general auditory and cognitive abilities.

By this description, the key points for the first account are (a) phonetic-level representation, and (b) specialized mechanisms. The key points for the second account are (a) no phonetic-level representation, and (b) mechanisms that are general.

Before going further, we need to decide what to call the two accounts. There are three dichotomous terms that have been used historically to characterize the two positions: *phonetic* versus *auditory, special* versus *general,* and *motor* versus *sensory.* The terms phonetic, special, and motor were used to characterize the first account; the terms auditory, general, and sensory, were used to characterize the second account.

The problem is that the terms associated with each position, while loosely associated, are not mutually exclusive. The term phonetic has been strongly associated with the *Motor Theory,* which argues that the phonetic-level representation can be specified only in motor terms (Liberman & Mattingly, 1985). However, others have not assumed that a phonetic-level representation must be specified in motor terms; instead, it has been argued that such a representation could be specified in auditory terms (Diehl & Kluender, in press), or in an abstract form not specific to either modality (i.e., in an amodal form) (Kuhl & Meltzoff, 1982, 1984; Studdert-Kennedy, 1986). Similarly, describing the alternative account as auditory restricts it to explaining behavior that is exclusively auditory in nature; the main postulate of the theory is that the underlying mechanisms are general rather than specialized. When referring to the two opposing views in this chapter, I will call the first account the Special Mechanism account (hereafter SMA). SMA argues for phonetic-level representations, and consequently for specialized mechanisms, but does not specify their exact form. I term the second account the "General Mechanism account" (hereafter GMA). GMA postulates general mechanisms and no phonetic-level representation.

Finally, it is worth noting that this debate about the nature of the mechanisms underlying the perception of complex signals is not restricted to speech. Ethologists have long favored the notion that complex perception, especially species-typical behavior, is accomplished by specialized neural mechanisms. Moreover, specialization has been advanced as a general theory of the perceptual processing of complex stimuli; it is a theory that now pervades all of the psychology of perception. The theory, advanced by Fodor (1983), centers on the concept of the *module*—the highly specialized neural architecture that does the computational work required to perceive eccentric stimuli. Modules do things like perceive speech, recognize objects, localize sound, track things that move in space, and detect color. Modules have a particular set of properties. They are first and foremost *modularized;* that is, they are separate from other modules, and they use specialized, rather than general-purpose mechanisms, to do their work. They operate only on stimuli of a particular kind (domain specific), their computations depend only on resources that are internal to the module (informationally encapsulated), and they are not accessible by higher-order mechanisms (cognitively impenetrable). Their operations are rapid and mandatory. Most pertinent to this discussion, they are *innate.*

It is not difficult to portray speech as a canonical case of an eccentric stimulus in need of a module. The problems inherent in the nature of speech, the extremely complex mapping between acoustic events and phonetic percepts, and the problem of segmenting the continuous stream of speech into linguistically appropriate units such as phonetic segments or features, appear to be intractable problems for computers (Klatt, 1986). Moreover, the complex equivalences detected by babies—between acoustic events that are physically different but phonetically similar, between the sight of a face and the sound of a voice when they both indicate the same phonetic unit, and between sounds articulated by someone else and then reproduced with our own mouths—are difficult to explain without reference to some kind of specialized mechanisms (Kuhl, 1986b).

A speech module for babies would indeed present a solution, but recent data suggest that the alternative be considered. Experiments on animals' perception of speech shows that they also demonstrate perceptual phenomena such as categorical perception, and that their categorical boundaries also move when the context is changed (Kuhl, 1987b). It is these phenomena that have been used as evidence for an innate speech module in humans. Moreover, recent data on infants' cognitive abilities suggest that they detect complex equivalences outside of the realm of speech, between sensory information presented to different modalities and even between sensory events and their motor equivalents. Thus, when the signal is speech, certain of the perceptual abilities thought to be species-specific are not; animals display them as well. And when the perceivers are human, complex perceptual abilities are not restricted to speech; stimuli in other domains evoke them as well.

The question is: What do we want to impute to the baby? Do infants come into the world equipped with special mechanisms that provide both a means for detecting phonetic equivalence and a means for segmenting the stream of speech into its component parts (SMA)? Or is there no phonetic-level representation of speech, in which case infants' abialities are attributed to their more general sensory and cognitive abilities(GMA)?

II. FOCUS OF THE DEBATE: THE BASIS OF INFANTS' ABILITIES

The two accounts just described do not take different positions regarding infants' capabilities. Both positions agree that infants' perception of speech shows remarkable sophistication. Instead, the differences lie in how they view the nature of the mechanisms that underlie infants' abilities. Thus the debate centers on the *basis* of behavior. The question is: Are infants' abilities based on special mechanisms (SMA) or more general ones (GMA)?

Traditionally, the basis question has been approached in two different ways. We consider these two ways and add a third.

Consider first the two traditional approaches. The first compares the perception of speech sounds with that of nonspeech sounds that are designed to mimic speech acoustically without being perceived as speech. The second compares the perception of speech by human and nonhuman listeners. I have argued elsewhere (Kuhl, 1986b, 1987a) that while both these traditional approaches address the SMA vs. GMA debate, they do not answer the same question. The distinction made here is a simple point of logic, which is offered to explain a point of view about the contributions of nonspeech tests.

I have argued that studies using nonspeech ask whether the mechanisms underlying speech perception are speech specific. No one disagrees with this point. But having determined the answer to this question we have to decide what we can conclude. Consider the easy case first. If speech and nonspeech findings completely diverge, as they did in early tests of speech perception (e.g., Mattingly, Liberman, Syrdal, & Halwes, 1971), it is sensible to conclude that the mechanisms underlying the phenomenon are speech-specific, and, thus, evolved especially for speech.

A problem emerges, however, if the opposite result obtains, with speech and nonspeech showing complete convergence (Miller et al., 1976; Pisoni, 1977; Pisoni, Carrell, & Gans, 1983). It is logical to conclude from such results that the mechanisms are *not* speech-specific. However, it cannot be argued unambiguously that such mechanisms did not evolve especially for speech. This argument cannot be made because the terms *speech-specific* and *especially evolved for speech* are not synonymous. Mechanisms could, in principle, have evolved especially for speech without being speech-specific.

Consider the following interpretation: Nonspeech sounds carefully designed to mimic the speech signal are processed as speech because they *fool* the special speech mechanism. Thus, the mechanisms that evolved especially for speech did so in such a way that they did not exclude nonspeech signals (Kuhl, 1978, 1986b). What this leaves us with is a situation in which results showing complete speech-nonspeech convergence can be explained by either alternative. Using the SMA, special mechanisms for speech have evolved but are fooled by nonspeech signals that mimic speech. The GMA argues that speech and nonspeech are processed similarly because there are no special mechanisms and both signals are handled by more general ones.

Therefore, studies involving nonspeech signals are most easily interpreted when the outcomes of the studies show a complete dissociation between speech and nonspeech, as they did in the early studies. Complete divergence of speech and nonspeech is easily interpreted as strong support for the theory that speech requires *special* mechanisms, ones different from those used in the processing of nonspeech signals. When studies on nonspeech demonstrate the opposite, that is, complete convergence between speech and nonspeech, the opposing claim cannot be unambiguously advanced.

Animal studies contribute to the debate in a different way. Tests of speech perception in animals answer a simple question: Can the perceptual phenomenon exist in the absence of mechanisms that evolved especially for speech? If animals replicate speech effects we can assert without ambiguity that special mechanisms are not *necessary* to account for the phenomenon. Animal replications do not prove that special mechanisms are not at work in humans, but the results eliminate the need for positing them to explain specific phenomena.

Both kinds of experiments help build theories. For example, if speech–nonspeech convergence is found with the same stimuli that animals succeed on, we have no reason to impute special processing of these stimuli. Furthermore, if both speech–nonspeech comparisons and animal tests fail at the same *level* of complexity the theoretical implications are strong. It would be at this level that evidence for special speech mechanisms would have been obtained. Taken together, the two approaches provide valuable complementary evidence for theory construction.

The speech phenomena demonstrated by infants will be discussed in the next section and studies done to investigate the basis of infants' abilities will also be described. In most instances studies on the basis of infants' abilities use nonspeech or animals to address the question. To these two traditional methods of testing the underlying basis of the effects in infants I add a third. This new approach involves asking whether or not similar phenomena have been observed with other than auditory stimuli. In other words, the broader issue of domain specificity will be addressed. If the detection of complex equivalences, such as those involving cross-modal or imitative abilities, are exclusive to speech, then this supports SMA. But if such abilities are demonstrated more generally in infants, and appear to be part of their native cognitive endowment, then there may be no reason to claim that the abilities are part of a specialized subsystem for speech.

III. INFANTS' DETECTION OF COMPLEX EQUIVALENCES

The most striking thing about infants' perception of speech is not their ability to detect fine differences between sounds that will eventually convey meaning, though they do that quite well. The most striking thing is their ability to detect similarity—equivalence—between stimuli that are phonetically equal but physically different. The detection of phonetic equivalence is in fact a critical problem for theory.

It is precisely this problem that causes computers to fail at speech recognition. Speech segments are coarticulated; this means that the acoustic cues for an individual unit vary dramatically depending on the context in which the unit appears. The phonetic unit /b/ in *bat* is not physically identical to the /b/ in *beet, bit, boat,* and *boot.* Yet, as adults we are good at recognizing its equivalence across these contexts—so good that it is difficult to view the detection of equivalence as a problem for theory. Similarly, when we perceive a phonetic unit as being the same regardless of whether the talker is a male, female, or young child, our recognition of the an equivalence is automatic. Yet neither of these perceptual feats can be performed by the most sophisticated computer (Klatt, 1986). The major point for this discussion is that infants are also good at equivalence detection. Solved by babies, but not by machines, the detection of equivalence is a central problem in speech perception; if we understood how it was done it would be a major breakthrough.

There are three classes of phenomena, each involving the detection of complex equivalences for phonetically similar but physically different stimuli, that have been demonstrated in infants. The three classes of phenomena include

(1). Auditory equivalence, the detection of equivalences between two auditory stimuli, as represented by the phenomena of categorical perception (Eimas, Siqueland, Jusczyk, & Vigorito, 1971) and of equivalence classification (Kuhl, 1979a, 1983, 1985a),

(2). Auditory-Visual equivalence, the detection of a correspondence between auditory and visual representations of the same phonetic unit (Kuhl & Meltzoff, 1982, 1984; MacKain, Studdert-Kennedy, Spieker, & Stern, 1983), and

(3). Auditory-Motor equivalence, as demonstrated by vocal imitation, wherein an auditory stimulus produced by someone else evokes the motor movements necessary to reproduce that signal oneself (Kuhl & Meltzoff, 1982, 1988; Lieberman, 1984).

Auditory Equivalence

There are two examples of auditory equivalence demonstrated by infants that theories regarding the initial state of perceptual mechanisms will have to explain. One is the classic phenomenon of *categorical perception* (CP), in which listeners are shown to be more sensitive to changes in a speech stimulus at the boundary between phonetic categories than they are in the middle of the category. The other, *equivalence classification,* is more like what cognitive psychologists classically refer to as categorization. It involves tests of infants' abilities to recognize equivalence between two auditory stimuli that they can easily discriminate.

Categorical Perception (CP)

One of the most significant early findings in favor of innate special mechanisms came from the discovery of categorical perception in infants (Eimas et al., 1971). In adults the phenomenon involved the following demonstration. A continuum of sounds was generated by computer along which an acoustic dimension was altered in small physically equal steps. Tests showed that while the acoustic dimension changed continuously along the continuum in a stepwise fashion, perception was discontinuous. The stimuli were heard as a series of stimuli (e.g., /ra/'s) that changed abruptly to a new series of stimuli (e.g., /la/'s) at some point on the continuum (Fig. 13.1, top). Moreover, the ability to discriminate between

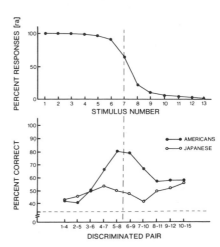

FIG. 13.1. Categorical perception in American and Japanese adults. From Miyawaki et al. (1975).

sounds taken from the series was constrained. Adults could discriminate quite easily between sounds that fell in different categories, but discrimination between sounds in the same category was quite difficult (Fig. 13.1, bottom) (Miyawaki et al., 1975).

Perception was shown to be categorical only for contrasts that were phonemic (made a difference between words) in the adult's language. Japanese adults, for whom the /ra-la/ distinction is not phonemic, did not produce the characteristic peak in the discrimination function for /ra-la/ stimuli (Miyawaki et al., 1975). Their ability to discriminate the stimuli hovered near chance (Fig. 13.1, bottom).

This phenomenon immediately raised a question about development: Do infants demonstrate CP initially, or only after experience with a specific language? The question was answered by Eimas et al.'s (1971) work on 1-month-old infants' perception of speech. Eimas showed that infants could discriminate computer-generated sounds that straddled the adult-defined phonetic boundary but failed to discriminate within-category stimuli (Eimas et al., 1971; Eimas, 1974, 1975). Infants' ability to do this in the absence of a protracted period of experience in producing or listening to speech suggested that the phenomenon was not learned. Infants appeared to partition the stimulus continuum just as adults did, right from the start. Further evidence against the learning account came from the finding that infants demonstrated the effect for all phonemic contrasts, whether native to the language environment in which they were raised or not (Aslin, Pisoni, Hennessey, & Perey, 1981; Streeter, 1976). These findings were extremely important because they were the first to suggest that infants might be innately endowed with mechanisms specialized for speech.

Other related phenomena such as *context effects* and *trading relations,* were also investigated with infants. These studies stemmed from early work focused on the acoustic analysis of speech. This early work showed that the acoustic cues underlying phonetic perception were context-dependent (Liberman et al., 1967). The phonetic units surrounding a target unit, the specific talker who produced it, the rate at which it was spoken, and its position in a syllable were shown to alter the acoustic cues that specified a particular phonetic unit. That adult listeners were sensitive to these contextual differences had been shown in studies of CP in adults (Best, Morrongiello, & Robson, 1981; Miller & Liberman, 1979; Summerfield & Haggard, 1977). These studies confirmed the perceptual effect of context by showing that the exact location of the phonetic boundary on a continuum was altered by the context in which the phonetic unit appeared.

An example of a context effect is that provided by a change in the rate of speech. Studies suggest that adult listeners may take rate-of-articulation information into account when making decisions about the phonetic identity of a particular phonetic unit. Miller and Liberman (1979) demonstrated that the location of the boundary between the consonants /b/ and /w/ changed as a function of the duration (and thus, to an adult, the perceived rate) of the syllable. In their first experiment, a /ba-wa/ syllable continuum was lengthened to indicate slower speech by increasing the duration of the vowel. For this *long* syllable continuum, the boundary was located at a longer transition duration than it was for the *short* syllable continuum. In a second experiment, the syllable was lengthened in a different way, one not associated with a slower rate of articulation. The syllable was lengthened by adding formant transitions to the end of the original vowel, which created the perception of a final consonant on the syllables (/bad-wad/) but did not signal a slowed rate of speaking. Here the effect was reversed; the perceptual boundary moved toward shorter transition durations.

Eimas and Miller (1980) showed that 2- to 3-month-old infants demonstrate one part of this effect. Using the same stimuli used by Miller and Liberman (1979), these authors selected syllables from the long and short /ba-wa/ continua. Syllables were chosen to create four stimulus pairs, including both within-category pairs and between-category pairs from each continuum. Infants were tested using the HAS (high amplitude sucking) technique. The results demonstrated that infants discriminated only the between-category pairs on both continua, thus suggesting that infants are sensitive to contextual information.

Trading relations effects are similar to context effects, but take the argument one step further. In these cases, the cues that are necessary to achieve a particular phonetic percept not only change with the context, but in a specific compensatory way. The value along one acoustic dimension determines the value that is required along a second dimension. The effects of the two dimensions appear to be additive, such that an increased value on the first dimension must be accompanied by a decreased value on the second dimension.

There are two examples of trading relations in infants. Both support the claim that infants are sensitive to compensatory effects. The first case involves a trading relation between the duration of the first formant and the VOT required to perceive a voiceless stop (Summerfield & Haggard, 1977). Miller and Eimas (1983) tested this trading relation on 2- to 3-month-olds using the HAS technique. They created two continua varying in VOT from 5 ms to 55 ms. This variation in VOT is sufficient to change an adult's percept from /ba/ to /pa/. One continuum was constructed with short (25 ms) transitions and the other with long (85 ms) transitions. For adults, the boundary value between voiced and voiceless stops on the short continuum occurred at about 25 ms, while on the long continuum the boundary occurred at about 45 ms. The infants were tested with four pairs of stimuli: 5 ms vs. 35 ms short (perceived as /b/ and /p/ respectively by adults); 35 ms and 55 ms short (both perceived as /p/ by adults); 5 ms vs. 35 ms long (both perceived as /b/ by adults); 35 ms vs. 55 ms long (perceived as /b/ and /p/ respectively by adults). The infants provided evidence of discriminating only the 5 ms vs. 35 ms *short* pair and the 35 ms vs. 55 ms *long* pair. Thus, the data suggest that the location of enhanced discriminability on these two continua occurs at different places for infants, as well as adults, thus providing evidence of trading relations in infants.

A second example of trading relations that has been tested with infants involved the contrast *say* vs. *stay*. Adult studies show that inserting a silent gap between the /s/ and the vowel in the word *say* induces the perception of a voiceless stop, so as to create the word *stay*. More importantly, the length of the silent gap inserted in these situations interacts with the spectral aspects of the remainder of the syllable. Best et al. (1981) synthesized two continua ranging from say to stay. One continuum was synthesized with formant transitions appropriate for /t/ and one was synthesized without these transitions. Best et al. showed that the silent duration required to perceive *stay* varied for the two continua. When the spectral information for ''t'' was more complete, less silence was required to produce *stay* than when the spectral information for ''t'' was less well specified. Best et al. argued that this perceptual trading relation was due to the listener's knowledge of the association of these two cues in the production of the sound.

Recently Eimas (1985) provided evidence for this trading relation in infants. He tested 2- to 4-month-olds using stimuli from the two continua. Pairs of stimuli were drawn such that adults perceived the stimulus pair as containing two *say* stimuli, two *stay* stimuli, or one of each. In all cases, discrimination was evidenced to be similar to an adult's; that is, infants failed to detect the difference between two syllables heard by adults to be equivalent (two versions of say, or two of stay), but always provided evidence of discriminating two syllables heard as different by adults.

In summary, the data that are available on context effects and trading relations in infants provide support for the notion that infants are sensitive to these effects. These effects are important to theory because they show that the perceptual boundary between phonetic categories moves. The fact that the boundary is not fixed makes it difficult to attribute these effects to a simple mechanism, and suggests the possibility that the perceived equivalence between acoustic events derives from their common articulatory origin. But infants have not yet produced these sounds, and therefore such motor knowledge has to be argued to be built-in. An alternative view (the GMA) is that these perceptual effects are the result of the functional characteristics of the auditory system. That is to say, it is possible that these perceptual effects derive from the complex way in which the auditory system combines acoustic information in perception, irrespective of its status as speech (Kuhl & Padden, 1983).

The Basis of CP

Tests on Nonspeech Signals.   Studies on adults have shown that CP can be replicated using stimuli that mimic speech sounds varying in VOT (Miller et al., 1976; Pisoni, 1977) and for nonspeech analogs mimicking the /ba-wa/ rate effect (Pisoni et al., 1983). The agreement between the speech and nonspeech data for adult listeners naturally led to a strong interest in the performance of infants in discrimination tasks involving nonspeech stimuli. Two of the studies cited above have been examined in young infants, one involving the nonspeech correlate of VOT, tone-onset time (TOT), and the other, the nonspeech correlate of /ba/ and /wa/ in tests of the context effect of rate. Jusczyk, Pisoni, Walley, and Murray (1980) tested the discrimination of sounds varying in tone-onset time (TOT). The stimuli were synthesized to duplicate those used by Pisoni (1977) on adults. Jusczyk et al. predicted that infants, like adults, would discriminate only those stimuli that straddled the −20 ms or +20 ms TOT boundaries. They tested a number of stimulus pairs: −70 ms vs. −40 ms; −40 ms vs. −10 ms; −30 ms vs. 0 ms; −20 ms vs. +10 ms; −10 ms vs. +20 ms; 0 ms vs. +30 ms; +10 ms vs. +40 ms; and +40 ms vs. +70 ms.

Contrary to their prediction, the sucking recovery scores indicated that only the −70 ms vs. −40 ms and +40 ms vs. +70 ms contrasts were discriminated. The data provided support for the notion that infants perceive three categories on the TOT continuum, but the data suggested that the boundaries for these categories were located in different places for infants than for adults, and that in infants the TOT nonspeech boundary does not coincide with the VOT speech boundary. The fact that discrimination was symmetrical, that on both sides of the continuum discrimination was not evidenced until the tones were temporally offset by at least 40 ms, suggests that infants may require a longer interval between the onsets of two tones before perceiving them as nonsimultaneous. The result is an important one, because it shows a dissociation between speech and nonspeech in infants that is not present in adults.

In a recent report, Jusczyk, Pisoni, Reed, Fernald, and Myers (1983) replicated with infants the context effect involving rate using the nonspeech analogs of /ba/ and /wa/. The results demonstrated that, just as when listening to speech, infants needed a shorter transition duration to detect a change in *short* stimuli, and a longer transition duration for detecting a change in *long* stimuli. This means that infants are sensitive to overall duration in nonspeech as well as in speech, and that transition duration is processed relationally for both signals.

Thus, the results for infants' perception of nonspeech are mixed, with the study of the context effect of rate (Jusczyk et al., 1983) supporting a close agreement between speech and nonspeech, and the TOT study (Jusczyk et al., 1980) failing to do so. A strong conclusion about the agreement between speech and nonspeech data by infants is not possible at this time; further experiments addressing this issue are needed.

Tests on CP in Animals.   The research completed on animals' perception of speech is at present quite extensive (Kuhl, 1986b); three examples are cited here to illustrate the findings. The first data are from the first study that examined an animal's ability to categorize sounds from a speech-sound continuum (Kuhl & Miller, 1975). This test focused on the characteristic labeling functions obtained in speech. The question for animals was whether the boundary between the two categories on the continuum coincided with the phonetic one, or appeared someplace else. The second data are more recent and focus directly on tests of the "phoneme boundary effect" (Kuhl & Padden, 1982, 1983). The question here is whether or not in the absence of any experience in *labeling* the stimuli on the continuum, an animal will demonstrate enhanced discriminability at the boundaries between phonetic categories, like human infants do. The third is our most recent result (Stevens, Kuhl, & Padden, 1988) and it concerns the context effect of rate demonstrated with the syllables /ba/ and /wa/.

The Kuhl and Miller (1975) study resembled an adult categorization experiment, only with animals. The question was: Where would an animal place the boundary on a phonetic continuum? Chinchillas were trained to distinguish computer-synthesized versions of the two endpoint stimuli on a /da-ta/ continuum, 0 msec VOT and +80 msec VOT. During training, they were not given any exposure to the rest of the test continuum. When performance on these endpoint stimuli was near perfect, a generalization paradigm was used to test the intermediate stimuli, those between /da/ and /ta/ on the continuum (+10 msec VOT to +70 msec VOT, in 10-msec steps). The design of the experiment was that during generalization testing, half of the trials would involve the endpoint stimuli. On these trials, all of the appropriate feedback was given, just as it had been during the training phase. On the other half of the trials, the intermediate stimuli were presented.

The intermediate trials were the ones most critical for theory. On trials involving intermediate stimuli, the feedback was arranged to indicate that the animal was always correct, no matter what the response. There was no training on these stimuli, and thus no clue was provided to the animal telling him how to respond and thus where to place the boundary on the continuum.

The data are shown in Fig. 13.2 (top). The mean percentage of /da/ responses to each stimulus on the continuum are plotted for chinchillas and human adults. The curves were generated by the same least-squares method. The resulting phonetic boundaries, located at 35.2 msec VOT for humans and 33.3 msec VOT for animals, did not differ significantly. A subsequent study using a totally different procedure and monkeys rather than chinchillas demonstrated that the location of the boundary on a /da-ta/ continuum was located at +28 msec, in good agreement with the chinchilla data (Waters & Wilson, 1976).

Kuhl and Miller (1978) extended these tests to continua involving other voiced-voiceless pairs, namely bilabial (/ba-pa/) and velar (/ga-ka/) contrasts. These stimuli were of interest because human listeners' boundaries differ with the place of articulation specified by the particular voiced-voiceless pair. The new tests involving the bilabial and velar stimuli were run exactly as the previous ones. The endpoint VOT values were 0 and +80 msec. The intermediate stimuli (+10 to +70 msec in 10-msec steps) were presented with feedback indicating that the animal was correct regardless of his performance. Thus, no training occurred on these stimuli. The results again demonstrated excellent agreement between the human and animal categorization data. The boundary values for the

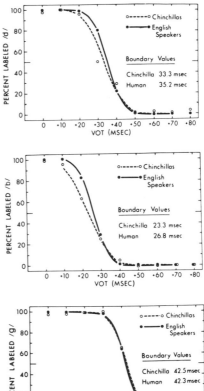

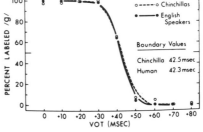

FIG. 13.2. Discrimination of sounds from speech continua by animals and human adults tested on /d-t/ (top), /b-p/ (middle), and /g-k/ (bottom) stimuli. The locations of the boundaries for the two groups did not differ significantly. From Kuhl and Miller (1978).

bilabial stimuli were 26.8 msec VOT for humans and 23.3 msec VOT for animals (Fig. 13.2, middle), which were not significantly different. The boundary values for the velar stimuli were 42.3 msec VOT for humans and 42.5 msec VOT for animals (Fig. 13.2, bottom). Again, the values did not differ significantly.

Taken together, the data suggested that animals' natural boundaries coincided with humans' phonetic ones, but to this point no studies had been done on animals' discrimination of specific pairs of stimuli from the continuum. Since it is the enhanced discriminability between categories—the phoneme boundary effect—that sets speech apart from other phenomena in psychophysics and in cognitive psychology, and since infants appear to demonstrate this effect without learning to experience (Eimas et al., 1971) discrimination tests were considered important.

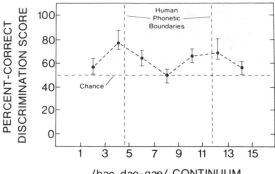

FIG. 13.3. Discriminability of pairs of speech stimuli taken from a place-of-articulation (/b-d-g/) continuum. The bars indicate the entire *range* of performance across animals for each stimulus pair. Performance was enhanced at the locations of humans' phonetic boundaries. From Kuhl and Padden (1983).

We conducted two studies that directly addressed discriminability of stimulus pairs from a speech-sound continuum (Kuhl & Padden, 1982, 1983). (See also Kuhl, 1981; Sinnott, Beecher, Moody, & Stebbins, 1976; and Morse & Snowdon, 1975, for different types of speech discrimination tests on animals). The technique used in our studies involved training a monkey on a same-different task. During training, stimuli that were easily discriminable like a tone versus a noise or a click versus a buzz, were used. Eventually the monkey had to discriminate various vowel sounds, some of which differed only in intensity or pitch. The experiment involved testing stimulus pairs from a speech sound continuum to examine their discriminability, just as is done in tests on infants. The CP model predicts differential discriminability across the continuum, with pairs that straddle the phonetic boundary being most discriminable. Kuhl and Padden (1982) used stimuli from three different voicing continua and Kuhl and Padden (1983) used stimuli from a place continuum. The results of the two experiments were identical—in both cases animals demonstrated the discrimination typical of CP.

The results from the /bæ-dæ-gæ/ experiment are shown in Fig. 13.3. The average percentage correct discrimination score is given for each pair. The locations of the human phonetic boundaries are marked by dashed vertical lines. As shown, the best performance occurred on stimulus pairs 3 vs. 5, 9 vs. 11, and 11 vs. 13. These are the only pairs that differ significantly from chance, and involve stimuli from different phonetic categories for humans. Thus, while stimulus pairs were always separated by an equal physical distance on the continuum, their perceived differences were not equivalent. Discriminability was poor when the stimuli involved pairs taken from the same involved pairs taken from different phonetic categories.

Most recently, our tests on animals have been extended to the phenomenon of "context effects." The particular example that we have tested involved the /ba-wa/ distinction and its dependence on rate (Stevens, Kuhl, & Padden, 1988). Recall that when the two syllables /ba/ and /wa/ are produced at *fast* as opposed to *slow* rates of speech, the boundary between them is located at two different places on the respective continua. On the fast continuum, shorter transition durations are required to change the percept from /ba/ to /wa/; on the slow continuum, longer transition durations are required to change the percept from /ba/ to /wa/. The problem for a theory of speech perception is to explain how the underlying mechanisms specify a different boundary for fast versus slow speech.

Our tests on macaques used the same stimuli used to test infants by Eimas and Miller (1980). The stimulus pairs had been chosen by these authors so as to include pairs that straddled the adult-defined boundaries on both the fast and slow /ba-wa/ continua, and pairs that fell within a single phonetic category. These same pairs were used to test macaques. Our results mirrored those found with infants. Macaques discriminated only the pairs that straddled adult human boundaries, while failing to show discrimination of pairs of stimuli that fell within a single phonetic category (Stevens, Kuhl, & Padden, 1988). Thus, it appears that macaques also show context effects for speech; their boundaries on speech continua move when the context is changed.

Taken as a whole, these data lend support to the notion that enhanced discrimination near phonetic boundaries can be demonstrated in mammals other than man. I have argued elsewhere that this finding supports two conclusions, one about evolution and the other about infant performance (Kuhl, 1986b; Kuhl & Padden, 1983). First, in the evolution of language, the choice of the particular phonetic units used in communication was strongly influenced by the extent to which the units were ideally suited to the auditory system (Kuhl, 1988; Stevens, in press). It has been argued (Kuhl, 1979b, 1981; Kuhl & Padden, 1983; Stevens, 1972, 1981) that the perception of certain auditory properties, such as spectral shape, detection of rapid formant change, and temporal order, served as a set of constraints on the acoustics of language. The second conclusion is that since animals demonstrate these speech phenomena, the fact that infants do so is not sufficient evidence *by itself* to support the notion that the mechanisms underlying the effects in infants are ones that evolved especially for speech. Animals demonstrate these effects in the absence of special mechanisms; infants may do so as well.

Equivalence Classification

A second kind of auditory equivalence is demonstrated by infants, one more like what cognitive psychologists call "categorization"—the ability to "render discriminably different things equivalent" (Bruner, Goodnow, & Austin, 1956).

Categorization is a phenomenon that characterizes all of perception. As stimuli typically vary along many dimensions, categorization requires that we recognize similarities in the presence of considerable variance. Often the exact criteria used to categorize are not obvious. Consider the categories *cat* and *dog*. Describing what distinguishes them, and thus what uniquely categorizes them, is not simple. They both have two eyes, two ears, four legs, fur, a tail, and so on. Configurational properties of the face probably distinguish them, but trying to describe these features is difficult. Yet we would not expect an adult to mistakenly identify a cat as a dog, or vice versa.

In speech, a similar categorization problem exists. Take a simple example, such as the vowel categories /a/ as in "cot" and /æ/ as in "cat." The differences between the two vowels are not subtle to the human ear; they are clearly different. But trying to program a computer to identify these vowels correctly when they are spoken by different individuals demonstrates it to be a very difficult problem. When different talkers produce these two vowels, there is overlap in the physical cues, the formant frequencies, that represent the two categories. The explanation for this has to do with the fact that people with different-sized vocal tracts (like males, females and children) produce different resonance frequencies when they create the same mouth shape. Thus far, no one has successfully described an algorithm that correctly recovers which of the vowels a speaker produced when acoustic information (the formant frequency values) is the only thing provided. In humans, various attempts to explain the processes by which we normalize the speech produced by different talkers have been offered; most of them involve computation of some kind (Lieberman, 1984, for review).

The critical question for the current discussion is whether infants recognize equivalence when the same vowel is produced by different talkers. Are all /a/'s the same to the baby, regardless of the talker who produced them? It is of no small import to the child that such an ability exists early in life. Vocal-tract normalization is critical to the infant's acquisition of speech. Their vocal tracts cannot produce the frequencies produced by the adult's vocal tract, so infants must normalize speech to imitate it.

How can the question be posed to the infant? We want to know if they can sort vowel sounds into two categories. When we ask whether infants can categorize, we want evidence that they can perceptually group a variety of instances into Type A and Type B events, even though the various A's (or B's) are clearly differentiable. To perform such a task requires that infants recognize similarity among discriminably different instances representing the A (and B) category, while ignoring the irrelevant differences between the various A's (and B's). Thus, categorization requires a process in which the perceiver perceptually establishes two groups of stimuli; in each category equivalence must be detected while irrelevant variations (though discriminable) must be ignored.

Two main features distinguish tests of "equivalence classification" from the tests of CP. First, the stimuli representing the categories are discriminably different. In tests of CP, the stimuli differ on a single acoustic parameter, and thus evidence of categorization is taken from infants' failure to evidence discrimination. In tests of equivalence classification, the stimuli vary along a number of dimensions and are clearly discriminable. Thus, categorization, if it occurs, cannot be attributed to a failure to discriminate the stimuli. In the first speech experiment on equivalence classification with infants, Kuhl (1979a) examined infants' discrimination of two vowel categories, /a/ (as in *pop*) and /i/ (as in *peep*). The stimuli used in the experiment varied along three dimensions, phonetic identity (/a/ versus /i/), pitch contour (rising versus falling), and talker identity (male, female, or child). Stimuli belonging to the same category (all /a/'s for example) were shown to be easily discriminable from one another by infants. The question was: Can infants perceptually group all of the /a/'s and all of the /i/'s?

Second, the categorization approach requires the infant to produce an equivalent response to stimuli that are perceived to be equivalent, rather than to produce a response based on the detection of a difference between two stimuli. In order to explore infants' abilities to categorize, a technique had to be developed that required the infant to report the perception of *similarity* rather than to report the perception of a *difference*. Because every member of the category is perceptually different, having infants' responses depend on their perception of a difference would not allow one to address the categorization question. Instead, we wanted infants to signal that they heard a similarity between a novel stimulus and a stimulus they heard previously. Moreover, we wanted this perception of *sameness* not to be based on a failure to discriminate the two stimuli.

A technique was developed by Kuhl (1985b) that achieves this goal. It uses a simple conditioning procedure that is shown in Fig. 13.4. The infant sits on a parent's lap and is visually engaged by an assistant, who manipulates toys silently. A speech sound, such as the vowel sound /a/, plays repeatedly from the loudspeaker at the infant's left. The infant quickly learned that when the sound changes from the vowel /a/ to the vowel /i/ a bear playing a drum inside a black box on top of the loudspeaker is turned on for a short period of time. Eventually the infant anticipates the occurrence of the bear and produces a head-turn in the direction of the box when the sound /i/ is played.

Once trained, the infant produces head-turning responses only when /i/ vowels occur, and does not turn during presentations of the vowel /a/. We want to know what infants will do when they are presented with new instances of /a/ and /i/vowels, instances clearly different from the /a/ and /i/ stimuli heard during training. To find out, infants were initially trained to make a response when an /a/ vowel, produced by a male voice with a falling pitch contour, was changed to an /i/ vowel. The two stimuli were acoustically matched in every other detail. After this initial training, infants were tested with novel stimuli representing the two categories, ones produced by female and child talkers, with either rising or falling pitch contours. All of the novel stimuli differed perceptually from the two initial training stimuli, and infants were shown to be capable of discriminating all of the /a/'s from one another. The hypothesis was that the infant's initial training to respond to a single /i/ sound would generalize to all members of the category; that is, we argued that if infants perceived all /i/'s as

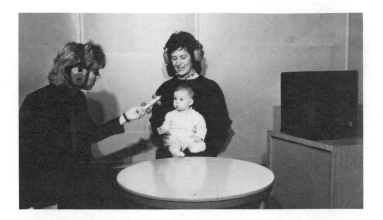

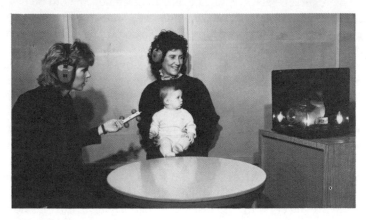

FIG. 13.4.   A head-turn technique used to test infants' categorization of speech sounds. Infants are trained to produce a head turn toward the loudspeaker on the infant's left when a speech sound from one phonetic category is changed to a sound from a second phonetic category. If infants do so at the appropriate time, a visual reinforcer is presented. Once training is complete, novel stimuli from both categories are presented to test infants' abilities to categorize them. From Kuhl (1986b).

perceptually equivalent, then if the infant had been trained to produce a head-turn response to the male's /i/ vowel, but not to his /a/ vowel, the infant would produce that response to all novel /i/'s (ones produced by females or children), but not to equally novel /a/'s.

The results show that this hypothesis was correct (Kuhl, 1979a). Infants responded correctly to the novel vowels. If the infant had been trained to turn to the male's /a/, then all novel /a/'s evoked the response, while none of the novel /i/'s did. The same was true if infants were trained to turn to the male's /i/—all novel /i/'s evoked the response, but not the novel /a/'s. Figure 13.5 shows the

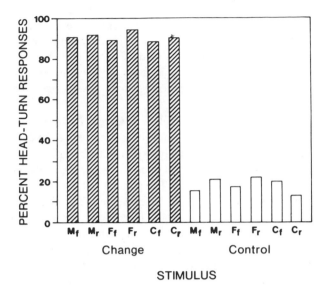

FIG. 13.5.   Group data for the /a-i/ vowel categorization experiment. Per cent head-turn responses to each novel stimulus that belonged to the phonetic category that was initially reinforced (Change stimuli) and the phonetic category that was not initially reinforced (Control stimuli). The training stimuli were the far left "Change" stimulus and the far left "Control" stimulus, each produced by a male (M) voice with a falling (f) pitch contour. After training, novel vowels produced by female (F) and child (C) talkers, with either rising (r) or falling pitch contours, were introduced. The data show excellent generalization from the training stimuli to novel stimuli representing the same phonetic category. From Kuhl (1987).

per cent head-turn responses to all of the stimuli introduced in the experiment. As shown, infants produced head-turn responses only to the stimuli that were members of the phonetic category that they were initially trained to respond to. They failed to produce head-turn responses to equally novel stimuli that were not members of the phonetic category that they were trained to respond to. More surprisingly, an analysis of infants' first-trial responses showed that infants performed correctly on the very first trial. These results suggest that six-month-old infants categorize all /a/'s (and all /i/'s) as the same.

Kuhl (1983) extended these results to vowel categories that are much more similar from an acoustic standpoint and therefore much more difficult to categorize. The vowels were synthesized versions of /a/ (as in *cot*) and /ɔ/ (as in *caught*). In naturally produced words containing these vowels, the overlap in the first two formant frequencies is so extensive that the two categories cannot be separated on this acoustic dimension (Peterson & Barney, 1952). Moreover, in most dialects used in the United States, talkers do not distinguish between the two vowels. The experiment was run just as before. Infants were trained on the

/a/ and /ɔ/ vowels spoken by a male talker. Then, novel vowels spoken by female and child talkers, with additional random changes in the pitch contours of these vowels, were introduced. Results of the /a–ɔ/ study showed that most of the infants performed as well as infants in the /a–i/ experiments had performed. For these infants correct performance to the novel vowels occurred on the first trial (Kuhl, 1983).

In a study just completed (Kuhl, Wolak, & Green, in preparation) we examined another difficult vowel contrast, /a/ as in cot and /æ/, as in cat. To make the test more similar to the situation typically experienced by infants growing up, all of the vowels were spoken naturally, as opposed to our previous tests, in which the vowels were computer-synthesized. The number of talkers was also increased from three (previous studies) to twelve. The twelve talkers included 5 males, 5 females, and 2 children. The variation in voices was quite astounding, even to the adult ear, and this made it all the more difficult to attend to the essential differences between the vowels /a/ and /æ/. Adults who were tested in this task told us that they had to pay attention in order to perform perfectly. How did infants fare? Six-month-olds tested on this task performed at about 76% correct, significantly above the 50% chance level ($p < 0.01$).

Thus, studies of vowel categories show that by six months of age infants recognize equivalence classes that conform to the vowel categories of English. Given the demonstration that infants categorize variants for an easily discriminable contrast (/a-i/), as well as for difficult contrasts (/a-ɔ/ and /a-æ/), infants probably demonstrate this vowel constancy for all vowel categories in English.

How do infants recognize speech categories? We have obtained preliminary evidence that infants' vowel categories may be organized around a central "good" stimulus—a prototype of the category (Grieser & Kuhl, 1989). Our evidence consists of the results of studies that show that infants' spontaneous tendencies to generalize to new instances of a vowel category are affected by the perceived goodness (to an adult ear) of the stimulus that infants were initially trained to respond to.

The experiment was conducted in the following way. We synthesized a variety of stimuli that conformed to points in a two-formant coordinate vowel space within the /i/ vowel category. We asked adults to rate the *goodness* of these vowels on a scale of 1 to 7. Based on these ratings, we chose one stimulus that was rated as a good version of the /i/ vowel and another rated as a poor version of /i/. Even the poor one was always classified as an /i/ rather than as some other vowel. We then synthesized 32 variants around the good and poor /i/ vowel stimuli. These variants formed "rings" around the stimuli. Each ring was a specified distance in mels[2] from these points (30, 60, 90 and 120 mels). On each ring, eight stimuli were synthesized, for a total of 32. Once again, adults were

---

[2]The mel scale equates for perceived changes in pitch at a variety of different frequencies. Using a mel scale to specify the vowel's formants was an attempt to make all stimuli on each of the rings equally different from the target vowel.

asked to rate the goodness of each of the variants (N = 64) around both the good and poor versions of /i/.

The tests on infants were designed to examine whether generalization around a good stimulus differed from generalization around a poor stimulus. The head-turn technique was used to examine infants' generalization to variants around the two points. The results showed that generalization around the good stimulus was significantly broader than generalization around the poor stimulus. When trained on a good variant of /i/, infants responded to many more stimuli in vowel space than they did when trained on a poor variant of /i/. In fact, the same /i/ stimuli were responded to differently depending upon whether the infant had been trained to respond to a good as opposed to a poor /i/ stimulus.

These studies suggest that some points in vowel space are ideal candidates for category centers, because they are associated with perceptual stability over a broad array of category variants. Other points in vowel space are poor candidates, as perception is not stable and generalization to novel exemplars is weak. These data support the notion first expressed by Stevens (1972), who argued that vowel categories were organized so as to take advantage of the quantal nature of perception. This phenomenon is consistent with prototype theory (Medin & Barsalow, 1987; Rosch, 1975), and is the first data that we are aware of that suggest that infants' speech categories demonstrate internal structure and organization by 6-months-of-age—and, in particular, that speech may be represented by prototypes in infants.

We turn now to studies of equivalence classification on consonant classes. They are of great interest theoretically. Because consonants cannot occur in isolation, and have to be coarticulated with vowels, the acoustic cues to a particular consonant vary a great deal depending on the vowel that precedes or follows it (Öhman, 1966, but see Stevens & Blumstein, 1981, for a description of cues that may be invariant across context). Thus, while we hear the /b/ in *bat, but, boot,* and even those in *tab, tub,* and *tube* as the same segment /b/, there is no theory that explains this, and computers are unable to identify a given segment as the same across different contexts. We therefore want to know whether infants perceive the similarity between consonants across vowel contexts.

Studies of equivalence classification for consonant classes have been undertaken in our lab (Hillenbrand, 1983, 1984; Kuhl, 1980). These experiments used the same basic design as the tests on vowels just described. Infants were trained to differentiate two CV syllables, whose initial consonants differed. In Kuhl (1980), we reported experiments on fricatives in which syllables beginning with /s/, as in *sell,* were contrasted with syllables beginning with /ʃ/, as in *shell.* During training the consonants were spoken by a female talker and they appeared in an /a/ vowel context (/sa/ vs. /ʃa/). Once training on these syllables was complete, novel /s/ and /ʃ/ syllables were introduced. These new syllables differed both in the talker who produced them (2 male and 2 female talkers) and the vowel context in which the consonants appeared (/a/, /i/, and /u/). Thus, infants not only had to recognize the consonant regardless of the talker, they also had to recognize the consonant regardless of the vowel context in which it appeared.

In all, 22 novel syllables were introduced. The infant's task was to categorize the novel syllables by producing a head-turn response to those beginning with one of the consonants (either /s/ or /ʃ/) and to inhibit the head-turn response to the opposite category. The experiments were also run with the fricatives /f/ and /θ/, and in the initial as well as in the final positions of syllables. (See Kuhl, 1980, for full details.)

It was a challenging task, more difficult than any of the vowel categorization tests in which the within-category variation was not as extreme. Yet infants performed well in the task, with some of them producing a near-errorless performance (Kuhl, 1980). It was clear that infants were capable of recognizing that the /s/'s in /si/, /sa/, and /su/ were the same and that all were distinct from the /ʃ/'s in /ʃi/, /ʃa/, and /ʃu/, which were themselves the same.

A complete discussion of the issues raised by the data is beyond the scope of this chapter. The main issue posed concerns segmentation: Do these results suggest that infants segment the syllables into two component parts, consisting of a consonant (/C/) and a vowel (/V/), and that the basis of category recognition is the common consonantal segment contained in each? If so, it would provide strong evidence in support of a phonetic level of representation for infants. Such an explanation is consistent with their performance, but we cannot go this far in explaining infants' performance on these tests (Kuhl, 1985a, 1986c). The conservative posture claims only that infants hear similarities between the initial (or final, since we tested both) "portions of the syllables" (Kuhl, 1985a). We do not know that infants hear two segmental events in these syllables, and that one of them, the consonant, is the same. It will take further experiments to decide this. For now, however, we can say that there is some evidence that infants can cope with the extreme variations in the acoustic cues underlying consonants, and this is impressive.

Experiments on equivalence classification have thus demonstrated infant's abilities to perceive a constancy of sorts for speech sounds. Infants recognize auditory equivalence for vowels spoken by different people, and for consonants in different contexts. At least in the case of vowels, we have evidence to suggest that infants' speech categories are organized around a *good* stimulus. These abilities are remarkable, and must be of enormous help in the infant's acquisition of phonology.

The Basis of Equivalence Classification

There are no nonspeech studies analogous to equivalence classification. There are, however, some data on animals' abilities to perform in tasks of this kind. In addition, there are data suggesting that equivalence classification is not restricted to the domain of speech, but occurs for other classes of stimuli as well.

Early studies on animals (Baru, 1975; Burdick & Miller, 1975; Kuhl &

Miller, 1975) involved tests that were similar to "equivalence classification." In these tests, animals were trained on a subset of sounds from two different categories and then tested for generalization to novel members of both categories. Kuhl and Miller used chinchillas to test categories of CV syllables differing in voicing (/t/ vs. /d/), with the talker and vowel context varying. Burdick and Miller and Baru reported on the perception of the vowels /a/ and /i/, with talker varying. These studies were the first to demonstrate that animals could learn to respond correctly to discriminably different instances representing a phonetic category, including novel ones.

Recent studies have provided additional support for the idea that non-human animals perceptually group speech sounds from a given phonetic category together. Kluender and Diehl (1987), for example, have shown that Japanese quail learn to categorize natural consonant-vowel syllables beginning with /d/, as opposed to /b/ or /g/, and that this learning generalizes to syllables having different vowels.

It is also worth noting that the ability to detect equivalences between discriminably different members of a category by infants has been shown for stimuli outside the domain of speech. Cohen and Strauss (1979) showed that 7-month-olds could form a category of a specific female, regardless of her orientation, or of female faces in general. Infants can form categories based on stimulus configuration (Milewski, 1979), the general characteristics of human faces (Fagan, 1976), and possibly even number (Starkey, Spelke, & Gelman, 1983). In other words, infants' abilities to recognize equivalence among discriminably different stimuli that belong to a category are not specific to speech; they are illustrated in many different perceptual domains.

Auditory-Visual Equivalence

Thus far infants' detection of equivalence for diverse auditory events has been discussed. Now we extend the discussion to the detection of cross-modal equivalence for speech, wherein categorization abilities go beyond those involving auditory perception. Recent studies on adults from our own lab (Green & Kuhl, in press; Kuhl, Green, & Meltzoff, 1988; Grant, Ardell, Kuhl, & Sparks, 1985) and others (McGurk & MacDonald, 1976; Massaro & Cohen, 1983; Green & Miller, 1985; Summerfield, 1979) show that the perception of speech is strongly influenced by information gleaned from watching the face of a talker. This raises profound problems for a theory of speech perception because it means that visual information, such as watching a talker's lips come together to produce the consonant /b/, is somehow equated in perception to acoustic information that auditorially signals the consonant /b/. (See Kuhl & Meltzoff, 1988, for discussion.) One important question about such complex "cross-modal" equivalences is how information as different as the sight of a person producing speech, and the auditory speech event that is the result of production, come to be related in development.

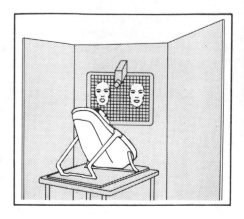

FIG. 13.6. Experimental set-up used to test the cross-modal perception of speech in infants. Infants view two faces producing the vowels /a/ and /i/ while a single sound (either /a/ or /i/) is presented from a loudspeaker located midway between the two facial images. (From Kuhl and Meltzoff, 1982.)

We designed an experiment to pose this problem to infants. We asked whether infants could relate the sight of a person producing a speech sound to the auditory concomitant of that event (Kuhl & Meltzoff, 1982). Infants were shown two filmed faces, side by side, of a woman articulating two different vowel sounds (Fig. 13.6). One face displayed productions of the vowel /a/, the other of the vowel /i/. While viewing the two faces, a single sound, either /a/ or /i/, was presented from a loudspeaker located midway between the two facial images. This eliminated any spatial cues as to which of the two faces produced the sound. The two facial images articulating the sounds moved in perfect synchrony with one another; the lips opened and closed at the exact same time, thus eliminating any temporal cues. The only way an infant could solve the problem was by recognizing a correspondence between the sound and the mouth shape that normally caused that sound. In other words, infants had to perceive a cross-modal match between the auditory and visual representations of speech.

Thirty-two infants ranging in age from 18 to 20 weeks were tested. They were placed in an infant seat facing a three-sided cubicle (Fig. 13.6). The experiment had two phases, a familiarization phase and a test phase. During familiarization, infants saw each of the two faces for 10 sec in the absence of sound. Following this, both faces were presented side by side, and the sound was turned on. Infants were video- and audio-recorded. An observer who was uninformed about the stimulus conditions scored the videotaped infants' visual fixations to the right or left stimulus.

The hypothesis was that infants would prefer to look at the face that *matched* the sound. The results confirmed this prediction; infants looked longer at the face that matched the vowel they heard. Infants presented with the auditory /a/ looked longer at the face articulating /a/; those who heard /i/ looked longer at the face articulating /i/. The effect was strong—of the total looking time, 73% was spent on the matched face ($p < 0.001$) and 24 of the 32 infants demonstrated the effect ($p < 0.01$). There were no other significant effects—no preference for the face located on the infant's right as opposed to the infant's left side, or for the /a/ face as opposed to the /i/ face. There was no significant difference in the strength of the effect when the matching stimulus was located on the infant's right as opposed to the infant's left. (See Kuhl & Meltzoff, 1984a, for full details.)

We then replicated the findings with 32 additional infants and a new research team (Kuhl & Meltzoff, 1984b). All other details of the experiment were identical. The results again showed that infants looked longer at the face that matched the sound they heard. Of the total fixation time, infants spent 62.8% fixating the matched face ($p < 0.05$), and 23 of the 32 infants demonstrated the effect ($p < 0.01$). Recently another team of investigators has also replicated this cross-modal matching effect for speech using disyllables such as *mama* versus *lulu* and *baby* versus *zuzi* in a design similar to ours (MacKain et al., 1983).

Most recently we have extended the tests to another vowel pair (/i-u/), thus including the third "point" vowel in the set of vowels tested. The point vowels are maximally distinct, both acoustically and articulatorily, and occur at the three endpoints of the triangle which defines "vowel space" (Peterson & Barney, 1952). The test was conducted just as it had been previously, only this time infants watched faces producing the vowels /i/ and /u/, and listened to either /i/ or /u/ vowels. The results showed that the effect could be extended to a new vowel pair. The mean percentage of fixation time to the matched face was 63.8% ($p < 0.05$), and 21 of the 32 infants looked longer at the matched face ($p < 0.05$) (Kuhl & Meltzoff, 1984b).

Thus, 4-month-olds perceive auditory-visual equivalents for speech. They recognize that /a/ sounds "go with" wide-open mouths, /i/ sounds with retracted lips, and /u/ sounds with pursed lips. What accounts for infants' cross-modal speech perception abilities? Have infants learned to associate an open mouth with the sound pattern /a/ and retracted lips with /i/ simply by watching talkers speak? Does some other kind of experience play a role in this ability? Our tests are now being conducted on younger infants to examine the learning account; we are specifically interested in whether or not experience in babbling plays a role in the effect (Kuhl & Meltzoff, 1984a).

Presuming for the moment that these effects can be demonstrated quite early, thus reducing the possibility that learning explains them, two theoretical possibilities were suggested (Kuhl & Meltzoff, 1984a). One is that the effect derives from a phonetic representation of speech such as that suggested by the SMA, the other that the effect is independent of speech, and based on infants' more general cognitive abilities (GMA). The main postulate of SMA is that the perceived match between the auditory and visual information is based on mediation by a representation of the phonetic unit, in this case, the vowels /a/ and /i/ in a form that specified both their auditory and visual instantiations. These representations would account for the detection of equivalence in the phonetic information perceived through the two modalities; the representation links the two stimuli.

Our second account, similar to the GMA, was very different. We argued that it was possible that the auditory and visual speech information was related by some other property, one that directly tied information such as the formant frequencies of the sound /a/ to the sight of a wide-open mouth. This account held that mediation at the phonetic level was not necessary to perceive a match between the two stimuli; it might be done on the basis of simple physics (Kuhl & Meltzoff, 1984b). A series of experiments aimed at separating the two explanations was designed.

The Basis of Auditory-Visual Equivalence

Our first question about the effect was whether or not a nonspeech sound that mimicked certain features of the auditory stimulus could replace it in the cross-modal test. We argued that the use of nonspeech stimuli helped identify what aspect of the auditory signal was necessary and sufficient to evoke the matching response. Was it necessary that the auditory signal contain enough information to identify the vowel or was a single feature of the vowel, presented in a nonspeech context, sufficient?

The nonspeech tests were conducted in two steps. The first was to verify that the cross-modal matching effect depended upon the spectral information in the vowels rather than temporal information. Vowels are defined primarily in terms of spectral information (formant frequencies) rather than in terms of temporal or amplitude information, so it was important to test whether the spectral information in the vowels was essential. Because the auditory and visual vowel stimuli had been matched on all temporal and amplitude parameters, we assumed that infants' matches must be based on the spectral differences between the /a/ and /i/ vowels. We thus hypothesized that if we altered this spectral information, taking the formant frequencies out of the sounds, infants could no longer succeed on the cross-modal task.

To test this directly, the /a/ and /i/ vowels used in our original study were altered to remove their formant frequencies while leaving whatever temporal and amplitude information remained. Using computer analysis techniques, we extracted the amplitude envelopes of the vowels and their precise durations. Then we computer synthesized pure-tone stimuli with a frequency of 200 Hz (the average value of the female talker's fundamental frequency), one for each of the 40 original /a/ and /i/ vowels. Each pure-tone stimulus exactly followed the amplitude envelope of its speech-stimulus original.

These pure-tone stimuli could not be identified as /a/ or /i/, yet when they were played while looking at the faces, the resulting display was quite engaging. Because the temporal properties of the tones matched the original vowels, the tones became louder as the mouths grew wider and softer as the mouths drew to a close. Thus, if infants in our task could discover a match between auditory and visual stimuli on time-intensity cues alone, they should succeed. If, however, the spectral properties of the vowels were necessary, the results should drop to chance. Arguing that the temporal-envelope properties of the stimuli were insufficient for success in our original experiment, we favored the spectral hypothesis.

The results were in support of the spectral hypothesis; infants' cross-modal performance dropped to chance. The mean percentage fixation time to the matched stimulus was 54.6% ($p > 0.50$), with only 17 of the 32 infants demonstrating the effect. Inspection of the looking data revealed that infants spent just as long looking at the faces in this experiment as they had in the previous three experiments in which they heard speech sounds rather than tones, so it was not as though they found these stimuli uninteresting. However, they could not detect a match between the tones and the faces. We had shown, then, that the temporal envelope of the vowel stimuli used in our experiment was not sufficient to produce the cross-modal effect. Some aspect of the spectral information was necessary, as we had hypothesized.

But what aspect of the spectral information was needed? Did the information in the auditory stimulus have to be sufficient to identify it as an /a/ or an /i/ in order for the match to be detected? Or would a simpler spectral property be sufficient? As a second step, we undertook a variety of tests involving nonspeech stimuli that captured spectral features of the /a/ and /i/ vowels. Additional tests using pure tones were conducted to see whether representing just the "grave-acute" distinctive feature (i.e., the low versus high tonal quality of the vowels) would be sufficient. Our tests had shown that pure tones can reliably be related to auditorily or visually presented vowels by adults; in both cases, they associate low tones with /a/ and high tones with /i/ (Kuhl & Meltzoff, 1988). We used nine different pure tones ranging from 250 Hz to 4000 Hz. We also used three-formant analog stimuli. These were made up of three pure tones whose frequencies matched the formant frequencies; thus, the 3-tone analogs more closely resembled the spectral properties of speech than did the simple pure tones. The results of these tests showed that neither simple distinctive features of the vowels (as represented by pure tones), nor our three-tone analog representations of the vowels were sufficient for infants. They could not detect a match between a nonspeech auditory stimulus and a face mouthing speech (Kuhl & Meltzoff, 1988). Only when the full signal was presented did infants relate the auditory and visual concomitants of speech.

Thus our studies on the basis of the effect suggest that nonspeech analogs do not work. Infants do not detect matches between auditory nonspeech events and faces that make speech movements; they may already know that mouths produce speech, rather than tones or chords. The fact that we have identified a dissociation between speech and nonspeech is intriguing, in light of the fact that nonspeech experiments on categorical perception have replicated the results of speech experiments.

Finally, it is clear that cross-modal perception in infants is not unique to speech. Meltzoff and Borton (1979) conducted experiments on cross-modal perception in 4-week-olds, showing that they could detect equivalences between information delivered tactually and visually. In this study infants were given one of two pacifiers, either one with nubs on it or a smooth one. The pacifier was then removed and two visual stimuli were presented, a sphere with nubs on it and a smooth one. The results showed that infants who sucked on the smooth pacifier looked at the smooth sphere while those who had sucked on the nubby pacifier fixated the nubby sphere. We can not claim, then, that cross-modal perception in infants is speech-specific.

Auditory-Motor Equivalence

Thus far in discussing the infant's detection of equivalences in speech we have focused on the perception of speech through different sensory modalities—auditory and visual. We now turn our attention to speech production to examine another aspect of equivalence that infants detect for speech.

As adults, we can produce a specific auditory target, such as a vowel, on the first try; it is not a trial-and-error process. Auditory signals are directly related to the motor commands necessary to produce them because adults have rules that dictate the mapping between articulation and audition. This mapping is quite sophisticated. Experiments show that if an adult speaker is suddenly thwarted in the act of producing a given sound by the introduction of a sudden load imposed on his lip or jaw, compensation is essentially immediate (Abbs & Gracco, 1984). The adjustment can occur on the very first laryngeal vibration, prior to the time the adult has heard anything. Such rapid motor adjustments suggest a highly sophisticated and flexible set of rules relating articulatory movements to sound.

How do auditory-articulatory mapping rules develop? Evidence suggests that at least one important mechanism for learning them is vocal imitation.

Among mammals, humans are the only animals who give evidence of vocal learning, that is, learning the species vocal repertoire by hearing it and mimicking it. We share this ability with a few select species of passerine birds (Marler, 1973). Presumably it is the mechanism of imitation that guides vocal learning. The power of its effects can be seen in the fact that early auditory exposure to a specific language pattern puts an indelible marker on one's speech patterns. Foreigners try to rid themselves of their language-specific phonetic errors and their foreign accents, but it is notoriously difficult to do so.

We presume then that at some point young infants must mimic the speech patterns that they hear others produce. But how early are infants capable of doing this? Some relevant data can be adduced from the earliest age at which infants from different language environments produce phonetic units that are unique to their own native language. The data on infant babbling show that infants produce sounds that are not specific to any one language (Oller, 1986; Stark, 1980). But by the time first words emerge, infants will begin to produce sounds that are typical of their language, but are rare in other languages. Moreover, these infants will have an accent. They will have adopted the prosodic features of the language—its cadence, rhythm and tempo, as well as its characteristic intensity and intonation contours. There is some research suggesting that as early as 12-months-of-age these differences are discernible (de Boysson-Bardies et al., 1984). The data thus suggest that at some point prior to the onset of speech and perhaps as early as 12-months-of-age, infants have acquired enough information about the phonetic units and prosody of their native language to produce it in a way that is characteristic of their native tongue. Thus, by this time, evidence of vocal learning exists.

A more direct approach to the question is to examine vocal imitation experimentally. From Piaget on, reports have appeared that are highly suggestive of vocal imitation of at least one prosodic aspect of speech, its pitch (Kessen, Levine, & Wendrich, 1979; Lieberman, 1984; Papousek & Papousek, 1981; Piaget, 1962); however, all but one of these studies (Kessen et al., 1979) involved natural interactions between adults and infants, and as such are subject to methodological problems (Kuhl & Meltzoff, 1988). Natural observations of mothers and their infants are usually subject to the question "who is imitating whom?" The Kessen et al. study tested infants in multiple sessions over several months, giving them repeated practice and feedback, so the issue of training is unresolved in the study.

With these issues in mind we sought evidence of vocal imitation in our own experiments on infants' cross-modal perception of speech (Kuhl & Meltzoff, 1982; 1988). The cross-modal studies provided a controlled setting in which to study vocal imitation. Recall our experimental set-up. Infants sat in an infant seat facing a three-sided cubicle. They viewed a film of a female talker producing vowel sounds. Half of the infants were presented with one auditory stimulus while the other half were presented with a different auditory stimulus. The stimuli were totally controlled, both visually and auditorially. There were no human interactions with the infant during the test, and thus no chance for spuriously shaping and/or conditioning of a response. The room was a soundproof chamber and a studio-quality microphone was suspended above the infant to obtain clear recordings that could be perceptually or instrumentally analyzed. Finally, the stimulus on film being presented to the infant occurred once every 3 sec, with an interstimulus interval of about 2 sec. This was ideal for encouraging turn-taking on the part of the infant. We found that infants in this setting were calm and highly engaged by the face-voice stimuli. They often listened for a while, smiled at the faces, and then started "talking back." Our question was: Do infants' speech vocalizations match those they hear?

In our initial report we described data that were highly suggestive of infants' imitation of the prosodic characteristics of the signal (Kuhl & Meltzoff, 1982). We observed infant matching of the pitch contour of the adult model's vowels. Both the adult's and infant's responses are shown in Figure 13.7. Instrumental analysis showed that the infant produced an almost perfect match to the adult female's rise-fall pattern of intonation. While the infant has shorter vocal folds and therefore produces a higher fundamental frequency the pitch pattern of a rapid rise in frequency followed by a more gradual fall in frequency duplicates

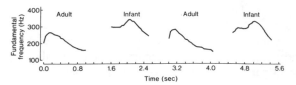

FIG. 13.7.   Pitch matching in tests of vocal imitation in infants. From Kuhl and Meltzoff (1982).

that of the adult. The two contours were perceptually very similar. The infant's response also matched the adult's in duration. Because vocalizations with this rise-fall pattern and of this long duration are not common in the utterances of four-month-olds, it was highly suggestive of vocal imitation. But because we had not varied the pitch pattern of the vowel in the experiment it was not possible to conclude definitively that infants could differentially match the pitch contour of vowels.

A more rigorous test of the young infant's ability to imitate relates to their matching of the phonetic segments of speech. Half of the infants in our experiments had heard /a/ vowels while the other half had heard /i/ vowels. This allowed a good test of the differential imitation of speech sounds. All of the vowel-like vocalizations produced by the infants in the /a-i/ studies were analyzed. Vowel-like sounds were defined on the basis of acoustic and articulatory characteristics typical of vowels. The sounds had to be produced with an open mouth, rather than one that was closed. They had to have a minimum duration of 500 msec. They had to be *voiced,* that is, vocalized with normal laryngeal vibration, and could not be aspirated or voiceless sounds. They could not be produced on an inhalatory breath. Vocalizations that occurred while the infant's hand was in his mouth could not be reliably scored and were excluded. Consonant-like vocalizations were also scored, but they occurred rarely and were always accompanied by vowel-like sounds.

Once identified, the sounds were submitted to analysis. Perceptual scoring was done by having a trained phonetician listen to each infant's productions and judge whether, on the whole, they were more ''/i/-like'' or /a/-like.'' Infants at this age cannot produce perfect /i/ vowels, due to anatomical restrictions. They can, however, produce other high front vowels such as /ɪ/ or /ɛ/. Similarly, a perfect /a/ is rare in the vocalizations of the 4-month-old, but similar central vowels, such as /æ/ and /ʌ/ are producible by infants at this age. Thus, the judgment made by the observer was a forced-choice one concerning whether an infant's vocalizations were more /a/-like or more /i/-like.

We then asked judges to predict whether infants had been exposed to /a/ as opposed to /i/, based on the infant's vocalizations. If judges can do so with greater than chance (50%) accuracy, then there is evidence for vocal imitation. The results confirmed this prediction. Infants produced /a/-like vowels when listening to /a/ and /i/-like vowels when listening to /i/, allowing the judges to predict accurately in 90% of the instances the vowel heard by the infant. These results were highly significant ($p < 0.01$) (Kuhl & Meltzoff, 1988).

We are now involved in the instrumental analysis of the sounds. Using distinctive feature theory to guide our instrumental analyses, we measured the graveness and compactness of the infants' vowel productions. The results demonstrated that infants' vocal responses to /a/ were significantly more grave, that is, they had a lower center of gravity, than their responses to /i/. Similarly, their responses to /a/ were significantly more compact, that is, they had formants spaced more closely together, than their responses to /i/. Taken together, the two analyses provide some evidence that 4-month-old infants are engaged in vocal imitation of the phonetic segments of speech.

The Basis of Auditory-Motor Equivalence

Our first question was again related to the effectiveness of nonspeech sounds. Could the auditory stimulus in vocal imitation studies be replaced by a nonspeech stimulus? The specific questions we were interested in were these: What happens when infants listen to speech as opposed to nonspeech sounds? Do vocalizations occur as frequently as they do when infants listen to speech? And if they occur, do these vocalizations sound like those given in response to the speech stimulus mimicked by the nonspeech analog?

Recall that in our cross-modal studies involving speech infants heard one of the three point vowels, /a/, /i/, or /u/. In two other studies infants heard nonspeech stimuli consisting of either pure tones or a three-tone analog stimulus. In the pure-tone study (Kuhl, Wolak, & Meltzoff, in preparation), nine pure tones were used, varying from 125 Hz to 4000 Hz. In the three-tone analog study, the tones matched the formant frequencies of the vowels. In neither of these nonspeech studies could any of the sounds be identified as speech.

Our original study included a nonspeech test in which a single pure tone was presented (Kuhl & Meltzoff, 1982). The results of the study suggested that nonspeech sounds were not effective elicitors of vocalization. We reported that the infants tested in the speech condition versus those tested in the tone condition produced a differential amount of vocalization. Infants who heard speech produced cooing sounds typical of speech. The infants who were presented with the nonspeech tone did not produce speech-like vocalizations. They had watched the same faces, heard sounds of the same duration and intensity, and were given just as long to reply. But they did not produce speech. In the 1982 paper we reported that 10 of the 32 infants hearing speech produced speech-like vocalizations whereas only a single infant hearing nonspeech produced speech-like vocalizations, and this difference was significant ($p < 0.01$).

We can now extend these results to a much larger sample. To date we have analyzed the vocalizations of all of the infants who participated in the two /a-i/ studies for a total of 64 infants. In addition, we have analyzed the vocalizations of the first half (72 infants) of the 144 infants tested in the pure-tone study (Kuhl

& Meltzoff, 1988). The results strongly show the superiority of human speech in eliciting infant vocalizations. Infants listening to speech produce speech, while infants listening to tones do not. Fully 40 of the 64 infants listening to speech in our sample produce vocalizations that are typical of speech, while only 5 of the 72 infants hearing nonspeech produce sounds of this type ($p < 0.001$). Infants listening to nonspeech do not tend to produce speech-like vocalizations; instead, they squeal, gurgle, grunt, or produce raspberries. Apparently, infants talk only to faces that are talking to them. Thus we see a dissociation between speech and nonspeech in our studies of vocal imitation.

Having these data on vocal imitation in hand, we can now ask whether the tendency to mimic human acts is unique to speech? Once again, the answer from cognitive development is clear. Meltzoff's work on facial and gestural imitation has shown quite convincingly that very young infants (in some instances newborns) imitate adult facial and manual gestures such as tongue protrusion, mouth opening, and the opening and closing of the hand (Meltzoff & Moore, 1977, 1983). Thus, we cannot claim that infants' imitative capacity regarding vocalization is a specialization that is speech specific.

IV. A RETURN TO THEORY

We began this chapter by noting the fact that for both animal and human species, the notion of "special mechanisms" has been offered to explain infants' early responsiveness to species-specific signals (SMA). For the case of human infants acquiring speech, however, a second account was described that is a viable alternative. The second account holds that general mechanisms may be sufficient to account for infants' abilities (GMA). Both accounts attempt to explain infants' detection of complex equivalences in speech: between auditory events that are physically different and easily discriminable, between speech stimuli presented to different modalities, as in auditory-visual speech perception, and between an auditory speech stimulus and its motor equivalent.

How do our two models account for the equivalence data? Recall that SMA argues that in each of the cases a phonetic representation of speech units mediates perception. This is its key point; without higher-order representations, these events cannot be equated in perception. They are not linked to each other in any other way. Auditory equivalence is perceived because two different speech events (such as the vowel /a/ spoken by two different people) are tied to the same phonetic representation. Thus, even though their surface acoustic properties are not the same, their common representation renders them equal. When auditory and visual versions of /a/ are detected, or when sounds are equated to the motor movements used to produce them, this account holds that it is because the two stimuli have a common underlying phonetic representation (Kuhl & Meltzoff, 1984a). The auditory and visual instantiations of speech are not themselves directly tied. Nor are sounds and the motor movements that produce them. They are linked up by virtue of the fact that they are both independently tied to the higher-order representation of the phonetic segment. Without higher-order representations, these events cannot be linked, and equivalence would not be detected (Kuhl & Meltzoff, 1984a).

What of GMA? How does it explain the data on infants' detection of equivalence? The mainstay of its argument is that infants' detection of equivalence for speech does not depend on a representation of phonetic units. On this view, perception of equivalence is not mediated by pre-existing representations of phonetic units because innately stored representations of phonetic units do not exist. Infants' capabilities are explained by their general auditory and cognitive abilities.

Regarding infants' detection of auditory equivalence, the GMA holds that this is due purely to the perception of auditory similarity. This is true both for two vowels spoken by different people, and for cues that "trade" in perception. On this view, these stimuli can be perceived to be auditorily equivalent in the absence of any other speech-specific processing. Critical data for this position are provided by the animal studies reviewed earlier; they show that animals detect auditory equivalences for speech.

According to the GMA higher-order equivalences involving cross-modal and imitative abilities are also not dependent upon preset phonetic representations. Critical data here are those provided by studies of infants' general cognitive abilities. Research on infants' cognitive development clearly demonstrates that these abilities exist outside the domain of speech. Thus, the key point argued by the GMA is that infants do not need special mechanisms to accomplish cross-modal and imitative tasks for speech; such mechanisms already exist for the perception of objects and faces.

Having summarized each account's approach to the data on equivalence detection, we address the evidence presented from tests on the basis of the effect. The SMA is most forcefully supported as an explanation for an effect when nonspeech tests fail, when animals fail, and when no other domain but speech gives evidence of the effect. The GMA is supported for effects in which nonspeech tests succeed, animals succeed, and other domains provide evidence of similar effects. What pattern of results was obtained? Did clear support for one or the other account emerge?

Consider first the pattern of results with nonspeech. There is evidence that CP effects in infants can be replicated with nonspeech, although the difference between VOT results and TOT results remains puzzling. Context effects and trading relations have also been demonstrated using nonspeech analogs with infants. The only effects that have clearly failed using nonspeech are complex tasks like cross-modal speech perception and vocal imitation. These effects appear to require the whole stimulus. We might therefore draw a line between the detection of auditory equivalence and the detection of equivalence for higher-order intermodal relations. Perhaps the detection of intermodal equivalences is indeed based on more specialized mechanisms.

We look for confirmation of this hypothesis in tests on animals. CP effects can be replicated in animals. Moreover, context effects have now been replicated, though only one example has been tested. Tests of equivalence classification also show that animals are capable of perceiving speech categories. Tests of cross-modal perception and imitation have not been completed, but a reasonable guess would be that these tests would fail. Animals are not known to be proficient on these tasks, particularly on imitation (Meltzoff, 1988). If we imagine, for the sake of argument, that animals will fail on these tasks, then a similar pattern of results with nonspeech and animals would have emerged, with both suggesting that *auditory* equivalence is less likely to require special mechanisms than are more complex *intermodal* equivalences.

Lastly, we look at the evidence for domain specificity. Are any of these equivalences detected by infants unique to speech? Here we have to conclude that speech is not unique. Equivalence classification, cross-modal perception, and imitation are cognitive abilities that appear to be quite robust in infants. One might have thought that evidence of such sophisticated talent would be rare in infants. It is not. Is speech a special case of these more complex skills? It may turn out to be, but one need not posit this, given infants' apparent cognitive capacity for the detection of higher-order equivalences.

V.   SUMMARY AND CONCLUSIONS

There are two distinct characterizations of infants' initial state for speech processing. Both conceed that infants demonstrate speech phenomena that are extremely sophisticated. Infants' detection of complex equivalences—between discriminably different auditory events, between speech information delivered auditorially and visually, and between the auditory and motor instantiations of a speech event—suggest an initial organization of speech that is highly conducive to the acquisition of an intermodally represented speech system. The Specialized Mechanism Account explains this by imputing phonetic-level representations of speech to the infant at birth. On this view, infants' detection of equivalence is due to the mediating effects of a phonetic-level representation. The General Mechanism Account claims that phonetic-level representations do not exist at birth and that infants' capabilities are due to their more general sensory and cognitive abilities. This account holds that phonetic-level representations are built up only later as the child acquires language.

Experiments directed towards identifying the basis of these effects were reviewed. These experiments include tests on nonspeech signals, tests on animals' perception of speech, and tests on equivalence detection in domains other than speech. These experiments show that both nonspeech and animal tests replicate auditory equivalence effects. Importantly, though, nonspeech signals fail to reproduce the auditory-visual cross-modal effect and fail to induce vocal imitation. It is tempting to conclude, then, that these higher-order equivalences require special mechanisms. Yet, the detection of higher-order equivalences by infants is not restricted to speech; they are demonstrated in other domains as well. Thus, even complex behaviors such as these may not be due to a domain-specific speech module. It appears, then, that even if speech is intermodally represented in infants, it may not require "special mechanisms" to be organized in that way. Rather, speech may draw upon a natural proclivity to represent information intermodally. At present, no clear evidence in favor of a phonetic-level representation of speech has been presented. Until further tests have been conducted, claims about infants' phonetic representation of speech are most wisely offered and debated, but not yet acclaimed as definitely proven.

ACKNOWLEDGMENTS

The author and the work described here were supported by grants from the National Science Foundation (BNS 8316318) and from the National Institutes of Health (HD-18286 and HD 22514). I am indebted to Karen Wolak, Craig Harris, and Kerry Green for assistance in the experiments, Karen Wolak for helpful comments on the manuscript, Andy Meltzoff for discussions of the issues raised here, and KKM for inspiration.

REFERENCES

Abbs, J. H., & Gracco, V. L. (1984). Control of complex motor gestures: Orofacial muscle responses to lead perturbations of the lip during speech. *Journal of Neurophysiology, 51*, 705–723.

Aslin, R. N., Pisoni, D. B., Hennessey, B. L., & Perey, A. J. (1981). Discrimination of voice onset time by human infants: New findings and implications for the effects of early experience. *Child Development, 52*, 1135–1145.

Baru, A. V. (1975). Discrimination of synthesized vowels [a] and [i] with varying parameters (fundamental frequency, intensity, duration, and number of formants) in dog. In G. Fant & M. A. A. Tatham (eds.), *Auditory analysis and perception of speech* (pp. 91–101). New York: Academic Press.

Best, C. T., Morrongiello, B., & Robson, R. (1981). Perceptual equivalence of acoustic cues in speech and nonspeech perception. *Perception and Psychophysics, 29*, 191–211.

Bruner, J. S., Goodnow, J. J., & Austin, G. A. (1956). *A study of thinking.* New York: Wiley.

Burdick, C. K., & Miller, J. D. (1975). Speech perception by the chinchilla: Discrimination of sustained [a] and [i]. *Journal of the Acoustical Society of America, 58*, 415–427.

Cohen, L. B., & Strauss, M. S. (1979). Concept acquisition in the human infant. *Child Development, 50*, 419–424.

de Boysson-Bardies, B., Sagart, L., & Durand, C. (1984). Discernible differences in the babbling of infants according to target language. *Journal of Child Language, 11*, 1–15.

Diehl, R. L., & Kluender, K. R. (in press). On the objects of speech perception. *Ecological Psychology.*

Eimas, P. D. (1974). Auditory and linguistic processing of cues for place of articulation by infants. *Perception and Psychophysics, 16*, 513–521.

Eimas, P. D. (1975). Auditory and phonetic coding of the cues for speech: Discrimination of the [r-l] distinction by young infants. *Perception and Psychophysics, 18*, 341–347.

Eimas, P. D. (1985). The equivalence of cues in the perception of speech by infants. *Infant Behavior & Development, 8*, 125–138.

Eimas, P. D., & Miller, J. L. (1980). Contextual effects in infant speech perception. *Science, 209,* 1140–1141.

Eimas, P. D., Siqueland, E. R., Jusczyk, P., & Vigorito, J. (1971). Speech perception in infants. *Science, 171,* 303–306.

Fagan, J. F., III. (1976). Infants' recognition of invariant features of faces. *Child Development, 47,* 627–638.

Fodor, J. A. (1983). *The modularity of mind.* Cambridge, MA: MIT Press.

Grant, K. W., Ardell, L. H., Kuhl, P. K., & Sparks, D. W. (1985). The contribution of fundamental frequency, amplitude envelope, and voicing duration cues to speechreading in normal-hearing subjects. *Journal of the Acoustical Society of America, 77,* 671–677.

Green, K. P., & Kuhl, P. K. (in press). The role of visual information in the processing of place and manner features in speech. *Perception and Psychophysics.*

Green, K., & Miller, J. L. (1985). On the role of visual rate information in phonetic perception. *Perception and Psychophysics, 38,* 269–276.

Grieser, D., & Kuhl, P. K. (1989). The categorization of speech by infants: Support for speech-sound prototypes. *Developmental Psychology.*

Hillenbrand, J. (1983). Perceptual organization of speech sounds by infants. *Journal of Speech and Hearing Research, 26,* 268–282.

Hillenbrand, J. (1984). Speech perception by infants: Categorization based on nasal consonant place of articulation. *Journal of the Acoustical Society of America, 75,* 1613–1622.

Jusczyk, P. W., Pisoni, D. B., Reed, M. A., Fernald, A., & Myers, M. (1983). Infants' discrimination of the duration of a rapid spectrum change in nonspeech signals. *Science, 222,* 175–177.

Jusczyk, P. W., Pisoni, D. B., Walley, A., & Murray, J. (1980). Discrimination of relative onset time of two-component tones by infants. *Journal of the Acoustical Society of America, 67,* 262–270.

Kessen, W., Levine, J., & Wendrich, K. A. (1979). The imitation of pitch in infants. *Infant Behavior and Development, 2,* 93–99.

Klatt, D. (1986). Problem of variability in speech recognition and in models of speech perception. In J. S. Perkell & D. H. Klatt (Eds.), *Invariance and variability in speech processes* (pp. 300–324). Hillsdale, NJ: Lawrence Erlbaum Associates.

Kluender, K. R., Diehl, R. L., & Killeen, P. R. (1987). Japanese quail can learn phonetic categories. *Science, 237,* 1195–1197.

Kuhl, P. K. (1978). Predispositions for the perception of speech-sound categories: A species-specific phenomenon? In F. D. Minifie & L. L. Lloyd (Eds.), *Communicative and cognitive abilities— Early behavioral assessment* (pp. 229–255). Baltimore: University Park Press.

Kuhl, P. K. (1979a). Speech perception in early infancy: Perceptual constancy for spectrally dis-similar vowel categories. *Journal of the Acoustical Society of America, 66,* 1668–1679.

Kuhl, P. K. (1979b). Models and mechanisms in speech perception: Species comparisons provide further contributions. *Brain, Behavior and Evolution, 16,* 374–408.

Kuhl, P. K. (1980). Perceptual constancy for speech-sound categories in early infancy. In G. H. Yeni-Komshian, J. F. Kavanagh, & C. A. Ferguson (Eds.), *Child Phonology, Vol. 2, Perception* (pp. 41–66). New York: Academic Press.

Kuhl, P. K. (1981). Discrimination of speech by nonhuman animals: Basic auditory sensitivities conducive to the perception of speech-sound categories. *Journal of the Acoustical Society of America, 70,* 340–349.

Kuhl, P. K. (1983). Perception of auditory equivalence classes for speech in early infancy. *Infant Behavior and Development, 6,* 263–285.

Kuhl, P. K. (1985a). Categorization of speech by infants. In J. Mehler & R. Fox (Eds.), *Neonate cognition: Beyond the blooming, buzzing confusion* (pp. 231–262). Hillsdale, NJ: Lawrence Erlbaum Associates.

Kuhl, P. K. (1985b). Methods in the study of infant speech perception. In G. Gottlieb & N. A.

Krasnegor (Eds.), *Measurement of audition and vision in the first year of postnatal life: A methodological overview* (pp. 223–251). Norwood, NJ: Ablex.

Kuhl, P. K. (1986a). Infants' perception of speech: Constraints on characterizations of the initial state. In B. Lindblom & R. Zetterstrom (Eds.), *Precursors of early speech* (pp. 219–244). New York: Stockton Press.

Kuhl, P. K. (1986b). Theoretical contributions of tests on animals to the special-mechanisms debate in speech. *Experimental Biology, 45,* 233–265.

Kuhl, P. K. (1986c). Reflections on infants' perception and representation of speech. In J. S. Perkell & D. H. Klatt (Eds.), *Invariance and variability of speech processes* (pp. 19–30). Hillsdale, NJ: Lawrence Erlbaum Associates.

Kuhl, P. K. (1987a). Perception of speech and sound in early infancy. In P. Salapatek & L. B. Cohen (Eds.), *Handbook of infant perception: From perception to cognition* (Vol. 2 pp. 275–382). Orlando, Fl.: Academic Press.

Kuhl, P. K. (1987b). The special-mechanisms debate in speech research: Categorization tests on animals and infants. In S. Harnad (Ed.), *Categorical perception: The groundwork of cognition* (pp. 355–386). Cambridge, England: Cambridge University Press.

Kuhl, P. K. (1988). Auditory perception and the evolution of speech. *Human Evolution, 3,* 19–43.

Kuhl, P. K., Green, K. P., & Meltzoff, A. N. (1988). Factors affecting the integration of auditory and visual information in speech: The level effect. *Journal of the Acoustical Society of America. 83,* Suppl. 1, S86(A).

Kuhl, P. K., & Meltzoff, A. N. (1982). The bimodal perception of speech in infancy. *Science, 218,* 1138–1141.

Kuhl, P. K., & Meltzoff, A. N. (1984a). The intermodal representation of speech in infants. *Infant Behavior and Development, 7,* 361–381.

Kuhl, P. K., & Meltzoff, A. N. (1984b). *Imitation, representation, and cross-modal perception in infants.* International Conference on Infant Studies, New York.

Kuhl, P. K., & Meltzoff, A. N. (1988). Speech as an intermodal object of perception. In A. Yonas (Ed.), *The Minnesota symposia on child psychology: Perceptual development in infancy* (Vol. 20, pp. 235–266). Hillsdale, NJ: Lawrence Erlbaum Associates.

Kuhl, P. K., & Miller, J. D. (1975). Speech perception by the chinchilla: Voiced-voiceless distinction in alveolar plosive consonants. *Science, 190,* 69–72.

Kuhl, P. K., & Miller, J. D. (1978). Speech perception by the chinchilla: Identification functions for synthetic VOT stimuli. *Journal of the Acoustical Society of America, 63,* 905–917.

Kuhl, P. K., & Padden, D. M. (1982). Enhanced discriminability at the phonetic boundaries for the voicing feature in macaques. *Perception and Psychophysics, 32,* 542–550.

Kuhl, P. K., & Padden, D. M. (1983). Enhanced discriminability at the phonetic boundaries for the place feature in macaques. *Journal of the Acoustical Society of America, 73,* 1003–1010.

Kuhl, P. K., Wolak, K. M., & Green, K. P. (in preparation). Infants' detection of auditory equivalences in speech: Vowel categories.

Kuhl, P. K., Wolak, K. M., & Meltzoff, A. N. (in preparation). Infants' cross-modal perception of speech: Studies on the basis of the effect.

Liberman, A. M., Cooper, F. S., Shankweiler, D. P., & Studdert-Kennedy, M. (1967). Perception of the speech code. *Psychological Review, 74,* 431–461.

Liberman, A. M., & Mattingly, I. G. (1985). The motor theory of speech perception revised. *Cognition, 21,* 1–36.

Lieberman, P. (1984). *The biology and evolution of language.* Cambridge, MA: Harvard University Press.

MacKain, K., Studdert-Kennedy, M., Spieker, S., & Stern, D. (1983). Infant intermodal speech perception is a left-hemisphere function. *Science, 219,* 1347–1348.

Marler, P. (1974). Constraints on learning: Development of bird song. In N. F. White (Ed.), *Ethology and Psychiatry: The Clarence M. Hincks Memorial Lectures for 1970.* (pp. 69–83). Toronto: University of Toronto Press.

Massaro, D. W., & Cohen, M. M. (1983). Evaluation and integration of visual and auditory information in speech perception. *Journal of Experimental Psychology: Human Perception and Performance, 9,* 753–771.

Mattingly, I. G., Liberman, A. M., Syrdal, A. K., & Halwes, T. (1971). Discrimination in speech and nonspeech modes. *Cognitive Psychology, 2,* 131–157.

McGurk, H., & MacDonald, J. (1976). Hearing lips and seeing voices. *Nature, 264,* 746–748.

Medin, D. L., & Barsalou, L. W. (1987). Categorization processes and categorical perception. In S. Harnad (Ed.), *Categorical perception:* The ground work of cognition (pp. 455–490). Cambridge, England: Cambridge University Press.

Meltzoff, A. N. (1988). The human infant as *homo imitans.* In T. R. Zentall & B. G. Galef (Eds.), *Social learning: Psychological and biological perspectives* (pp. 319–341). Hillsdale, NJ: Lawrence Erlbaum Associates.

Meltzoff, A. N., & Borton, R. W. (1979). Intermodal matching by human neonates. *Nature, 282,* 403–404.

Meltzoff, A. N., & Moore, M. K. (1977). Imitation of facial and manual gestures by human neonates. *Science, 198,* 75–78.

Meltzoff, A. N., & Moore, M. K. (1983). Newborn infants imitate adult facial gestures. *Child Development, 54,* 702–709.

Milewski, A. E. (1979). Visual discrimination and detection of configurational invariance in 3-month infants. *Developmental Psychology, 15,* 357–363.

Miller, J. L., & Eimas, P. D. (1983). Studies on the categorization of speech by infants. *Cognition, 13,* 135–165.

Miller, J. L., & Liberman, A. M. (1979). Some effects of later-occurring information on the perception of stop consonant and semivowel. *Perception and Psychophysics, 25,* 457–465.

Miller, J. D., Wier, C. C., Pastore, R. E., Kelly, W. J., & Dooling, R. J. (1976). Discrimination and labeling of noise-buzz sequences with varying noise-lead times: An example of categorical perception. *Journal of the Acoustical Society of America, 60,* 410–417.

Miyawaki, K., Strange, W., Verbrugge, R., Liberman, A. M., Jenkins, J. J., & Fujimura, O. (1975). An effect of linguistic experience: The discrimination of /r/ and /l/ by native speakers of Japanese and English. *Perception and Psychophysics, 18,* 331–340.

Morse, P. A., & Snowdon, C. T. (1975). An investigation of categorical speech discrimination by rhesus monkeys. *Perception and Psychophysics, 17,* 9–16.

Öhman, S. E. G. (1966). Coarticulation of VCV utterances: Spectrographic measurements. *Journal of the Acoustical Society of America, 39,* 151–168.

Oller, D. K. (1986). Metaphonology and infant vocalizations. In B. Lindblom & R. Zetterström (Eds.), *Precursors of early speech* (pp. 21–35). New York: Stockton Press.

Papousek, M., & Papousek, H. (1981). Musical elements in the infant's vocalization: Their significance for communication, cognition, and creativity. In L. P. Lipsitt & C. K. Rovee-Collier (Eds.), *Advances in infancy research* (Vol. 1, pp. 164–224). Norwood, NJ: Ablex.

Peterson, G. E., & Barney, H. L. (1952). Control methods used in a study of the vowels. *Journal of the Acoustical Society of America, 24,* 175–184.

Piaget, J. (1951). *Play, dreams and imitation in childhood.* New York: W. W. Norton.

Pisoni, D. B. (1977). Identification and discrimination of the relative onset time of two component tones: Implications for voicing perception in steps. *Journal of the Acoustical Society of America, 61,* 1352–1361.

Pisoni, D. B., Carrell, T. D., & Gans, S. J. (1983). Perception of the duration of rapid spectrum changes in speech and nonspeech signals. *Perception and Psychophysics, 34,* 314–322.

Rosch, E. (1975). Cognitive reference points. *Cognitive Psychology, 7,* 532–547.

Sinnott, J. M., Beecher, M. D., Moody, D. B., & Stebbins, W. C. (1976). Speech sound discrimination by monkeys and humans. *Journal of the Acoustical Society of America, 60,* 687–695.

Stark, R. (1980). Stages of speech development in the first year of life. In G. Yeni-Komshian, J.

Kavanagh, & C. Ferguson (Eds.), *Child phonology: Production* (Vol. 1, pp. 73–92). New York: Academic Press.

Starkey, P., Spelke, E. S., & Gelman, R. (1983). Detection of intermodal numerical correspondences by human infants. *Science, 222,* 179–181.

Stevens, E., Kuhl, P. K., & Padden, D. (1988). Macaques show context effects in speech perception. *Journal of the Acoustical Society of America, 84,* Suppl. 1, 577(A).

Stevens, K. N. (1972). The quantal nature of speech: Evidence from articulatory-acoustic data. In E. E. David, Jr. & P. B. Denes (Eds.), *Human communication: A unified view* (pp. 51–66). New York: McGraw-Hill.

Stevens, K. N. (1981). Constraints imposed by the auditory system on the properties used to classify speech sounds. Evidence from phonology, acoustics, and psychoacoustics. In T. Myers, J. Laver, & J. Anderson (Eds.), *Advances in psychology: The cognitive representation of speech.* Amsterdam: North-Holland.

Stevens, K. N. (in press). On the quantal nature of speech. *Journal of Phonetics.*

Stevens, K. N., & Blumstein, S. E. (1981). The search for invariant acoustic correlates of phonetic features. In P. Eimas & J. Miller (Eds.), *Perspectives on the study of speech.* Hillsdale, NJ: Lawrence Erlbaum Associates.

Streeter, L. A. (1976). Language perception of 2-month-old infants shows effects of both innate mechanisms and experience. *Nature, 259,* 39–41.

Studdert-Kennedy, M. (1986). Development of the speech perceptuomotor system. In B. Lindblom & R. Zetterström (Eds.), *Precursors of early speech* (pp. 205–217). New York: Stockton Press.

Summerfield, Q. (1979). Use of visual information for phonetic perception. *Phonetica, 36,* 314–331.

Summerfield, Q., & Haggard, M. (1977). On the dissociation of spectral and temporal cues to the voicing distinction in initial stop consonants. *Journal of the Acoustical Society of America, 62,* 435–448.

Waters, R. S., & Wilson, W. A., Jr. (1976). Speech perception by rhesus monkeys: The voicing distinction in synthesized labial and velar stop consonants. *Perception and Psychophysics, 19,* 285–289.

Editor's Comments on Dooling

In the study of complex auditory perception, species comparisons, especially human and animal comparisons, are notoriously difficult. It is never certain that the tasks are equivalent or that complex stimuli have equal salience for the organisms being compared. Yet such comparisons must be made if we are to understand the basic biological processes involved in complex acoustic perception. Otherwise said, it just as important to know whether animals and humans perceive speech sounds in a similar manner as it is to know whether they perceive complex, animal communication sounds in a similar manner.

In this chapter, Dooling reviews five comparative experiments involving birds and humans. The data reveal ways in which birds and humans differ on the perception of complex bird calls and on the perception of human speech sounds. In spite of dramatically different peripheral and central auditory systems and differences in critical band filtering properties of the auditory systems of birds and humans, both species show similar perceptual categories for different classes of budgerigars vocal signals and human speech sounds. These data argue that perceptual categories for complex sounds including speech involve mechanisms or processes at a basic enough level to be common to both the avian and mammalian auditory systems.

14 Perception of Complex, Species-Specific Vocalizations by Birds and Humans

Robert J. Dooling
University of Maryland

INTRODUCTION

The songs of birds have soothed and entertained human beings throughout the ages. Aside from the historic and aesthetic fascination with bird song there is a more recent and more alluring, scientific attraction. Modern signal analysis techniques confirm that bird vocalizations are some of the most complex biological signals known to man. The mystery of bird song deepens with the realization that birds communicate fairly complex messages with these vocal signals and that, in many species, these communication signals develop through learning.

Students of bird song have long suspected that birds are capable of producing, perceiving, and learning, subtle features of complex vocal signals to which the human auditory perceptual machinery seems insensitive. Comparing birds and humans on the perception of bird vocalizations provides perhaps the most appropriate test of this hypothesis. Because humans are the most rigorously tested organisms in the realm of psychoacoustics they also provide the best mammalian standard for comparison in trying to understand differences in auditory perception between birds and mammals. Another powerful motivation for comparing birds and humans on the perception of bird vocalizations is that we can always ask humans to describe exactly what they hear when listening to these complex sounds, which provides a unique tool for understanding the cues that birds use in acoustic communication.

The comparative strategy also represents the best approach to some of the most interesting scientific issues that have emerged from the study of bird vocalizations. These isuses include the coding of information in vocal signals and perceptual adaptations for the processing of species-specific vocalizations. In species that learn their vocalizations, there is, of course, the exciting possibility of parallels with human vocal learning. The focus of this chapter is on comparative psychoacoustics involving complex stimuli with the principle comparison between humans and birds. All of the experiments reviewed here were selected to illustrate the value of the comparative psychological approach to addressing scientific questions and generating hypotheses in the study of complex auditory perception.

Definition of Complex Acoustic Signals

There is no clear-cut, precise agreement on what constitutes a *complex* sound but there does seem to be a general consensus, at least in psychoacoustic work (Ehret, this volume; Yost & Watson, 1986). A pure tone having a constant frequency and intensity over its entire duration is a simple sound. By contrast, noise and pure tones that change in frequency or intensity or in their temporal characteristics are considered complex sounds. There is probably universal agreement on the most common examples of complex sounds including most natural sounds, animal vocalizations, human speech, and music.

Methods for Psychoacoustic Study of Hearing in Birds

The data reviewed here were all collected using the traditional methods of animal psychophysics (Stebbins, 1970). Birds were trained by positive reinforcement techniques to respond by pecking a key to the presence of (or change in) an acoustic stimulus. Two general procedures were employed in these experiments. The first procedure is often used for the measurement of absolute thresholds, masked thresholds, or difference thresholds. Here a threshold value for detection or discrimination is sought. This value is most often defined as the stimulus value at which 50% correct responding occurs in combination with an appropriately low false alarm rate.

Some of the data reviewed in this chapter were collected with a second, more elaborate procedure called the Same/Different procedure. The bird pecks an observation key to begin a trial. Immediately following this peck, two sounds are presented separated by only a few hundred msec. If the two sounds are different, the bird must peck a report key to obtain access to food. If the two sounds are the same, the bird must withhold responding. With the task structured in this way, response latency or reaction time becomes a sensitive measure of stimulus similarity. In other words, when two sounds are very different, the bird responds quickly. When two sounds are more similar, the bird responds more slowly.

This relation between response latency and stimulus similarity can be empirically determined using pure tones that vary in only one dimension (e.g., frequency). Tones close together in frequency result in longer response latencies while tones far apart in frequency result in shorter latencies. A similar relation is obtained for tones that vary only in intensity or only in duration (Dooling, Brown et al., 1987).

The use of response latency as a dependent variable in auditory operant detection tasks is not new. Response latency has proven useful in constructing equal loudness scales in both mammals (Stebbins, 1970) and birds (Dooling, Zoloth, & Baylis, 1978). The present procedure is similar to that used in these other studies but with several important differences. Here, response latencies are collected for all possible pair-wise comparisons drawn from a set of complex sounds. An important consequence of this strategy is that it provides a metric by which each sound in a set of sounds can be compared with every other sound in the set. Once such a metric is established, response latencies can then be used as input to multidimensional scaling algorithms to produce a spatial representation of the similarities among complex sounds (Howard & Silverman, 1976; Kruskal & Wish, 1978; Murry & Singh, 1980). These procedures provide an efficient, direct, and quantitative way to compare perception of complex sounds between species.

Another important advantage of the Same/Different procedure is that the birds are not trained to a particular class of sounds. In typical studies of natural concepts (see, for example, Herrnstein, 1984) or perceptual categories (see Kuhl & Miller, 1975), animals are trained to respond one way to a particular stimulus or class of stimuli and different way (or to withhold responding in the case of a Go/Nogo paradigm) to another stimulus or class of stimuli. Once trained, the animals are tested for responses to novel or intermediate instances of complex stimuli. The response pattern is used to demonstrate the existence of a concept or category and define its boundaries. It is sometimes difficult to eliminate perceptual learning during training as an explanation for category effects in these procedures. By contrast, in the Same/Different procedure birds are trained to respond to the *difference* between any two complex stimuli. Category effects that emerge from analysis of these latency data are not induced or influenced by asymmetries in conditioning procedures.

Human Same/Different data were collected by having subjects listen to stimulus pairs and then rate the similarity of each pair by entering a number on the computer keyboard. A scale of 1–5 was used with 1 representing very different and 5 representing very similar (Dooling, Park et al., 1987).

Avian Psychoacoustics—Five Comparisons

The last several decades have seen renewed interest in the study of hearing in birds using rigorous, modern psychophysical techniques (see, for review, Dooling, 1982). To summarize briefly, there are differences among birds and between birds and humans in both detection and discrimination of simple sounds. On average, birds hear best in the frequency region of 2–5 kHz with relatively poor absolute thresholds at frequencies below and above this spectral region. In detecting acoustic change in the frequency, intensity, or duration of simple pure tones in this same spectral region, birds show thresholds that are only slightly worse than humans and similar to most other vertebrates (Dooling, 1980, 1982).

The following experiments involve species and stimulus comparisons especially relevant to the theme of comparative psychoacoustics and for which human data are available.

I. DETECTION OF TONES IN NOISE

The perception of tones in noise can probably be characterized as the *simplest* example of the perception of a complex acoustic stimulus. The critical ratio (i.e., the ratio of tone power to noise power at masked threshold) is an important measure of signal processing and a valuable basis for comparison of human/bird perception because it bears directly on perception of vocal signals under natural conditions, it has significance as a measure of frequency selectivity or spectral resolving power (Ehret, this volume; Scharf, 1970), and it is very easy to obtain comparative data.

It has been known for some time that budgerigars have an unusual critical ratio function compared with most other vertebrates (Dooling & Saunders, 1975). But, it has also been the case that the budgerigar was the only avian species for which critical ratio data were available. Thus, it was not known whether all birds had nonmonotonic critical ratio functions or whether only budgerigars were unusual. One of my students, Kazuo Okanoya, undertook a project to measure critical ratios in several different species of birds all tested in the same apparatus with the exact same behavioral procedures. Okanoya's data along with recent data on blackbirds and pigeons (Hienz & Sachs, 1987), bring to 10 the number of avian species in which critical ratios have been measured (Okanoya & Dooling, 1987a). Critical ratio functions for budgerigars and six other avian species tested in the same apparatus are shown in Fig. 14.1.

This comparison reveals large differences in the size of the critical ratio among birds. At 2 kHz for instance, the canary (*Serinus canarius*) has a critical ratio of 30 dB while that of the swamp sparrow (*Melospiza georgiana*) is 24 dB (Okanoya & Dooling, 1987a). Even more intriguing, the critical ratios of budgerigars are dramatically different from other birds both in the slope of the critical ratio function and the size of the critical ratio between 2–4 kHz. It is worthwhile to note that the cockatiel (*Nymphicus hollandicus*), also a psittacine, has a critical ratio function like other birds rather than like the budgerigar.

Figure 14.2 compares critical ratio functions of the chinchilla, cat, rat, and human with the critical ratio function of the average bird and the budgerigar. This comparison reinforces the point that the critical ratios of most birds are similar to most mammals both in absolute value and in showing a 3 dB/octave slope. A sufficient number of vertebrates have now been tested that we can conclude with some confidence that budgerigars are different from mammals and different from other birds. There is only one highly specialized mammal, the Horseshoe bat, whose critical ratio function departs from the 3 dB/octave rule at

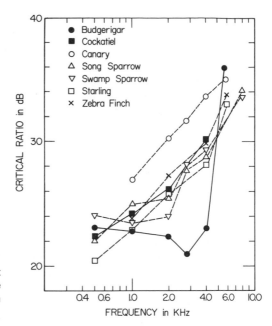

FIG. 14.1. Critical ratios for six species of small bird and the budgerigar. Reprinted from Okanoya and Dooling (1987a).

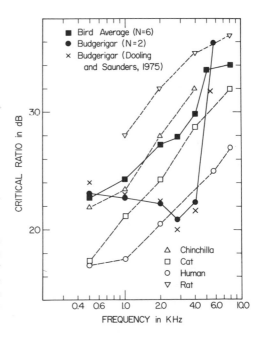

FIG. 14.2. Critical ratio data for the budgerigar (closed circles) are compared with similar data from four species of mammals (open symbols). Also shown are the average data for the other six species of birds tested in the same apparatus used to test the budgerigars. Reprinted from Okanoya and Dooling (1987a).

the very high frequencies used for echolocation (Long, 1977). Few data are available for other vertebrates but some frogs may also show unusual critical ratio functions at low to middle frequencies (Moss & Simmons, 1986; Gerhardt, this volume).

The mechanism(s) underlying masking bandwidths are probably also involved as well in the processing of complex acoustic stimuli (Scharf, 1970; Ehret, this volume). It is likely, therefore, that small critical ratios in the budgerigar between 2–4 kHz are related to the perception and learning of species-specific vocal signals. Many budgerigar vocalizations have energy in this spectral region and at least one call—the contact call—falls exclusively in the spectral region of 2–4 kHz (Dooling, 1986). To determine whether there is a relation between masking bandwidths and vocal signals, one must examine the perception of vocal signals.

II. PERCEPTION OF BUDGERIGAR VOCAL CATEGORIES

The most fascinating challenge in hearing is to delineate the role that auditory perceptual processes play in the development and maintenance of vocal learning and communication. This question is as crucial for understanding bird song (Marler, 1982) as it is for understanding human speech (Kuhl, 1986, this volume; Mullenix & Pisoni, this volume;).

The budgerigar vocal repertoire consists of a number of functionally and acoustically distinct call types some of which develop through learning (Brockway, 1964, 1965, 1969; Dooling, 1986; Dooling, Gephart, Price, McHale, & Brauth, 1987). The following is not an exhaustive list, but these call types include contact calls (given by birds when separated), alarm calls (given by birds when disturbed), nest defense calls (given only by females in the nest box), thwart calls (given by males following a rebuffed attempt at mounting during courtship), solicitation calls (given by females to solicit courtship feeding by the male), and food-begging calls given by young birds (Brockway, 1969, Dooling, 1986).

The following experiment uses the Same/Different procedure followed by a multidimensional scaling analysis of response latencies to examine whether budgerigars perceive these vocal signals as belonging in different categories and whether these categories are different for budgerigars and humans. Multidimensional scaling algorithms produce a spatial representation or "perceptual map" of a set of complex sounds on the basis of similarity measures (e.g., confusion scores, response magnitudes, error rates, or response latencies). In a spatial plot produced by MDS, stimulus similarity is represented by spatial proximity. In the following experiments, a group or cluster of stimuli in multidimensional space is taken to indicate the existence of a perceptual category.

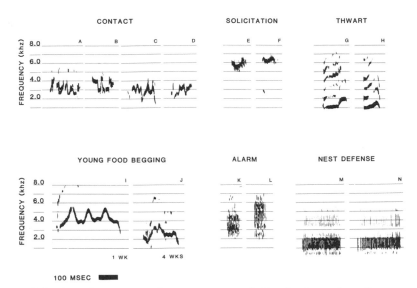

FIG. 14.3. Sonagrams of an assortment of 14 calls drawn from the budgerigar vocal repertoire. Reprinted from Dooling, Park, et al. (1987).

The stimuli in this experiment were four contact calls and two calls from each of the other major categories of calls. Sonagrams of these stimuli are shown in Fig. 14.3. Three birds and four humans were tested on these 14 stimuli.

The two-dimensional spatial representation generated by SINDSCAL of the perceptual similarity among these calls for the three budgerigars is shown in Fig. 14.4. The results from the Symmetric INdividual Differences SCALing (SIN-DSCAL) analysis reveal stimulus clusters expected from a functional and sonagraphic analysis of the vocal repertoire (Dooling, 1986) with just one exception. The food-begging call from the 4-week-old bird is very near the cluster of contact calls while the food-begging call from the 1-week-old bird is off by itself. It is also apparent that the cluster of contact calls is much more spread out than the clusters of other calls. This means that differences among contact calls are more salient to budgerigars than are the differences among calls within other categories.

The two dimensional spatial representation of these stimuli based on human direct rating data is shown in Fig. 14.5. The results show that these complex stimuli are grouped in similar ways by humans and budgerigars but the relation among the stimulus groupings is somewhat different for the two species.

For both species, the first dimension correlates roughly with the concentration of energy in the spectral region of 2–4 kHz. Contact calls with energy concentrated in the 2–4 kHz region are at one end of the first dimension while nest-defense calls having energy concentration outside this spectral region are at the

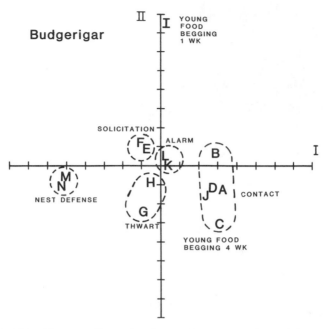

FIG. 14.4. The two dimensional spatial representation of these 14 calls as perceived by three budgerigars. Reprinted from Dooling, Park, et al. (1987).

other end of the first dimension. Human listeners report that contact calls sound both high-pitched and whistled while nest-defense calls sound low-pitched and raucous.

One noticeable difference between the spatial plots of budgerigars and humans is that the contact call cluster is more spread out for budgerigars than for humans. In other words, budgerigars find the differences among contact calls more salient than humans do. Another difference between budgerigars and humans is that budgerigars clearly hear a difference between the calls of 1-week-old and 4-week-old birds. In the human spatial plot, both of these calls from young birds are very near the cluster of contact calls. An intriguing possibility is that calls of very young birds have particular salience for adult budgerigars much like the cries of young infants for adult humans.

In general, however, the slight differences between budgerigar and human, though they may turn out to be quite important, are overshadowed by the obvious similarities. In spite of dramatic differences in the peripheral and central auditory systems of budgerigars and humans (Brauth, McHale, Brasher, & Dooling, 1987; Smith, 1985), and known differences in the filtering properties of the auditory system (Okanoya & Dooling, 1987a; Saunders, Rintelmann, & Bock, 1979), the perception of these complex sounds is roughly similar for the two species.

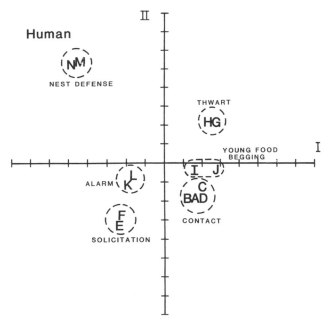

FIG. 14.5. The two dimensional spatial arrangement of the perceptual similarity among these same stimuli for four humans. Reprinted from Dooling, Park, et al. (1987).

These results provide objective, quantitative, psychophysical evidence for the existence of perceptual categories for species-specific vocal signals in birds. These comparisons, of course, have particular significance for understanding vocal learning and communication in budgerigars. The similarity between budgerigars and humans in the perceptual organization of budgerigar calls shows that, to a very large extent, the determinants of natural perceptual categories for these calls in budgerigars do not involve *special* or species-specific processes. To be sure, the similarity between budgerigars and humans does not rule out the possibility that special processes are involved in more subtle ways or invoked with only certain vocalizations. One likely candidate for special processing effects, for instance, is the category of contact calls.

III. PERCEPTION OF CONTACT CALLS

Recent work by one of my students, Thomas Park, supports the notion that the contact call occupies a special place in the auditory world of the budgerigar (Dooling, 1986). Park showed that budgerigars can learn and remember, for long periods of time, an acoustic discrimination problem involving a large number of contact calls and that high levels of performance can be maintained even when

CONTACT CALLS

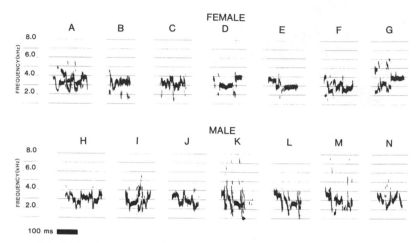

FIG. 14.6.   Sonograms of 14 contact calls from individual budgerigars (7 male, 7 female). Reprinted from Brown, Dooling, and O'Grady (1988).

these stimuli are highly degraded (Park & Dooling, 1985, 1986). The previous experiment using MDS has shown that while human and budgerigars show similar perceptual categories for the major classes of budgerigar calls, contact calls may be perceived differently by the two species.

One promise of multidimensional scaling is the possibility of uncovering the acoustic dimensions that animals (or humans) use in discriminating among complex sounds. Individual differences scaling offers the specific advantage that comparisons can be made between subjects or between species tested on the same set of sounds. Another of my students, Susan Brown, has explored this problem by examining the acoustic basis of contact call discrimination in budgerigars and compares budgerigars and humans on the perception of this category of calls.

Brown compared humans and budgerigars on a set of 14 contact calls (7 from male and 7 from female birds) (Brown, Dooling, & O'Grady, 1988). Sonograms of these calls are shown in Fig. 14.6. Five budgerigars and five humans were tested on this set of calls using the Same/Different procedure described earlier followed by multidimensional scaling of response latency matrices. A powerful feature of SINDSCAL is that the data for both birds and humans can be analyzed together and the subject weights compared as a measure of species differences.

The three-dimensional spatial arrangement of these contact calls is shown in Fig. 14.7. The first dimension is relatively more important for the human sub-

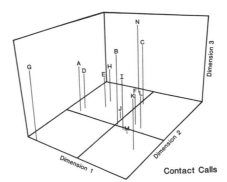

FIG. 14.7. The three dimensional spatial representation of set of 14 contact calls representing a joint solution from 5 humans and 5 budgerigars. Replotted from Brown et al. (1988).

Contact Calls

jects accounting for 79% of the variance in the human data and only 24% of the variance in the budgerigar data. The second dimension is more important for the budgerigars accounting for 64% of the variance in the budgerigar data and only 20% of the variance in the human data. The third dimension is weighted roughly the same by budgerigars and humans accounting for 30% and 42% of the variance, respectively.

Subject weights describe the amount of variance in each subject's data accounted for by distances along each dimension in the spatial arrangement of stimuli. The subject weights for all subjects are shown two-dimensional space in Fig. 14.8. The subject weights for humans and birds form two separate groups showing humans and budgerigars place different emphasis on the stimulus dimensions represented. In addition, the subjects weights for budgerigar are not as tightly clustered as those of the human subjects suggesting greater variability between budgerigars than between humans.

To identify stimulus characteristics accounting for the spatial arrangement, the acoustic properties of the calls were compared with the coordinates for each dimension using multiple regression analysis. Acoustic properties were found which corresponded to the distances along two of the three dimensions in the

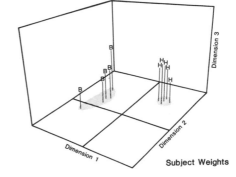

FIG. 14.8. The three dimensional representation of the subject weights corresponding to the previous MDS solution. Replotted from Brown et al. (1988).

Subject Weights

stimulus space. A measure of the predominant frequency of the call (the mean peak frequency of serial power spectra) correlated well with all coordinates on the first dimension—that weighted most by humans. The correlation coefficient for predominate frequency and the first dimension call coordinates was .70. The measure of spectral energy concentration (the ratio of energy between 2.8 and 3.2 kHz to the total amount of energy in the call) correlated well with call coordinates on the second dimension—that weighted most by budgerigars. The correlation coefficient for spectral energy concentration and the second dimension call coordinates was .74 (Brown et al., 1988).

This comparison reveals how budgerigars and humans differ in the perception of complex vocal signals. Rather than perceiving *different* aspects or acoustic features of these complex stimuli, humans and budgerigars differentially weight the *same* acoustic features. Peak frequency is most salient for humans and the concentration of spectral energy in the 2–4 kHz region is most salient for budgerigars.

The correlations between acoustic properties and spatial coordinates are significant but they are not perfect. Thus, the concentration of spectral energy certainly does not provide a complete account of contact call perception in budgerigars or humans. These results do suggest, though, that in the search for special mechanisms, the basis of acoustic categorization, or species differences in the coding of important information, factors related to energy concentration in the region of 2–4 kHz will be important.

IV. PERCEPTION OF SYNTHETIC SPEECH SOUNDS

Experiments on the perception of synthetic speech by humans have contributed tremendously to our understanding of speech communication (see, for example, Kuhl, 1986; Liberman, 1982). The comparisons of humans and animals tested on the same synthetic speech sounds directly address the issue of whether humans are specialized for the perception of speech (see, Kuhl & Miller, 1975, 1978; Kuhl, this volume; Mullenix & Pisoni, this volume). One enduring issue is whether the categorical effects observed with these synthetic speech series are the result of general psychoacoustic properties of the mammalian auditory system or whether they are a reflection of more specialized processes possessed only by humans who have the capacity to produce and understand these sounds (Kuhl, 1986). Previous studies show that humans, monkeys, and chinchillas perceive the voicing distinction among stop consonants in a similar way (Kuhl, 1981, 1986; Sinnott, Beecher, Moody, & Stebbins, 1976).

In a recent study, my students and I trained two budgerigars on the endpoints of an alveolar plosive VOT synthetic speech series (i.e., /da/–/ta/) and tested their ability to classify intermediate VOT tokens using a testing paradigm very similar to that used to test chinchillas (Kuhl & Miller, 1975). The results were

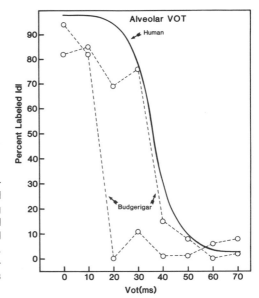

FIG. 14.9. Identification functions for two budgerigars tested on the /da-ta/ continuum using a Go/Nogo procedure (dashed lines) and the human. Replotted from Dooling, Soli, et al. (1987). Data for the human were collected using similar procedures used to test the budgerigars.

interesting in several ways. First, the 50% point or category boundaries for the two budgerigars were different from each other. On average, the two budgerigars showed a boundary at a shorter VOT value than chinchillas and humans (Kuhl & Miller, 1975). For one bird the category boundary was near that of mammals. For the other bird, the category boundary was at a much shorter VOT (Dooling, Soli et al., 1987). These results are shown in Fig. 14.9. We interpreted these limited results as demonstrating a failure of budgerigars to code the relevant acoustic information for discrimination, but there is another possibility.

It was surprisingly difficult to train budgerigars to respond to the endpoints of the /da/–/ta/ series in a GO-NOGO task. The difficulty experienced by budgerigars on this task stands in marked contrast to their performance on similar tasks involving discrimination of bird calls. Other budgerigars have been easily trained and tested on acoustic discriminations involving pure tones or bird calls using the same apparatus and a very similar training and testing paradigm (Park, Okanoya, & Dooling, 1985). A budgerigar requires approximately 1000 to 1400 trials (10–14 days at 100 trials per day) to learn to discriminate between two pure tones (e.g., 2 kHz and 3 kHz), two budgerigar calls, or two canary calls (Dooling, 1986; Park & Dooling, 1985; Park et al., 1985). Acquiring the discrimination between /da/ (0 ms VOT) and /ta/ (+70 ms VOT) required well over 10,000 trials. We concluded from this that budgerigars either could not code or could not remember the phonemically relevant acoustic changes that are occurring in the alveolar VOT series (Dooling, Soli et al., 1987).

The following experiment supports the notion that the problem lies somewhere other than in the sensory coding of relevant information. Here an approach

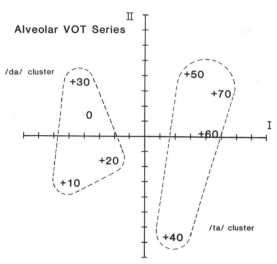

FIG. 14.10. The two dimensional spatial representation from two budgerigars tested on the /da–ta/ synthetic speech series using a discrimination paradigm followed by MDS analysis of response latencies.

to the study of speech perception by budgerigars was used which minimizes memory load. Two birds were tested on the same /da/–/ta/ described earlier using a repeating background procedure and response latencies were taken as a measure of stimulus similarity. These latencies were used as input to a multidimensional scaling algorithm (Okanoya & Dooling, 1988).

The two dimensional spatial representation of the results of two budgerigars tested in the /da/–/ta/ series is shown in Fig. 14.10. These 8 stimuli are clearly

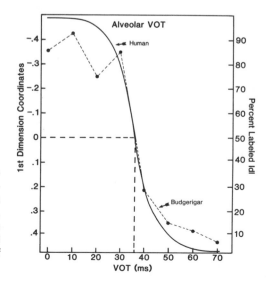

FIG. 14.11. MDS data for budgerigars plotted with coordinates along the first dimension (left axis) as a function of VOT. For comparison, human data are plotted as percent labeled /d/ (right axis) as a function of VOT.

separated into two groups along the first dimension showing that budgerigars experience an abrupt change in percept along this continuum. The results of a cluster analysis confirm that budgerigars group these stimuli into two large categories with a "boundary" between 30 and 40 ms. For comparison with more conventional psychometric functions, these data can be plotted as coordinates along the first dimension in the MDS plot versus VOT. The average results for the two birds are shown in Fig. 14.11. For comparison, data are also shown for the humans. These data show that budgerigars perceive the voicing distinction among stop consonants in the same way as humans and chinchillas (Kuhl & Miller, 1975).

V. STRAIN DIFFERENCES IN AUDITORY SENSITIVITY IN THE CANARY

There is in the study of perception the temptation to assume that the perception of simple stimuli engages less of an organism's central nervous system machinery than the perception of complex stimuli and therefore is less interesting. But as is obvious from the work of Ehret (Chapter 1, this volume) and Saunders and Henry (Chapter 2, this volume), most of what we know about hearing—especially about the auditory periphery—is based on experiments aimed at understanding the processing of simple sounds such as pure tones. It's hard to imagine reaching an understanding of the perception of complex sounds without first understanding the perception of simple sounds. For this reason, the final comparison involves simple rather than complex sounds. The basis of comparison is the pure tone audiogram in two strains of canaries.

The domestic canary, a cardueline finch, has been bred for hundreds of years for the quality of its song and plumage (Guttinger, 1985). More recently, canaries from a closebred colony of the Belgian Waterslager strain in Millbrook, NY have been the focus of both behavioral and neuroanatomical studies of vocal learning (see, as examples, Marler & Waser, 1977; Nottebohm, Nottebohm, & Crane, 1986; Nottebohm, Nottebohm, Crane, & Wingfield, 1977; Waser & Marler, 1977).

Psychoacoustic studies of hearing in Belgian waterslager canaries from this colony and other colonies has recently shown that, at high frequencies (i.e., above 2.0 kHz), absolute thresholds for pure tones in the strain are between 30 and 40 dB (SPL) higher than those of other song birds—including other strains of canaries (Okanoya & Dooling, 1985, 1987a, 1987b). Audiograms for Belgian waterslager canaries and non-waterslager canaries are compared in Fig. 14.12. Non-Belgian waterslager canaries show a typically avian audiogram with a narrow range of maximum sensitivity in the spectral region of 1–5 kHz with decreasing sensitivity at lower and higher frequencies. By contrast, Belgian waterslager canaries show similar thresholds to non-waterslagers at low frequencies but at frequencies above 2 kHz, thresholds are markedly elevated.

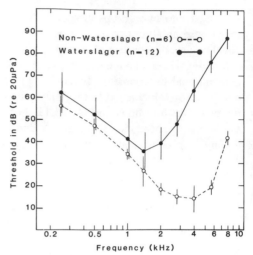

FIG. 14.12. Audiograms from 12 Belgian waterslager canaries and 6 non-Belgian waterslager canaries. Replotted from Okanoya, Dooling, and Downing (in preparation).

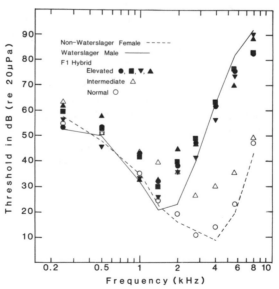

FIG. 14.13.   Audiograms from a male Belgian waterslager canary and a female, non-Belgian Waterslager canary and six of their offspring. The thresholds of four the F1 hybrids are elevated at high frequencies. Replotted from Okanoya, Dooling, and Downing (in preparation).

Because Belgian waterslager canaries have been bred for loud, low-pitched song and because they must learn this song by reference to auditory information, this comparison may prove to be particularly interesting. A number of possible explanations for these strain differences in auditory sensitivity can be entertained but one is especially intriguing. Perhaps in artificially selecting for loud, low-pitched song, breeders were actually selecting for poor high-frequency hearing. Aside from the obvious significance for theories of selective vocal learning in song birds, this possibility also points in the direction of a simple genetic component to elevated thresholds in Belgian waterslager canaries.

As one test of this possibility, Okanoya and I examined the thresholds of young birds produced from cross-breeding a Belgian waterslager canary with elevated thresholds and a common, mixed-strain canary with a normal pure tone audiogram. Figure 14.13 shows the audiograms of both parents and 6 of their offspring (Okanoya, Dooling, & Downing, in prep). Four of these F1 hybrids have elevated thresholds characteristic of Belgian waterslager canaries. One F1 hybrid clearly has normal thresholds for pure tones and the remaining F1 hybrid has mildly elevated thresholds at high frequencies. Clearly, more hybrids need to be tested to fully address the question of how elevated high-frequency thresholds might be inherited. Nevertheless, it is not hard to imagine that the large differences in basic auditory sensitivity in these two canary strains could exert a profound influence on the selection of complex song syllables for learning.

VI. DISCUSSION

The comparisons drawn in this chapter demonstrate the value of the comparative approach in making discoveries and generating hypotheses by highlighting specific differences between birds and humans.

The comparative data on masking thresholds provide one illustration of the value of this approach. The concept of a critical band is central to a host of human psychoacoustic phenomena including loudness, pitch, musical consonance, and speech perception. But the 3 dB/octave increase in critical bandwidth is a characteristic that humans share with most other mammals and birds that have been tested. Budgerigars are different from these other vertebrates. It will be interesting to see whether the budgerigar critical ratio function, with its unusual shape, proves to be as unifying a concept for auditory perception in this species as critical bandwidths have been for human hearing. There is evidence that critical ratio, critical band, and psychophysical tuning curve functions vary in a similar way across frequency for budgerigars (Dooling & Searcy, 1985; Saunders et al., 1979). If this correspondence holds for other auditory perceptual phenomena, the budgerigar may provide an interesting and unique test of the auditory filter hypothesis.

The comparative approach to masked auditory thresholds raises several questions. How is it that most birds and mammals with dramatically different central and peripheral auditory systems show such similar critical ratio functions? On the other hand, given the similarity among birds in peripheral and central auditory system anatomy and physiology, why are budgerigars so different? Does the fact that the spectra of contact calls in budgerigars are matched to the region of smallest critical ratios have significance for the acoustic communication system of this species? If so, then why is there no similar match in other birds that communicate with complex, learned vocal signals. All of the birds for which we now have critical ratio data also have vocal signals that fall in restricted spectral regions between roughly 1–8 kHz yet only budgerigars show the curious match between critical ratio and vocalization spectra.

The experiments using species-specific vocal signals and multidimensional scaling represent a direct, quantitative measurement of perceptual categories for species-specific vocal signals. The perceptual categories described for budgerigars are *natural* categories both in the sense that the stimulus objects are natural (i.e., vocal signals) and that the categorization effects are not influenced or induced by asymmetries in the conditioning procedures. Important questions remain about how these categories come about, at what level the categorization is occurring, and what role these categories play in the development of vocal behavior in budgerigars. But, what is most revealing is the comparison—the fact that humans and budgerigars show similar perceptual categories for these same sounds.

This comparison has considerable significance for the role that perceptual processes play in vocal learning in budgerigars. As with many songbirds, both deafened (Dooling, Gephart et al., 1987) and isolate-reared (Dooling, unpublished data) budgerigars develop abnormal contact calls so auditory experience plays a critical role in the normal vocal development in this species. The present results show that the perceptual organization of complex, species-specific, vocal signals in budgerigars relies on mechanisms common to both the mammalian and avian auditory systems. Thus, in the sense that only very general auditory mechanisms are involved (i.e., those common to human and avian auditory systems), the budgerigar auditory system may be said to be *hardwired* for the major categories of vocal signals with experience playing little or no role.

This is not to minimize the role of experience as a factor in fine-tuning the auditory perceptual system particularly for intracategory discriminations. Recent work has shown that while budgerigars caged together develop similar contact calls, they nevertheless can discriminate among the calls of their cagemates. When budgerigars unfamiliar with these cagemates are tested on the same calls, they fail to discriminate among the calls of different individuals (Brown et al., 1988).

Experiments on contact calls are also beginning to reveal the nature of differences between human and budgerigar perception of this particular category of calls. The acoustic correlates of the perceptual dimensions obtained from MDS show that budgerigars and humans may use the same acoustic cues but the salience of these cues is different for the two species. The comparison raises several important questions: Where is the mechanism(s) that results in the differential perceptual weighting of the same acoustic features by humans and budgerigars? Is this mechanism innate or does it develop through learning? If learning is involved, what kind of experience with contact calls is required to alter perception?

Not surprisingly, the questions that arise from comparing budgerigars and humans on the perception of bird calls are also at the heart of experiments on the perception of synthetic speech sounds by animals (Kuhl, 1986). If budgerigars and humans hear the major classes of budgerigar calls in a similar fashion, it should be expected that these two species might, at least under some conditions, perceive synthetic speech sounds the same way.

The two experiments comparing budgerigars and humans on the perception of speech are important for theories of speech perception for the following reasons. The results from the multidimensional scaling analysis of response latencies indicate that budgerigars hear an abrupt perceptual change in the /da–ta/ continuum between 30 ms and 40 ms VOT. Thus, these data demonstrate that perceptual discontinuity in the /da/–/ta/ continuum—once thought to be a uniquely human characteristic—is not even unique to the mammalian auditory system. Clearly, this suggests that categorical perception of the /da/–/ta/ continuum is due to even more basic processes common to both the mammalian and avian auditory systems.

But, in assessing the impact of these results on the perception of speech by budgerigars, an equally important finding is the difficulty encountered in training budgerigars on the extremes of the /da–ta/ continuum in a classification task where memory load was high. The results from this study suggest that budgerigars are quite different from humans, chinchillas, and monkeys (Dooling, Soli et al., 1987). In the budgerigar experiments, difference between the MDS procedure and the classification task is primarily one of memory load. Thus, species differences may emerge at a more central or integrative level of processing beyond the simple coding of information by the auditory periphery. It appears that budgerigars have trouble remembering the salient acoustic features required for distinguishing among individual tokens in the /da/–/ta/ synthetic speech series.

The final comparison—that of elevated thresholds in the Belgian Waterslager strain of canary—is relevant in yet another way. Years of selective breeding of canary strains certainly open the possibility for a relation between strain differences in vocalizations and strain differences in hearing sensitivity. The mixed auditory sensitivity of F1 hybrids suggests the phenomenon of elevated thresholds in Belgian Waterslager canaries may have a relatively, simple inheritance mechanism. Because so few F1s have been tested, this conclusion is at best, very tentative. There are still many questions to be answered about this phenomenon and its relevance, if any, for vocal learning in canaries. It is not too difficult to imagine how elevated thresholds might have a profound influence on the learning of song in Belgian Waterslager canaries. Indeed, a comparative study of vocalization properties, song learning, and auditory discrimination in different strains of canary could provide an unusually clear and direct example of how innate perceptual mechanisms might guide the vocal learning process.

In summary, the five comparative studies cited herein on birds and humans serve at once to deepen the mystery of bird song but also to underscore the value of the comparative approach to the perception of complex sounds. This approach stands at the nexus of three scientific disciplines: comparative psychology with its theoretical underpinnings in developmental and evolutionary processes, psychoacoustics with its emphasis on threshold measurement and stimulus control, and vocal learning, which focuses attention on the perhaps unique relation between sensory processing of vocal signals and motor control of the vocal production apparatus.

ACKNOWLEDGMENTS

Preparation of this chapter was supported by NIH grants NS19006 and HD00512 to R. Dooling. I thank S. Brown, S. Hulse, K. Okanoya , and T. Park for comments on earlier drafts.

REFERENCES

Brauth, S. E., McHale, C. M., Brasher, C. A., & Dooling, R. J. (1987). Auditory pathways in the budgerigar, I. Thalamo-telencephalic projections. *Brain, Behavior, and Evolution, 30,* 174–199.

Brockway, B. F. (1964). Ethological studies of the budgerigar (*Melopsittacus undulatus*): Non-reproductive behaviour. *Behaviour, 22,* 192–222.

Brockway, B. F. (1965). Ethological studies of the budgerigar (*Melopsittacus undulatus*): Reproductive behaviour. *Behaviour, 23,* 294–324.

Brockway, B. F. (1969). Role of budgerigar vocalizations in the integration of breeding behavior. In R. Hinde (Ed.), *Bird vocalizations* (pp. 131–158). Cambridge, England: Cambridge University Press.

Brown, S. D., Dooling, R. J., & O'Grady, K. (1988). Perceptual organization of acoustic stimuli by budgerigars (*Melopsittacus undulatus*): III. Contact calls. *Journal of Comparative Psychology, 102,* 236–247.

Dooling, R. J. (1980). Behavior and psychophysics of hearing in birds. In A. N. Popper & R. R. Fay (Eds.), *Comparative studies of hearing in vertebrates* (pp. 261–288). New York: Springer-Verlag.

Dooling, R. J. (1982). Auditory Perception in Birds. In D. E. Kroodsma, & E. H. Miller (Eds.), *Acoustic communication in birds, Vol. 1* (pp. 95–130). New York: Academic Press.

Dooling, R. J. (1986). Perception of vocal signals by budgerigars (*Melopsittacus undulatus*). *Experimental Biology, 45,* 195–218.

Dooling, R. J., Brown, S. D., Park, T. J., Soli, S. D., & Okanoya, K. (1987). Perceptual organization of acoustic stimuli by budgerigars: I. Pure tones. *Journal of Comparative Psychology, 101,* 139–149.

Dooling, R. J., Park, T. J., Brown, S. D., Okanoya, K., & Soli, S. D. (1987). Perceptual organization of acoustic stimuli in budgerigars *(Melopsittacus undulatus)*: II. Vocal signals. *Journal of Comparative Psychology, 101,* 376–381.

Dooling, R. J., Gephart, B. F., Price, P. H., McHale, C., & Brauth, S. E. (1987). Effects of deafening on the contact call of the budgerigar *(Melopsittacus undulatus)*. *Animal Behaviour, 35,* 1264–1266.

Dooling, R. J., & Saunders, J. C. (1975). Hearing and vocalizations in the parakeet *(Melopsittacus undulatus)*: Absolute thresholds, critical ratios, frequency difference limens, and vocalizations. *Journal of Comparative and Physiological Psychology, 88,* 1–20.

Dooling, R. J., & Searcy, M. H. (1985). Nonsimultaneous auditory masking in the budgerigar *(Melopsittacus undulatus)*. *Journal of Comparative Psychology, 99,* 226–230.

Dooling, R. J., Soli, S. D., Kline, R. M., Park, T. J., Hue, C., & Bunnell, T. (1987). Perception of synthetic speech sounds by the budgerigar (Melopsittacus undulatus). *Bulletin of the Psychonomic Society, 25,* 139–142.

Dooling, R. J., Zoloth, S. R., & Baylis, J. R. (1978). Auditory sensitivity, equal loudness, temporal resolving power, and vocalizations in the house finch *(Carpodacus mexicanus)*. *Journal of Comparative and Physiological Psychology, 92,* 867–876.

Guttinger, H. R. (1985). Consequences of domestication on the song structures in the canary. *Behaviour, 92,* 255–278.

Herrnstein, R. J. (1984). Objects, categories, and discriminative stimuli. In H. L. Roitblat, T. G. Bever, & H. S. Terrace (Eds.), *Animal Cognition* (pp. 233–261). Hillsdale, NJ: Lawrence Erlbaum Associates.

Hienz, R. D., & Sachs, M. B. (1987). Effects of noise on pure-tone thresholds in blackbirds *(Agelaius phoeniceus* and *Molothrus ater)* and pigeons *(Columba livia)*. *Journal of Comparative Psychology, 101,* 16–24.

Howard, J. H., & Silverman, E. G. (1976). A multidimensional scaling analysis of 16 complex sounds. *Perception and Psychophysics, 19,* 193–200.

Kuhl, P. K. (1981). Discrimination of speech by nonhuman animals: Basic auditory sensitivities conducive to the perception of speech-sound categories. *Journal of the Acoustical Society of America, 70,* 340–349.

Kuhl, P. K. (1986). The special-mechanisms debate in speech: Contributions of tests on animals (and the relation of these tests to studies using non-speech signals). *Experimental Biology, 45,* 233–265.

Kuhl, P. K., & Miller, J. D. (1975). Speech perception by the chinchilla: Voiced-voiceless distinction in alveolar plosive constants. *Science, 190,* 69–72.

Kuhl, P. K., & Miller, J. D. (1978). Speech perception by the chinchilla: Identification functions for synthetic VOT stimuli. *Journal of the Acoustical Society of America, 63,* 905–917.

Kruskal, J. R., & Wish, M. (1978). *Multidimensional scaling.* Beverly Hills: Sage Publications.

Liberman, A. M. (1982). On finding that speech is special. *American Psychologist, 37,* 148–167.

Long, G. R. (1977). Masked auditory thresholds from the bat, *Rhinolophus ferrumequinum. Journal of Comparative Physiology, 116,* 247–255.

Marler, P. (1982). Avian and primate communication: The problem of natural categories. *Neuroscience and Biobehavioral Reviews, 6,* 87–94.

Marler, P., & Waser, M. S. (1977). Role of auditory feedback in canary song development. *Journal of Comparative and Physiological Psychology, 91,* 8–16.

Moss, C. F., & Simmons, A. M. (1986). Frequency selectivity of hearing in the green treefrog, *Hyla cinerea. Journal of Comparative Physiology, 159,* 257–266.

Murry, T., & Singh, S. (1980). Multidimensional analysis of male and female voices. *Journal of the Acoustical Society of America, 68,* 1294–1300.

Nottebohm, F., Nottebohm, M. E., & Crane, L. (1986). Developmental and seasonal changes in the anatomy of song-control nuclei. *Behavioral and Neural Biology, 46,* 445–471.

Nottebohm, F., Nottebohm, M. E., Crane, L. A., & Wingfield, J. C. (1987). Seasonal changes in gonadal hormone levels of adult male canaries and their relation to song. *Behavioral and Neural Biology, 47,* 197–211.

Okanoya, K., & Dooling, R. J. (1985). Colony differences in auditory thresholds in the canary (*Serinus canarius*). *Journal of the Acoustical Society of America, 78,* 1170–1176.

Okanoya, K., & Dooling, R. (1987a). Hearing in Passerine and Psittacine birds: A comparative study of absolute and masked auditory thresholds. *Journal of Comparative Psychology, 101,* 7–15.

Okanoya, K., & Dooling, R. J. (1987b). Strain differences in auditory sensitivity in the canary (*Serinus canarius*). *Journal of Comparative Psychology, 101,* 213–215.

Okanoya, K., & Dooling, R. J. (1988). Obtaining acoustic similarity measures from animals: A method for species comparisons. *Journal of the Acoustical Society of America, 83,* 1690–1693.

Okanoya, K., Dooling, R. J., & Downing, J. D. (in preparation). Hearing and vocalizations in hybrid Belgian Waterslager-German Roller canaries. *Hearing Research.*

Park, T. J., & Dooling, R. J. (1985). Perception of species-specific contact calls by budgerigars (*Melopsittacus undulatus*). *Journal of Comparative Psychology, 99,* 391–402.

Park, T. J., & Dooling, R. J. (1986). Perception of degraded vocalizations by budgerigars (*Melopsittacus undulatus*). *Animal Learning and Behavior, 14,* 359–364.

Park, T. J., Okanoya, K., & Dooling, R. J. (1985). Operant conditioning of small birds for acoustic discrimination. *Journal of Ethology* (Japan), *3,* 5–9.

Saunders, J. C., Rintelmann, W. F., & Bock, G. R. (1979). Frequency selectivity in bird and man: A comparison among critical ratios, critical bands, and psychophysical tuning curves. *Hearing Research, 1,* 303–323.

Scharf, B. (1970). Critical bands. In J. V. Tobias (Ed.), *Foundations of modern auditory theory* (Vol. 1). New York: Academic Press.

Sinnott, J. M., Beecher, M. D., Moody, D. B., & Stebbins, W. C. (1976). Speech sound discrimination by monkeys and humans. *Journal of the Acoustical Society of America, 60,* 687–695.

Smith, C. A. (1985). Inner ear. In A. King & J. MacLeland (Eds.), *Form and function in birds* (Vol. 3, pp. 273–310). New York: Academic Press.

Stebbins, W. C. (1970). *Animal psychophysics: The design and conduct of sensory experiments.* New York: Appleton-Century-Crofts.

Waser, M. S., & Marler, P. (1977). Song learning in canaries. *Journal of Comparative and Physiological Psychology, 91,* 1–7.

Yost, W. A., & Watson, C. S. (1986). *Auditory processing of complex sounds.* Hillsdale, NJ: Lawrence Erlbaum Associates.

Editorial Comments on Sinnott

In this chapter, Sinnott offers a fascinating and suggestive theoretical analysis of some data obtained when redwing blackbirds and cowbirds learned to discriminate among examples of their own conspecific song or among examples of song from an alien species. Human subjects were also included. In general, all species learned to discriminate complete songs equally well, although humans were somewhat faster than the birds in developing the discrimination. However, a second experiment broke songs into syllables and tested for differential discrimination of the syllables. Once again, birds and humans did equally well on the beginning introductory elements of the song, but their discrimination performance differed for terminal elements of the song. Redwings did better on their own song than did cowbirds, but cowbirds did better on their song than did redwings. Humans, once again, perform better than all birds in the final elements. Another experiment showed that all birds could learn to discriminate on the basis of the final elements of song if they were tutored and given practice in doing so—so differences in processing the terminal elements were not due to some inherent lack of perceptual capacity.

   An interesting set of results receives an interesting theoretical analysis. The analysis is based on several models drawn from human information processing. These range from the idea of automatic processing where well-practiced habits run off without any attention to detail (i.e., terminal syllables), through an analysis based on Garner's integral-separable distinction in perception to linguistic models based on syntactic and semantic constraints. The article is especially interesting because the application of these principles may lead to novel ways of analyzing complex acoustic structures like birdsong. The analysis also suggests that for the species under study, at least, some of the perceptual predilections of the birds may be innately controlled. That issue is an old and continuing controversy that is well represented in this book.

15 Internal Cognitive Structures Guide Birdsong Perception

Joan M. Sinnott
University of South Alabama

> *For to pass by other Instances, Birds learning of Tunes, and the endeavors one may observe in them to hit the Notes right, put it past doubt with me, that they have Perception, and retain Ideas in their Memories, and use them for Patterns.*
>
> John Locke
> Essay on the Human Understanding
> Book II, Chapter X, Paragraph 10

INTRODUCTION

Many animals use various "special" (species-specific) mechanisms to enhance the processing of information in biologically relevant communication signals. While frogs use low-level peripheral filtering in decoding conspecific vocalizations (Capranica, Frishkopf, & Nevo, 1973), monkeys use higher-level mechanisms that implicate semantic communication (Seyfarth, Cheney, & Marler, 1980) and selective attention (Petersen, 1982). As humans, we are most familiar with the special aspects of our own communication system, which uses internal cognitive structures (i.e., sentences) to impose grammatical relationships on speech (Chomsky, 1967; Miller, 1962). Human sentence formation is difficult, if at all possible, for nonhumans to acquire (Terrace, Petitto, Sanders, & Bever, 1979). Nevertheless, it seems appropriate from an evolutionary orientation to search for rudimentary internal cognitive structures in animals by examining the processing of their own conspecific communication signals.

The present research uses songbirds as subjects. Songbirds (oscines; Passeriformes) are distinguished taxonomically by a very complex syrinx, or sound

447

producing organ (Brackenbury, 1982). This anatomical specialization is reflected in the complex acoustic structure of birdsong, in which song elements and syllables are combined into intricate patterns of up to several seconds in duration (Greenewalt, 1968). Consider the chatter of a dawn chorus of songbirds, where many different species sing simultaneously. What mechanisms do birds use to enhance the processing of conspecific song in the midst of the presumably irrelevant and distracting noise from alien species? To what extent do they involve semantic or syntactic processing versus lower-level auditory processing? To what extent do they reflect innate versus learned components? Finally, to what extent can they be related to mechanisms involved in human speech perception?

In pursuing answers to these questions, the present research contributes to a relatively new area of animal communication that involves training animals to respond to vocal signals in the laboratory using operant conditioning techniques (Park & Dooling, 1985; Petersen, 1982; Sinnott, 1980), rather than using playback techniques in which the animals' responses are limited by their natural inclinations to respond. With operant techniques, the way is open to precise psychophysical analyses of communication signals. An added advantage is that the animals' responses to alien as well as conspecific signals can be examined. Thus processing measures can be compared for biologically "relevant" versus "irrelevant" signals and the differences between specialized versus generalized processing can be more clearly defined.

This chapter reviews data from a series of studies that indicate that songbirds use special mechanisms to guide their perception of conspecific song in a laboratory situation (Sinnott, 1980, 1987). In addition, I present new data that cast light on the questions of automatic and innate processing mechanisms. I then discuss several theoretical frameworks from human cognitive psychology and psycholinguistics to conceptualize the differences between conspecific and alien song perception. Finally, I discuss the value that animal models have for clarifying current controversial issues regarding species-specific coding of communication signals, including human speech.

I. GENERAL METHOD

Subjects and Stimuli

Bird subjects were red-winged blackbirds (*Agelaius phoeniceus*) and brown-headed cowbirds (*Molothrus ater*), both members of the North American blackbird family (Icteridae). According to Bent (1965), redwings originally inhabited marshlands, but as these were drained they readily adapted to other environments and in some cases have become agricultural pests. Cowbirds originally inhabited the Great Plains and followed buffalo herds in order to eat displaced insects. As the buffalo were killed off and the forests of eastern North America were cut down, the cowbirds spread eastward and transferred their affiliation to domesticated farm animals. Thus both species have proven to be highly adaptable in response to human encroachment and habitat destruction, and are now considered to be "trash" birds. In present times, redwings and cowbirds freely associate with each other in feeding, roosting, and migratory groups. Cowbirds are unusual in their habit of nest-parasitism; the females appropriate the nests of alien species to lay their eggs, which are then hatched and raised by foster parents.

For redwings, song plays an important role in male territoriality (Yasukawa, 1981), while, for cowbirds, song appears to function primarily in mate attraction (West, King, & Eastzer, 1981). In both species, song production is limited to males, who possess song "repertoires" that contain several clear and discrete song theme categories. Striking structural similarities exist between redwing and cowbird song. Both consist of a sequence of introductory notes ranging from 1–3 kHz, and followed by a longer, louder, higher-frequency, sustained portion. The most species-distinctive portion is this final part, which for redwings consists of a rapidly modulated trill centered near 4 kHz (Brenowitz, 1983; Marler, 1969), and for cowbirds consists of a high-frequency, pure-tone whistle ranging between 6–10 kHz (Greenewalt, 1968; West et al., 1981).

My experiments employed wild-caught adult redwings (four males, two females) and cowbirds (three males, two females) who were trapped at the Patuxent Wildlife Research Center in Laurel, MD. Once in the laboratory, redwings and cowbirds were housed together in a colony room in which the light–dark cycle was synchronized with the normal seasonal daylight cycle. Birds sang readily at dawn and dusk under these conditions. Other studies describe methods of maintaining these birds in captivity, adapting them to the experimental apparatus, and obtaining basic data concerning their psychoacoustic capacities (Hienz, Sinnott, & Sachs, 1977, 1980; Sinnott, Sachs, & Hienz, 1980).

Song stimuli were recorded in the laboratory from a captive male redwing and cowbird, during periods when each was removed from the colony room and introduced into a large cage with a conspecific female companion. Overt responses to song by the females (e.g., copulatory postures) were never observed. All four of these birds were subsequently used as subjects. Spectrographic analyses revealed that each male possessed a repertoire of 5–6 different song themes, differentiated from one another by the patterning of the introductory notes and the modulation in the final song portion. Two themes were chosen from each male to represent the song stimulus classes for the present experiments. The entire song stimulus set, which included two tokens of each theme, is shown in Fig. 15.1. Two pure tones of 500 Hz and 6 kHz were also recorded from an oscillator for use as control stimuli.

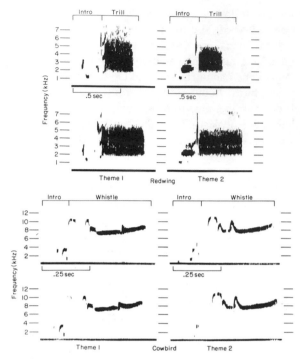

FIG. 15.1.   Song stimuli recorded from a male redwing (4 top songs) and a male cowbird (4 bottom songs). Two themes from each male's repertoire are shown, along with two tokens of each theme. Brackets indicate the points where introductory notes were separated from trills or whistles during song element test sessions. From Sinnott (1980), *Journal of the Acoustical Society, 68,* p. 495. Copyright 1980 by the American Institute of Physics.

Apparatus and Procedure

The bird test apparatus is shown in Fig. 15.2. Birds entered a wire-mesh test cage that was suspended in the center of a soundproof IAC booth and contained a perch, three response keys, and a grain feeder. A go-right/go-left procedure was employed for stimulus classification. A trial sequence was initiated by a peck on the center key, which caused a sound-stimulus to be repetitively presented from a loudspeaker mounted near the cage. Stimuli representing two classes (e.g., red-wing Theme 1 versus redwing Theme 2) were randomly presented with equal probability. If a stimulus was a token from Class 1, a right keypeck was immediately rewarded by 2-sec access to grain, and, if the stimulus belonged to Class 2, a left keypeck was similarly rewarded. In each case, the stimulus terminated only

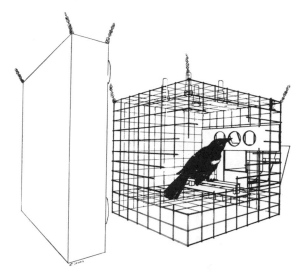

FIG. 15.2. Drawing of the three-key, go-left, go-right testing apparatus. From Hienz, Sinnott, and Sachs (1977), *Journal of Comparative and Physiological Psychology, 91*, p. 1366. Copyright 1977 by the American Psychological Association.

after its current readout was complete. A 1-sec intertrial interval followed each reward, and errors were punished by 6 sec timeouts. To eliminate biases to either key, a correction procedure caused missed stimuli to be repeated in subsequent trials (but not counted in the data analysis) until a correct response occurred. All experimental contingencies, including the readout of the digitized stimuli, were controlled by a Varian 620-I computer.

Speculation that humans may be insensitive to information in birdsong (e.g., Greenewalt, 1968) prompted the recruitment of two human subjects to be tested along with the birds. Humans sat on a stool to the right of the cage and extended their left hands inside the cage to press the keys with their fingers. One human (termed the "naive" human) was never informed of the purpose of the experiments nor of the nature of the stimuli: he was simply instructed to respond in the apparatus by making correct responses and avoiding errors. In contrast, the second human (termed the "sophisticated" human) was a 33-year-old auditory research scientist with extensive previous experience in psychoacoustic testing. He was shown spectrographs of the stimuli and was aware of how they were composed of various song elements. He was encouraged to be as quick and as accurate as possible in his responses. In short, he was given much feedback to ensure that he would display optimal human performance.

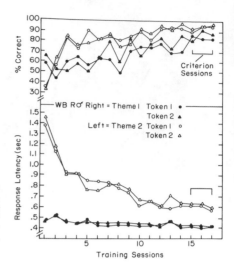

FIG. 15.3. Percent correct responses and median correct response latencies as a function of training sessions for a redwing learning to classify 4 cowbird songs.

II. DATA

Learning to Classify Tones, Redwing Songs and Cowbird Songs

The first experiment compared the abilities of redwings, cowbirds, and humans to learn to classify simple pure tones, redwing songs, and cowbird songs. The three stimulus sets were tested separately. For tone classification, a right response was correct for the 500 Hz tone and a left response was correct for the 6 kHz tone. For each song classification condition, the four song tokens were randomly presented with equal probability (0.25). A right response was correct for the two tokens of Theme 1, and a left response for the two tokens of Theme 2. For all conditions, the criterion for learning was 3 successive test sessions with a mean percent correct score of >85%. All subjects learned to classify all three types of stimuli. For example, Fig. 15.3 shows a learning curve from a redwing classifying cowbird songs. Performance started at close to chance levels (50% correct) and improved until the 85% correct criterion was reached at session 17. Throughout the learning process, this bird exhibited shorter right-side response latencies (400–500 ms) than left (>550 ms).

Figure 15.4 shows the mean number of sessions to criterion for redwings, cowbirds, and humans classifying tones, redwing songs and cowbird songs. Tones were learned most quickly, followed by redwing songs, and then cowbird songs. In general, birds learned equally well to classify conspecific and alien song themes. Humans learned more quickly than birds to classify all three types of stimuli, and the sophisticated human learned faster than the naive human.

Figure 15.5 shows mean response latencies averaged over the three criterion

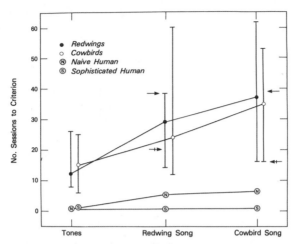

FIG. 15.4. Number of training sessions to criterion for tones, redwing songs and cowbird songs. For birds, means based on 5 redwings (filled symbols) and 5 cowbirds (open symbols) are shown along with the ranges of individual performance. Performance levels of the male birds who produced the stimuli (plain arrows) and of the females caged with them (crossed arrows) are indicated. Individual human data are shown: N = naive human, S = sophisticated human.

sessions. In general, birds responded equally fast to tones, redwing songs, and cowbird songs. In contrast to birds, both humans exhibited considerably longer latencies (by 120–200%) to song themes than to tones. The sophisticated human was overall faster to respond than the naive human.

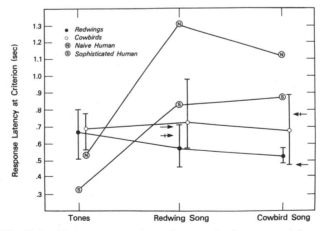

FIG. 15.5. Mean response latencies at criterion averaged over the right and left side stimuli for tones, redwing songs and cowbird songs. See Fig. 15.4 for subject legend.

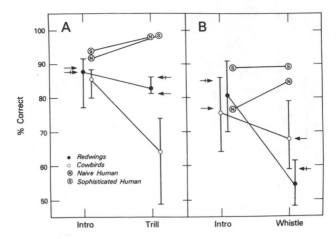

FIG. 15.6.   Percent correct responses of redwings, cowbirds, and humans for redwing song elements (A) and cowbird song elements (B), averaged over sessions 5–10 of testing. See fig. 15.4 for subject legend.

Song Element Test Sessions

A second experiment assessed which song elements the subjects used for their full-song classifications. Songs were edited into their introductory notes and final trills (or whistles) as indicated by the brackets in Fig. 15.1. Redwing and cowbird elements were tested separately. In each condition, the right-side stimuli were the two tokens of introductory notes and the two tokens of trills (or whistles) from Theme 1, and the left-side stimuli were the corresponding tokens of Theme 2, for a total of eight stimuli to be classified. Figure 15.6 shows at what levels of accuracy the subjects classified the isolated song elements. Redwings, cowbirds, and humans performed similarly for introductory elements, but there was strikingly clear differentiation among the three species for final (trill or whistle) song elements. For redwing trills (15.6A), redwings performed better than cowbirds, but for cowbird whistles (15.6B), cowbirds performed better than redwings. Humans performed better than all birds on final elements.

Trill and Whistle Tutoring

In view of these strikingly poorer performances of birds classifying alien final song elements, a third experiment investigated the effects of tutoring the birds with these same final elements. Tutoring sessions presented only trills (or whistles) in the stimulus set, without the added distraction of introductory notes, for a total of only four stimuli to be classified. With tutoring, the performance of alien birds rapidly improved, eventually reaching levels of accuracy comparable to

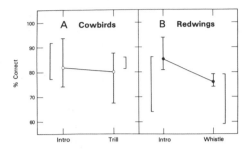

FIG. 15.7. Mean percent correct responses and ranges of performance for (A) five cowbirds classifying redwing song elements after
trill tutoring, and (B) for three redwings classifying cowbird song elements after whistle tutoring. For comparison, brackets indicate the
range of performance of untutored birds classifying conspecific elements during the original song element test sessions (from Fig. 15.6).

those of the conspecific birds. After tutoring, birds were again presented with
sessions consisting of both alien introductory notes and final trills (or whistles).
Figure 15.7 shows results for all tutored alien birds, compared with the non-
tutored performances of conspecific birds. There was less species differentiation
after tutoring than before, suggesting that the original deficits observed by alien
birds (compare with Fig. 15.6) were largely attentional, and did not stem from an
inability to discriminate the acoustic features of alien song.

Therefore, how to account for the superior processing of final song portions
by the untutored conspecific birds in Fig. 15.6? Perhaps, during the original full-
song training sessions, the two species were differentially processing the same
physical input. Birds classifying alien songs may have focused their attention
primarily on the introductory elements and discarded the final elements as irrelevant information. Animals can learn to ignore stimuli that have no bearing on
reinforcement (Mackintosh, 1973). It would be advantageous for any food deprived organism to use the minimal amount of information necessary to identify
the full song themes (i.e., the introductory information) and then respond as
quickly as possible to obtain food.

Examination of the learning curve of the redwing in Fig. 15.3, where the
stimuli were cowbird themes, seems to verify this hypothesis. This subject
consistently exhibited latencies on the right-side response key of less than 500
ms. Since the overall duration of the cowbird song stimuli was approximately
500 ms, this bird's latencies imply that his decision to respond must have been
made before the whistle portion of the song had ended. It is unlikely, therefore,
that he was actively attending to the complete whistle in learning to classify these
stimuli. Hulse and Cynx (1986) also report that songbirds (starlings) classifying
arbitrary tone patterns attend primarily to the introductory portions. In contrast,
birds classifying conspecific themes in the present study may have attended to

information in the entire song during learning, final as well as introductory, since the song was for them a biologically relevant stimulus and may have had reinforcing properties of its own (Stevenson, 1969).

According to this hypothesis, however, an examination of the latency data in Fig. 15.5 should reveal that birds classifying conspecific themes would exhibit longer latencies compared to alien themes, indicative of extra processing time resulting from extra attention focussed on the final song elements. But the data show that latencies (at criterion) were not any longer for conspecific themes, compared to alien themes. Furthermore, consider the latencies to the 200 ms tones as *baseline* data. Birds as a group devoted no more processing time to the 500–600 ms songs than to the 200 ms tones, suggesting that, in processing the songs, all birds attended primarily to the first 200 ms, which includes a portion of the introductory notes.

Nevertheless, the possibility remained that birds may have invested more time in processing conspecific themes relative to alien at some initial stage in the learning process. Therefore, latencies were also examined before criterion was reached, when correct detections reached levels of 55%, 65% and 75%. Results, shown in Fig. 15.8, also indicate no latency differences between birds classifying conspecific versus alien song themes during these times. Therefore, it does not appear that either redwings or cowbirds invested more processing time in any stage of learning to classify conspecific versus alien songs.

Note, however, that both humans, who performed better than all birds in classifying final elements (Fig. 15.6), appeared to invest significantly more processing time in order to attain this level of accuracy, as indicated by their criterion latency data to full song themes, which were 120–200% longer than to

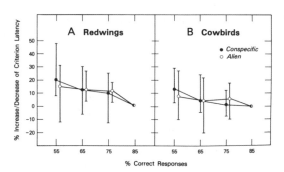

FIG. 15.8. Latencies to conspecific and alien song for (A) redwings and (B) cowbirds examined at four different stages in learning, when performance reached levels of 55, 65, 75, and 85% correct (criterion). Latencies were averaged over three successive test sessions at each learning stage and then normalized relative to each bird's criterion latency to yield a percentage increase or decrease. Error bars denote ranges of individual performance.

tones (Fig. 15.5). More detailed analyses of individual bird and human latency data that support these observations are presented in Sinnott (1987).

III. THEORY

Automatic versus Controlled Processing

Human cognitive psychology defines "automatic" (as opposed to "controlled") processes as requiring no attention, unavoidable, occurring without awareness, highly efficient, difficult to modify once learned, and not subject to capacity limitations (Eysenek, 1984). For example, when driving a car is automatic, it does not require attention, so that one can do something else (carry on a conversation) and drive at the same time. In the original full-song learning experiment, conspecific birds apparently processed the trills (whistles) automatically while pecking the keys to obtain rewards after listening to the introductory notes, whereas the alien birds did not process these elements until their controlled attention was specifically focused on them by tutoring.

However, it is the notion of "capacity limitation" that is most relevant to the present results, because it uses reaction time as an important measure in defining automaticity. For example, automaticity for humans is evident in the visual identification of highly overlearned symbolic classes such as letters versus numbers: Here no increases in reaction time accrue as more tokens are added to the classes, so the capacity for classification is said to be "unlimited" (Schneider & Shiffrin, 1977; Shiffrin & Schneider, 1977). Applying this framework to the present song classifications, the conspecific birds were clearly less capacity-limited than the alien birds, because they processed both the initial and final song portions without investing more time than the alien birds who processed primarily the initial song portions.

Integral versus Separable Dimensions

Human cognitive psychology uses the term "integral" to refer to stimulus compounds in which a subjects's perception of the elements resists individual analysis (e.g., hue and brightness), while "separable" refers to compounds in which the subject performs operations on some property of the stimulus without reference to other properties (e.g., form and size) (Garner, 1974). These phenomena are investigated in animals by using matching-to-sample experiments (Riley, 1984), and the present studies can also be analysed as such. Consider the full-song stimuli presented in the first experiment as a compound sample. After criterion was reached, the isolated song elements presented in the second experiment had to be matched to the original sample. For conspecifics, the trills (whistles) could not be separated from the previously associated introductory notes, while for aliens, these elements were dissociated. The terms integral and separable may therefore describe the song element processing modes of the conspecific and alien birds, respectively.

Riley (1984) has also shown that the external structure of a stimulus may influence how it is processed. For example, if pigeons are given two dimensions of color and line orientation in a compound sample, then their perception during the match tends to be integral if the two dimensions had been unified into one sample figure, but separable if they had been separated in space. If, in the present study, the two species processed the same physical input differentially, then this implies that conspecifics must have used an *internal* cognitive structure that unified the song elements into an integral percept, while the alien birds lacked such a structure. Human data also indicate that the perception of sequential phonemes involves integral processing, if the stimuli are perceived as speech, while the same stimuli are processed in a separable fashion if perceived as nonspeech (Tomiak, Mullennix, & Sawusch, 1987).

Syntactic and Semantic Constraints

It is a classic psycholinguistic observation that sentences are encoded and re-called much more easily than strings of nonsense syllables of comparable length, because humans can employ semantic and syntactic constraints to chunk the sentence elements (Miller, 1962). For example, after hearing a grammatical subject "a stitch in time," a human expects to hear an appropriate predicate "saves nine." Playback experiments with birds also suggest sequential con-straints operating in the introductory-note/trill structure found in several species of songbirds. For example, the introductory notes may serve an *alerting* function for the following trill either to (1) ensure accurate perception under degraded listening conditions (Wiley & Richards, 1982), (2) signal other males to stop singing to prevent mutual masking (Wasserman, 1977), or (3) simply gain the attention of other males (Beletsky, Chao, & Smith, 1980).

The present bird subjects, after hearing conspecific introductory notes, may have been alerted to hear trills or whistles, due to the sequential dependencies existing between the song elements and/or the "meaning" they understood in their conspecific signals. But redwings were not alerted to hear whistles after cowbird introductory notes, nor were cowbirds alerted to hear trills after redwing introductory notes, because the meaning of alien song was not understood. The performance of alien birds might be analogous to an attempt by humans to encode a list of nonsense syllables.

Marlsen-Wilson and Tyler (1980) propose a model of human speech percep-tion by which both sensory and contextual knowledge interact to provide an efficient decoding of speech. Their model is relevant to the present results because they use a reaction time measure to delineate automatic ("obligatory") speech-processing modes that allow humans to identify words before the stimuli have even ended. For example, subjects identifying target words have shorter RTs when the words occur in sentences, as opposed to unrelated lists. They report 270 ms RTs to words that are 370 ms long, implying that humans identify the words from the first two phonemes, and do not wait until the word has ended. Therefore, if the context is adequate, a complete sensory analysis of the word is not necessary for identification. Similar processes may have occurred for conspecific birds in the present study, who identified their final song portions without devoting extra processing time to a complete sensory analysis.

Limited data suggest that birds did not begin the experiment with a priori knowledge of which conspecific final elements were associated with which introductory notes. During a pilot study, one redwing was inadvertently trained to classify redwing themes using a different procedure that terminated the song stimulus at the time of the report response. This bird had very short RTs for one side key (similar to the bird in Fig. 15.3) which caused him to terminate the songs without hearing the trills. When subsequently tested for classification of song elements, his introductory note score was normal (85–90% correct), but his trill score was <70% correct, deficient for redwings although comparable to some of the better cowbirds in Fig. 15.6A. The results from this one pilot subject indicate that the final portion of conspecific song must at least physically impinge on the bird's sensory apparatus as a necessary prerequisite to accurate classification. According to the Marlsen-Wilson speech model, sensory data must also initiate the perceptual process ("bottom-up priority").

Innateness versus Learning

The mechanism that guided conspecific processing in the present study may be the "song template" hypothesized to control the selective attention of young songbirds to acoustic features in conspecific song and the rejection of alien models (Konishi & Nottebohm, 1969; Marler, 1976). Aspects of these proposed templates are studied in social-isolation experiments, where birds are raised without the opportunity to hear conspecifics. Some species, such as cowbirds, develop structurally normal songs when raised in isolation (West et al., 1981). On the other hand, isolate redwings develop normal song elements, but may use incorrect combinations, such that trills may be followed by introductory notes (Marler, Mundinger, Waser, & Lutjen, 1972). Such studies typically rely on the birds' productions as a measure of their perceptions. However, data from sparrows indicate that purely perceptual selectivities to conspecific song may operate before birds are capable of song production (Dooling & Searcy, 1980).

To shed light on the question of innate processes in the present purely perceptual experiments, an isolate-raised redwing was obtained from the Rockefeller University Field Research Center at Millbrook, NY. The bird had been removed from the nest at the age of 4 days and hand-reared in a room with canaries and sparrows. At the age of 6 months, he was brought to our laboratory and housed

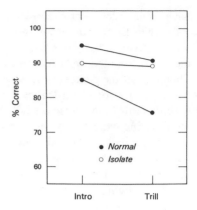

FIG. 15.9. Percent correct responses to redwing song elements for an isolate redwing male, compared with two wild-caught males.

apart from our wild birds. He was never heard to sing anything resembling redwing song. When 1-year-of-age, he was trained to classify the present redwing song stimuli and then tested with song elements, along with two normal wild-caught redwings. Results of these three birds' song element test sessions are shown in Fig. 15.9. The isolate responded in the same way as the wild birds, for both introductory and final (trill) elements. Although data from one isolate subject are necessary limited in scope, this result strongly suggests that the special perceptual mode of redwing trill processing uncovered here has a significant genetic component. Thus, even a socially deprived redwing has a more efficient trill processor compared to wild non-redwings (cowbirds).

As the present isolate-redwing had no functional experience with redwing song in nature, he presumably had no access to any coding strategies that required social learning from conspecifics. Semantic or syntactic constraints, however, may have a more innate basis. For example, cowbirds appear to have an innate recognition of the sexual and aggressive messages in their songs (West et al., 1981). In human speech development, the "deep structure" syntactic component is hypothesized to be largely innate, allowing the child to acquire the phonological and semantic structures of any language through mere exposure (Chomsky, 1967; Lenneberg, 1967).

Issues in Species-Specific Coding

Several other animal species have been examined in the laboratory for differential processing of conspecific versus alien signals. Parakeets appear to have specialized psychoacoustic capacities for dealing with conspecific sounds, but they also learn, with equal ease, the calls of alien birds, e.g., canaries (Park & Dooling, 1985). Japanese macaques are superior to other monkey species in discriminating classes of conspecific "coo" calls, especially when distracting variables, such as variations in fundamental frequency, are introduced into the stimuli (Petersen, 1982). For human speech, animals discriminate some isolated phonemes and even perceive them "categorically" (Kuhl, 1986), which suggests that the sensory mechanisms that humans use for speech sounds are not excessively specialized. On the other hand, animals appear unable to use the complex grammatical codes of speech, so human-specific coding is easier to demonstrate at the level of syntax or semantics (Terrace et al., 1979).

One major problem in attempting to delineate aspects of special coding in human speech is that there exists no animal that provides an adequate cognitive control for a human. If a chimp cannot "create a sentence" (Terrace et al., 1979), is this deficiency due to the lack of a speech processor, or does it simply reflect a generally inferior learning ability? Experiments with animals provide more controlled contexts with which to address such questions, as it is relatively easy to find species with similar learning abilities, but different communication systems. For example, the present redwings and cowbirds appeared similar in their learning abilities for tones and introductory notes, so specialized trill or whistle processing cannot be attributed to different general learning abilities.

Needless to say, there is currently considerable controversy concerning the nature of the mechanisms underlying species-specific coding in communication signals. Further research using additional species, stimulus manipulations, response latency measures, and human controls will help to clarify the nature of the mechanisms underlying special coding in animals and to what extent they are similar to those operating in human speech perception. The present results, taken together with other data that have uncovered parallels between birdsong and human speech involving sensitive periods, subsong, neural lateralization, and dialects (Marler, 1970; Nottebohm, 1970), suggest that songbirds provide excellent animal models for studying the evolutionary basis of many phenomena in human communication.

ACKNOWLEDGMENTS

This research was supported by NIH. Experiments were conducted in the Neural Encoding Laboratory at the Johns Hopkins Medical Institutions in Baltimore, MD. Special thanks to Murray Sachs and Robert Hienz for their interest, support, encouragement, and for conducting the experiment with the isolate redwing. The Patuxent Wildlife Research Center in Laurel, MD provided the wild bird subjects. Robert Dooling and Peter Marler provided the isolate redwing. Robert Hienz and Orlando Asuncion participated as human subjects. David Pisoni, Robert Hienz and Peter Marler provided comments on the manuscript.

REFERENCES

Beletsky, L., Chao, S., & Smith, D. (1980). An investigation of song-based species recognition in the redwing blackbird. *Behaviour, 73,* 189–203.

Bent, A. (1965). *Life histories of North American blackbirds, orioles, tanagers, and allies* (pp. 123–150, 421–453). New York: Dover.

Brackenbury, J. (1982). The structural basis of voice production and its relationship to sound characteristics. In D. Kroodsma & E. Miller (Eds.), *Acoustic communication in birds, Vol. 1*, (pp. 53–71). New York: Academic Press.

Brenowitz, E. (1983). The contribution of temporal song cues to species recognition in the redwing blackbird. *Animal Behaviour, 31*, 1116–1127.

Capranica, R., Frishkopf, L., & Nevo, E. (1973). Encoding of geographic dialects in the auditory system of the cricket frog. *Science, 182*, 1272–1275.

Chomsky, N. (1967). The formal nature of language. In E. Lenneberg, *Biological foundations of language* (pp. 397–442). New York: Wiley.

Dooling, R., & Searcy, M. (1980). Early perceptual selectivity in the swamp sparrow. *Developmental Psychobiology, 13*, 499–506.

Eysenck, M. (1984). *A handbook of cognitive psychology* (pp. 49–77). Hillsdale, NJ: Lawrence Erlbaum Associates.

Garner, W. (1974). *The processing of information and structure.* Hillsdale, NJ: Lawrence Erlbaum Associates.

Greenewalt, C. (1968). *Bird song: Acoustics and physiology.* Washington, D.C.: Smithsonian Institution Press.

Hienz, R., Sinnott, J., & Sachs, M. (1977). Auditory sensitivity of the redwing blackbird and brown-headed cowbird. *Journal of Comparative and Physiological Psychology, 91*, 1365–1376.

Hienz, R., Sinnott, J., & Sachs, M. (1980). Auditory intensity discrimination in blackbirds and pigeons. *Journal of Comparative and Physiological Psychology, 94*, 993–1002.

Hulse, S., & Cynx, J. (1986). Interval and contour in serial pitch perception by a Passerine bird. *Journal of Comparative Psychology, 100*, 215–228.

Konishi, M., & Nottebohm, F. (1969). Experimental studies in the ontogeny of avian vocalizations. In R. Hinde (Ed.), *Bird vocalizations* (pp. 5–18). Cambridge, England: Cambridge University Press.

Kuhl, P. (1986). Theoretical contributions of tests on animals to the special-mechanisms debate in speech. *Experimental Biology, 45*, 233–265.

Lenneberg, E. (1967). *Biological foundations of language* (pp. 371–395). New York: Wiley.

Mackintosh, N. (1973). Stimulus selection: Learning to ignore stimuli that predict no change in reinforcement. In R. Hinde & J. Stevenson-Hinde (Eds.), *Constraints on learning* (pp. 75–100). New York: Academic Press.

Marler, P. (1969). Tonal quality of bird sounds. In R. Hinde (Ed.), *Bird vocalizations* (pp. 5–18). Cambridge, England: Cambridge University Press.

Marler, P. (1970). Bird song and speech development: Could there be parallels? *American Scientist, 58*, 669–673.

Marler, P. (1976). Sensory templates in species-specific behavior. In J. Fentress, (Ed.), *Simpler networks: An approach to patterned behavior and its foundations* (pp. 314–329). New York: Sinauer.

Marler, P., Mundinger, P., Waser, M., & Lutjen, A. (1972). Effects of acoustical stimulation and deprivation on song development in redwing blackbirds. *Animal Behaviour, 20*, 586–606.

Marlsen-Wilson, W., & Tyler, L. (1980). The temporal structure of spoken language understanding. *Cognition, 8*, 1–71.

Miller, G. (1962). Some psychological studies of grammar. *American Psychologist, 17*, 748–762.

Nottebohm, F. (1970). Ontogeny of bird song. *Science, 167*, 950–956.

Park, T., & Dooling, R. (1985). Perception of species-specific contact calls by budgerigars. *Journal of Comparative Psychology, 99*, 391–402.

Petersen, M. (1982). The perception of species-specific vocalizations by primates: A conceptual framework. In C. Snowdon, C. Brown, & M. Petersen (Eds.), *Primate communication* (pp. 171–211). Cambridge, England: Cambridge University Press.

Riley, D. (1984). Do pigeons decompose stimulus compounds? In H. Roitblatt, T. Bever, & H. Terrace (Eds.), *Animal Cognition* (pp. 333–350). Hillsdale, NJ: Lawrence Erlbaum Associates.

Schneider, W., & Shiffrin, R. (1977). Controlled and automatic human information processing: I. Detection, search, and attention. *Psychological Review, 84,* 1–66.

Seyfarth, R., Cheney, D., & Marler, P. (1980). Vervet monkey alarm calls: Semantic communication in a free-ranging primate. *Animal Behaviour, 28,* 1070–1094.

Shiffrin, R., & Schneider, W. (1977). Controlled and automatic human information processing: II. Perceptual learning, automatic attending, and a general theory. *Psychological Review, 84,* 127–189.

Sinnott, J. (1980). Species-specific coding in birdsong. *Journal of the Acoustical Society, 68,* 494–497.

Sinnott, J. (1987). Modes of perceiving and processing information in birdsong. *Journal of Comparative Psychology,* 101, 355–366.

Sinnott, J., Sachs, M., & Hienz, R. (1980). Aspects of frequency discrimination in passerine birds and pigeons. *Journal of Comparative and Physiological Psychology, 94,* 401–415.

Stevenson, J. (1969). Song as a reinforcer. In R. Hinde (Ed.), *Bird vocalizations* (pp. 49–60). Cambridge, England: Cambridge University Press.

Terrace, H., Petitto, L., Sanders, R., & Bever, T. (1979). Can an ape create a sentence? *Science, 206,* 891–900.

Tomiak, G., Mullennix, J., & Sawusch, J. (1987). Integral processing of phonemes: Evidence for a phonetic mode of perception. *Journal of the Acoustical Society, 81,* 755–764.

Wasserman, F. (1977). Intraspecific acoustical interference in the white-throated sparrow. *Animal Behaviour, 25,* 949–952.

West, M., King, A., & Eastzer, D. (1981). The Cowbird: Reflections on development from an unlikely source. *American Scientist, 69,* 56–66.

Wiley, R., & Richards, D. (1982). Adaptations for acoustic communication in birds: Sound transmission and signal detection. In D. Kroodsma & E. Miller (Eds.), *Acoustic communication in birds. Vol. 1* (pp. 132–181). New York: Academic Press.

Yasukawa, K. (1981). Song repertoires in the redwing blackbird; A test of the Beau Geste hypothesis. *Animal Behaviour, 29,* 114–125.

Author Index

Subject Index